The

BEST LIFE GUIDE

to MANAGING DIABETES
and PRE-DIABETES

BOB GREENE

JOHN J. MERENDINO JR., M.D.
JANIS JIBRIN, M.S., R.D.

SIMON & SCHUSTER
NEW YORK   LONDON   TORONTO   SYDNEY

Simon & Schuster
1230 Avenue of the Americas
New York, NY 10020

For information about special discounts for bulk purchases,
please contact Simon & Schuster Special Sales at
1-866-506-1949 or business@simonandschuster.com

The Simon & Schuster Speakers Bureau can bring authors to your live event. For more information or to book an event contact the Simon & Schuster Speakers Bureau at 1-866-248-3049 or visit our website at www.simonspeakers.com

Designed by Joel Avirom and Jason Snyder

Manufactured in the United States of America

1   3   5   7   9   10   8   6   4   2

The Library of Congress has cataloged the hardcover edition as follows:
Greene, Bob (Bob W.)
The best life guide to managing diabetes and pre-diabetes /
Bob Greene, John J. Merendino, Janis Jibrin.
p. cm.
1. Diabetes—Popular works. 2. Diabetics—Life skills guides—Popular works.
I. Merendino, John Jerome. II. Jibrin, Janis. III. Title.
RC660.4.G737 2009
616.4'620654—dc22   2009024752
ISBN 978-1-4165-8838-2
ISBN 978-1-4165-8839-9 (pbk)
ISBN 978-1-4391-7304-6 (ebook)

ACKNOWLEDGMENTS

Just as good diabetes management depends on keeping up on a number of fronts—diet, exercise, and medication—putting together a truly comprehensive diabetes management book requires the input of a variety of experts. Chef Sidra Forman's recipes and meals prove that you don't have to sacrifice great taste and familiar favorites to stay healthy. We got meticulous research help from exercise physiologist Michelle Kennedy and from registered dietitians Beth Ehrensberger, Heather Kris Jones, Samina Riaz, and Susan Weiner—Susan is also an exercise physiologist and a certified diabetes educator. Two other certified diabetes educators—Kathleen Mahan and Linda Henderson—offered their insights into helping manage the disease. We're grateful to David R. Brown, M.D., PhD, for reviewing the manuscript; he's an endocrinologist skilled in the management of diabetes who is also plugged into the latest research. Some of the more fascinating research tidbits in the book are courtesy of two university professors, Bernard Venn, PhD, and Richard Mattes, PhD. Therapists Kristin Vickers Douglas, PhD, and Jody Brand Levine, LCSW-C, both work on the emotional aspects of diabetes—they've shared valuable counseling tips. You'll also get inspiration from the real life stories of Chip Hiden, Nicola Farman, and Lisa Provenzo, who have actually become healthier, fitter, and happier *after* their diagnoses. And helping us pull all the strings together is our incomparable editor, Donna Fennessy.

CONTENTS

INTRODUCTION

WHEN YOU FIRST FOUND out that you had diabetes or pre-diabetes, you probably experienced a wave of emotions: concern, fear, confusion, maybe even anger. But despite the fact that both are serious conditions, the good news is that there's a lot you can do to stay healthy and improve your quality of life; there are so many more treatment options and resources at your disposal than just fifteen years ago. This is, in large part, a reaction to the epidemic in this country—about 24 million Americans have been diagnosed with diabetes and another 57 million have pre-diabetes, a precursor of the disease. Though this may not be positive news for us as a country, it's placed diabetes high on the national health agenda. There are millions of people with these conditions, just like you, who are able to continue living a healthy and fulfilled life.

Always keep in mind that how well you fare after your diagnosis is largely up to you. Diabetes and pre-diabetes are conditions that you can manage well by making some important lifestyle changes. When you take the reins and do what you can to manage these conditions, you can dramatically improve your life. I've seen this firsthand—in family members who have diabetes as well as clients I've worked with over the years. *The Best Life Guide to Managing Diabetes and Pre-Diabetes* will map out a clear and practical plan for living your healthiest, happiest, fullest life. Once you know what diabetes and pre-diabetes are, how they affect you, and what you can do to stay healthy, you'll feel more in control and less afraid.

The Best Life program's design reflects the three pillars of diabetes management: diet, exercise, and medication. It's no accident that I've listed medication last—diet and exercise are the drivers here. Eat right and move enough, and you won't need as many drugs. In some cases, you can eliminate the drugs altogether, at least for a few years (diabetes is a progressive disease, so the need for medication usually arises again eventually). If you have pre-diabetes you're probably not on medication; the Best Life program can completely reverse this condition and prevent diabetes down the road.

Whether you have pre-diabetes or diabetes, the dietary and fitness guidelines in this book will help you bring your blood sugar into the best possible range, with a minimum of highs and lows. If you have diabetes you'll be using a blood glucose monitor to test your sugar and you'll be logging (see log on page 335) select blood sugar readings, meals, and bouts of exercise. This log will play a crucial role in your diabetes management—it will help you piece together important patterns that you can use to create an individualized program that fits with your disease and your lifestyle. The response to food and exercise varies from person to person; the log will uncover your unique reactions. For instance, you might note that your blood sugar is usually high after eating bread but not after eating pasta. Or that your blood sugar is in a great range after 30 minutes on the treadmill but a little too low after 40 minutes. Or that the dose of medication taken in the morning seems to send your blood sugar plummeting in the afternoon, which is something you and your doctor can adjust.

Not only will all of these tools help you manage the disease—and in some cases, eliminate it altogether—they will also reduce your risk of some of the serious complications of diabetes, such as heart disease, stroke, eye disease, kidney disease, nerve damage, and sexual problems. If you already have one or more of these complications, following this plan can slow their progression and potentially even reverse them. And you'll probably find that once you adopt this way of eating and exercising, you'll be slimmer and healthier than you've ever been before.

It doesn't matter how long you've had diabetes or pre-diabetes or how healthy you are right now. This plan works as well for someone who has just been diagnosed as it does for someone who has had diabetes for years and has a number of complications. This is as true of someone who's sedentary and overweight as of someone who's out running marathons. No matter how progressed your disease is or what your current health status is, this plan can be tailored to fit your needs and even your tastes. For instance, the diet plan, which is very flexible in terms of calories and types of meals, allows for easy substitutions. Hate broccoli but love zucchini? No problem! And the exercise plan meets you at your current level and helps you move up gradually, with useful, practical tips for increasing your activity at any level, from couch potato to ultimate athlete.

By taking the time to read and understand this book, you've already made a huge step toward living a healthier life, and I'm thrilled to guide you on this journey. For nearly three decades, I've been focused on helping people make meaningful changes in their lives, including being more active, overhauling their diet, losing weight, and discovering the issues that may be standing in the way of their happiness and well-being. Often the people who seek my help have a variety of ailments, including heart disease, arthritis, high blood pressure, and depression, but I'm seeing more and more people with pre-diabetes and diabetes. And because of their specific needs, I've partnered with two leading experts in their respective fields, John J. "Jack" Merendino Jr., M.D., and Janis Jibrin, M.S., R.D., to create a program that provides a multifaceted approach to managing the disease. As an exercise physiologist, I'll help you safely step up your physical activity. Dr. Merendino will explain the specifics of diabetes and pre-diabetes care. A Yale- and Harvard-trained physician, he was a researcher at the National Institutes of Health before becoming a prominent endocrinologist, and has been caring for people with diabetes and pre-diabetes for more than twenty years. Janis offers a nutrition prescription that is loaded with delicious and tasty foods. She has authored several books and hundreds of magazine articles on healthy eating. She has been the lead nutritionist of www.thebestlife.com for the last few years, and I've witnessed her passion for nutrition and the joy she gets from helping people.

Before you get ready to jump in and get started, I want to prepare you: you definitely have to commit to this plan for it to work. If you rise to the challenge, you'll be rewarded greatly, not only with good control of your diabetes or the reversal of your pre-diabetes, but also with more energy, a trimmer, fitter body, and better overall health. You can look at your diabetes or pre-diabetes diagnosis in one of two ways: as a strike against your health that's too great to overcome, or as an opportunity to really care for and nurture yourself.

This program isn't a quick fix. However, the gradual changes you'll make during the three phases of the plan will ensure long-term success. During each phase, you'll be given a number of goals to work on. After several weeks of practicing these healthy habits, you'll be given another set of goals, and so on, until you're leading a more active life, choosing more nutritious foods, and having consistently better control over your blood sugar. In my experience, the best way to change your diet and exercise habits is to do it gradually—it's those changes that tend to stick for life. Here's a quick snapshot of what the three phases look like:

- In Phase One, you'll work on putting the appropriate amount of carbohydrates on your plate. You'll be getting more exercise, using the Best Life Activity Scale as your guide. And all the while, you'll be regularly checking your blood sugar if you have diabetes. (Need to lose weight? You should see the pounds start to drop in this phase.)

- Four weeks later, you'll be ready to start Phase Two. At this point, you'll work on tightening control of your blood sugar even further. You'll be getting choosier about the carbs you eat; you'll also get some guidance on the best protein-rich foods and healthful fats to eat at meals and snacks. You'll use the Hunger Scale, a handy tool that will help you eat when you need to and stop when you should. And finally, many of you will add more physical activity. (Again, for those who need it, your weight should continue to drop.)

- Phase Three is about staying healthy for life. Of course, you'll still be keeping on top of your disease with all the lifestyle habits that have now become second nature, but in this phase you'll set other aspects of good, lifelong care into place. For instance, you'll be working on motivation and coping with the emotional side of your condition. You'll refine your diet even further, not only to keep blood sugar in check, but to combat cancer and other chronic illnesses. You'll become more confident at the doctor's office when you read our advice on how to get the most out of your health care.

Throughout the three phases we'll be filling you in on how medication (if you're taking any) fits into the picture. For instance, we'll explain how getting more exercise and eating fewer carbs might affect the dosage of your drugs. We've also devoted an entire chapter to medications, and this information will allow you to work with your doctor to make the best drug choices for you.

In addition to the information in this book, you can find ongoing support, more meals and recipes, and a handy online log at my Web site www.thebestlife.com. Dr. Merendino, Janis, and I, along with the team of Best Life nutritionists, exercise physiologists, and other health experts, have met with and exchanged e-mails with thousands of subscribers to the Web site; using their feedback and our knowledge, we've created a targeted diet plan for people with diabetes. As a member, you'll get daily and weekly meal plans as well as an electronic Best Life Diabetes Management Log; you'll also have access to other diabetes-related content to help you manage your condition better, as well as to a thriving community of people just like you who are trying to live more healthfully. You can share tips, offer encouragement, and get support whenever you need it.

I'm confident that the advice, facts, and guidance we offer in this book will put to rest the fears, confusion, and anxieties you first felt once you learned you had diabetes or pre-diabetes. And in time, I hope that you'll be able to look back at your diagnosis as a turning point in your life—and a positive one at that, because it was the day you started making your health and your needs a priority. It was the day you made the conscious decision to start living your Best Life.

1

WHAT ARE DIABETES AND PRE-DIABETES?

YOU KNOW YOUR SUGAR is too high, but you might be wondering: How did I get diabetes or pre-diabetes? What, exactly, has gone awry in my body? Is it curable? How does it affect my health now, and ten years down the road? Will I have to take insulin?

This chapter will answer all of these questions and more. Even if you know a lot about diabetes and pre-diabetes, you'll still probably learn a lot: this is the place to get straight talk and scientifically up-to-date information. We're going to start at the beginning, telling you just what these diseases are, how they play out in your body, the effects of diet and exercise, and the conditions that you're at an increased risk of developing, such as heart disease and nerve damage. We're going to be straight with you: diabetes is a serious medical problem and one that requires constant and consistent care. And more and more we're learning about the major health consequences of pre-diabetes. But if you understand what's going on in your body and the way diet, exercise, and drugs work together to keep you at your healthiest, you'll be more informed and motivated to manage your condition properly. The single most important thing to remember about diabetes is that if you can keep it under fairly good control, you are far less likely to develop any of the serious complications.

So where to start? You probably know the most basic fact about diabetes: it's a condition of high blood sugar. Sometimes people will even describe their diabetes by saying "I have sugar." Sugar refers to *glucose*, the main sugar your body uses as a fuel. (We'll fill you in on glucose in a short while.) Whenever someone talks about "blood sugar," they are really talking about "blood glucose," and in this book we'll use these terms interchangeably.

How did your doctor determine that you have diabetes or pre-diabetes? By measuring the amount of sugar in your blood. Perhaps your disease was caught through a routine blood test. In this case, when a patient comes in with no other symptoms, a doctor should order a second test for confirmation. Or, perhaps your doctor decided to test you for the disease after you came in with classic symptoms (excessive thirst, frequent urination, blurred vision, or fatigue) or because you have a strong family history of diabetes or pre-diabetes. He may have even ordered the test because he was concerned about your large belly, which predisposes you to these conditions. If there are clear symptoms of diabetes and the blood sugar test result is high enough to make the diagnosis, a repeat test is not necessary. These are the tests your doctor uses for diagnosis:

- *Fasting blood sugar test.* This blood test is done after you have fasted for eight or more hours (usually overnight). Normal fasting blood sugar is under 100 mg/dL. (This is shorthand for milligrams per deciliter. Throughout this book we'll simply use the number and skip the mg/dL.) If your blood glucose is between 100 and 125 then you meet the criteria for pre-diabetes; a glucose level of 126 or more meets the criteria for diabetes.

- *Non-fasting blood sugar test.* If your blood glucose level at any time exceeds 200, then you would also be diagnosed with diabetes. (There is no standard to indicate pre-diabetes.)

- *Oral glucose tolerance test (OGTT).* For this test, you go to the doctor's office and down a syrupy drink containing 75 grams of glucose. Normal blood sugar two hours later is under 140; between 140 and 199 qualifies as pre-diabetes; and if your blood sugar tops 200, you've tested positive for diabetes. This test is usually done when the doctor suspects that you have diabetes or pre-diabetes but standard blood sugar tests don't confirm the diagnosis.

In the near future, another test may become the preferred way of diagnosing both diabetes and pre-diabetes: the hemoglobin A1c test, which reflects average blood sugar over the previous two or three months (see page 31 for more details on the test). Doctors currently use this blood test to track the progression of your diabetes, but in 2009 a group of leading diabetes experts from around the world recommended using the A1c test for the diagnosis of diabetes as well. More on this in the "A1c's Got Your Number" box on page 32.

Although a sugar solution is used in the OGTT to diagnose diabetes, don't be misled into thinking that your diabetes came about from eating too much sugar. Although certain types of diets can increase the risk of diabetes (see "Sugar Does Not Cause Diabetes, But . . ." on page 18), the condition really develops because of a glitch in the way your body produces or handles the hormone insulin. To understand diabetes, you have to understand insulin—how it's supposed to regulate blood sugar and what happens when it doesn't.

IT'S ALL ABOUT INSULIN

Insulin is a hormone that is produced by cells in your pancreas and is essential for maintaining proper health. (A hormone is a chemical that is manufactured in one part of the body and travels through the bloodstream to other parts of the body, where it has powerful effects.) One of insulin's main jobs is to help transport glucose into your cells. Without insulin, you'd starve to death, because no matter how much you eat, if glucose and the energy it provides can't get into your cells, you can't survive.

From the Cereal Bowl to Your Cells

Food takes a remarkable journey from your plate to your cells, thanks in large part to insulin. Insulin is critical for ensuring that carbohydrates make the trip but also plays a role in the way cells handle protein and fat.

Carbohydrates are so important because your body converts them into glucose, its preferred fuel. It's what keeps your cells running most of the time. There are times they use fat for energy (for instance, muscle cells do during low-intensity exercise), but most of the time it's a steady diet of glucose, especially in the brain, which uses glucose almost exclusively. The carbohydrates in foods like cereal, milk, fruit, and candy come in three basic forms: sugars, starches, and fiber. Sugars are "simple" carbohydrate molecules—small in size and close in chemical form to how your body uses them for energy. Glucose is a sugar, as is table sugar or cane sugar, also called sucrose. Starches and fiber are termed "complex" carbohydrates because they are large molecules that consist of many sugars chemically attached to one another. Your body turns starch as well as sugar into glucose. But when you eat fiber, it simply passes through your body undigested because you don't have the enzymes to break it down. (That's a good thing. You'll learn more about fiber in Phase Two.) So sugar and starch provide glucose and calories, but fiber does not.

How is food broken down into glucose? Let's track the fate of the Day 1 breakfast, Steel-Cut Oats with Walnuts and Orange Zest and Silk Light Vanilla Soymilk (page 259). The carbs in this meal come from the sugar in the soy milk and the starch and fiber in the oatmeal. (Or, if you make this breakfast using milk, the sugar would come from the naturally occurring milk sugar, lactose.)

The soy milk's sugar takes a quick and easy ride into your bloodstream. Your body doesn't have to do much work; enzymes in the intestine break the sucrose into two simple sugar molecules that are then absorbed directly through the lining of your intestine into your bloodstream. We'll catch up with this sugar in just a bit, but first let's look at what's happening with the starch in the oatmeal. It takes longer to be absorbed because starches are large molecules and the digestive enzymes must break them down into many sugar molecules. These are then absorbed into the bloodstream through the lining of the intestine. The starch in the oatmeal is broken down slowly, but some starchy foods, such as white bread, turn into simple sugar much more quickly (more on this in Phase Two).

Blood from the intestine is now rich in sugar from the soy milk and the oatmeal's broken-down starch. This blood travels next to the liver and the pancreas. The liver metabolizes any simple sugars other than glucose and stores some of the glucose for later use. The remaining glucose stays in the bloodstream. In the pancreas, specialized cells known as beta cells detect the high glucose level and release insulin into your blood in response. If things are working properly, the more glucose there is in your blood, the more insulin is made by the pancreas.

The insulin and glucose then travel together throughout your body, reaching every single one of the hundreds of billions of cells. Think of insulin as the doorman in a fancy apartment building: insulin opens the cell's doors and lets glucose in. Without the doorman, glucose can't get into the cells, and without glucose, the cells can't function. Here's the key point to remember: *insulin is necessary for glucose to get inside most of your body's cells.* Without insulin, glucose accumulates in your blood but cannot be used to fuel cells. That's what happens when you have diabetes. The more out of control your diabetes is, the higher the amount of sugar in your blood that can't be used by your body; you're essentially starving.

In most cells, glucose is quickly used for energy: to keep your heart pumping, your lungs expanding, and the nerve cells in your brain firing. In liver and muscle cells, however, some of the glucose is converted into glycogen. Glycogen is a storage form of glucose, released as needed for fuel. For instance, when you start a workout, it's mainly glycogen feeding your muscles. When you haven't eaten anything for a while, the liver releases the glucose stored as glycogen and can also convert protein and fat into glucose if necessary to tide you over until the next meal. Whether the blood sugar comes from that sandwich you just ate or is released by the liver between meals, insulin is the ticket to getting it into cells to give you the energy you need.

Insulin does more than just regulate carbohydrates; it also affects the way your body processes protein and fat. For instance, the protein in the soy milk you had for breakfast is broken down into amino acids that are then absorbed into the blood. From there, the body reassembles those amino acids to create new proteins, such as hemoglobin, which carries oxygen to all your cells. Insulin lends a hand in constructing those new proteins, which are critical to our survival. Insulin also helps your body store the fat you absorb from your diet so you can use it for energy later.

Insulin, Interrupted

That's how it's all supposed to work, but diabetes throws a wrench into the way insulin operates. No matter what you have—pre-diabetes, type 1 diabetes, type 2 diabetes, or gestational diabetes (we'll explain the differences in a minute)—you have an insulin problem. In one way or another *pre-diabetes and all types of diabetes result from inadequate insulin action in the body*. This does more than simply raise blood sugar. Because of insulin's other roles, it means that proteins aren't properly produced, fat isn't properly stored, and many other metabolic processes are out of whack. The cumulative effect of these disruptions can hit you hard, resulting in complications of diabetes, such as diseases of the heart and kidneys.

Notice we said that diabetes and pre-diabetes result from inadequate insulin *action*, not necessarily from inadequate insulin *supply*. That's because there are two basic reasons that diabetes or pre-diabetes develops: either there is not enough insulin being produced or the body is not responding properly to the insulin being made. The second problem is called *insulin resistance*, and we'll have a lot to say about it a little later. Sometimes one problem exists almost exclusively, but in many situations, people are hit with both issues at once. When you get to the chapter on medications used to treat diabetes, you'll see how the various drugs are targeted to overcome one or the other of these problems.

PRE-DIABETES AND TYPES OF DIABETES

When we talk about diabetes in this book, we're using the shorthand for the medical term diabetes mellitus (*mellitus* means "honey" in Latin), which includes type 1, type 2, and gestational diabetes, the type that develops in pregnancy. All three types are characterized by high blood sugar. There is another condition, diabetes insipidus, that relates to kidney function and has nothing to do with high blood sugar. Below is an explanation of pre-diabetes and of the differences between type 1 and type 2 as well as an overview of diabetes in pregnancy.

WHO HAS DIABETES AND PRE-DIABETES?

The same issues that led to the obesity epidemic—huge portion sizes, overeating, an increasingly sedentary lifestyle—have created epidemics of diabetes and pre-diabetes. The diabetes epidemic is really a type 2 diabetes epidemic because one of the main triggers of type 2 diabetes is obesity. The number of people affected just keeps growing: newly diagnosed cases of diabetes rose 90 percent in just one decade from the mid-1990s to the mid-2000s. And from 1980 through 2006, the number of Americans with diabetes tripled. Take a look at these staggering statistics about Americans:

- 23.6 million children and adults—8 percent of the population—have diabetes.

- 5.7 million people with diabetes are not even aware they have the disease.

- 57 million people—nearly 1 person in 5—have pre-diabetes.

AMONG CERTAIN RACIAL AND ETHNIC GROUPS

- 3.7 million, or 14.7 percent, of all non-Hispanic black adults have diabetes, compared to only 9.8 percent of non-Hispanic white adults.

- Diabetes is at least two to four times as common among non-Hispanic black, Hispanic/Latin American, American Indian, and Asian/Pacific Islander women as among non-Hispanic white women.

IN YOUNG PEOPLE

- About 1 in every 400 to 600 children and adolescents has type 1 diabetes.

- 2 million adolescents (or 1 in 6 overweight adolescents) age 12 to 19 have pre-diabetes.

Type 1 Diabetes

If you have diabetes mellitus type 1, you'll need to take insulin, because with this type of diabetes, the body makes essentially no insulin at all. (People are often making some insulin when first diagnosed, but in nearly all cases it eventually dwindles down to virtually nothing.) Sometimes it happens because the pancreas, where insulin is made, is removed surgically or severely damaged by a disease such as pancreatitis. But by far the majority of type 1 cases are triggered by an autoimmune disease that destroys the insulin-producing beta cells in the pancreas. (An autoimmune disease occurs when a person's immune system attacks normal body tissue instead of protecting it. That's what happens in rheumatoid arthritis, multiple sclerosis, and some forms of thyroid disease, for example.) Experts aren't really sure what triggers autoimmune disorders. Many believe the most plausible theory is that a person is first hit with a virus, but instead of just fighting off the virus, the immune system starts attacking organs, such as the pancreas in the case of diabetes. Unfortunately, even after the virus has been completely destroyed, the immune response continues to damage the insulin-producing cells in the pancreas. Whether the virus theory pans out or whether other forces, such as environmental toxins or genes that go awry, are at play, the end result is clear: over time, most or all of the beta cells are destroyed and insulin production dries up. This causes type 1 diabetes.

The process of autoimmune damage to the body's insulin-producing cells usually takes years, and most people aren't even aware when it begins. It typically progresses to the point of diabetes sometime in childhood or adolescence. For this reason, diabetes mellitus type 1 used to be called *juvenile diabetes*. This term is still commonly used, but many people develop type 1 diabetes in their 30s, 40s, or even later, so this isn't really an accurate description. The term insulin-dependent diabetes mellitus or IDDM was also used in the past, but this really isn't an accurate term either, because many people with type 2 diabetes also need insulin.

It's easy to make the diagnosis of type 1 diabetes when a young child has high blood sugar, but it's not always easy to know whether an older adolescent or adult has it or whether it is type 2. The distinction is critical because the doctor needs to know whether to start insulin treatment— mandatory for type 1—or whether it is safe to try oral medication first. Sometimes blood tests such as the C-peptide test, which can tell whether the person is making any insulin, or tests for antibodies that are part of the immune attack against the pancreas, are helpful. But often the diagnosis becomes clear only over time, such as when a person fails to respond to oral medications.

Genetics can play a role in the development of type 1 diabetes, and in some cases you'll find a family with many members who have the condition, but that's not usually the case. It's thought that some people inherit a genetic susceptibility to something in the environment, such as a particular viral infection, which can trigger the autoimmune reaction. If they don't get the virus, that autoimmune reaction will never spring to life. Currently, there are no genetic tests that will reliably tell you if you're likely to develop type 1 diabetes.

Type 1 diabetes accounts for 5 to 10 percent of all people with the condition. There is some evidence that the incidence of type 1 diabetes may be increasing, but it still represents only a minority of cases. And even if it is increasing, it is doing so at a much slower rate than the other major form: diabetes mellitus type 2.

Type 2 Diabetes

Those headline-grabbing statistics—the 90 percent rise in diabetes prevalence in the last decade and the tripling of diabetes cases since the 1980s—are all about type 2 diabetes. And the staggering number of people with pre-diabetes doesn't bode well for an end to the epidemic. Type 2 diabetes makes up 90 to 95 percent of all diabetes cases. It used to be known as *adult-onset diabetes*—not any more; it has begun to strike children and adolescents at an alarming rate. Even though the prevalence is still much lower in young people than in the adult population, it has increased by 33 percent in the past fifteen years, especially among certain racial and ethnic groups, such as African Americans, American Indians, Hispanic/ Latin Americans, and some Asians and Pacific Islanders. Type 2 diabetes also used to be called non-insulin-dependent diabetes mellitus or NIDDM, but this is misleading as well because many people with type 2 need insulin treatment.

Type 2 diabetes is actually a bit more complicated than type 1. In type 2, both a deficiency of insulin and the body's lackluster response to insulin, known as insulin resistance, are at work. Let's focus on insulin resistance for a moment.

Earlier on, we compared insulin to a doorman in a fancy building. Well, if the door is stuck, even the doorman can't get it open. That's what happens when a person develops insulin resistance. The glucose is there, waiting to get into the cell, but insulin can't open the door. Now, if the doorman gets a couple of his buddies, all of them together might be able to open the door. It's the same thing in insulin resistance. Insulin resistance means that it takes a lot more insulin to do the job than in a normal situation.

That's exactly what your body does early on in the disease: your pancreas spews out high levels of insulin to normalize your blood sugar level. After a while, though, your body can't make enough insulin to corral all the glucose, and your blood sugar rises into the diabetic range. No one is sure why this happens. Some decline in insulin production is natural with aging, and it may be that the pancreas eventually just gets "worn out" from putting out all that extra insulin. Once the blood sugar level rises, the problem gets worse. High glucose levels further damage the pancreas's beta cells, a phenomenon called glucose toxicity, and insulin production plunges further. So, while most people with type 2 diabetes start out with insulin resistance, most also develop insulin deficiency as time goes on.

BLAME YOUR BELLY

For many years, the cause of insulin resistance has been one of the most pressing questions in diabetes research. There's one clear link: being overweight or obese. And there's an even clearer culprit: a large belly. Actually, a specific type of belly fat, called visceral or intra-abdominal fat, is to blame. This is fat in and around the liver and other organs inside the abdomen, and it differs from subcutaneous fat—fat under the skin. Liposuction can't reduce visceral fat because the procedure removes only subcutaneous fat. Subcutaneous fat does not seem to cause insulin resistance or the other problems that are part of the metabolic syndrome (page 20). If your jeans are too tight, subcutaneous fat might be somewhat to blame, but once you've hit the numbers outlined in "Get Out the Measuring Tape" on page 17, you most likely have too much visceral fat as well.

Why is visceral fat so toxic? It appears that visceral fat cells manufacture chemicals that prevent other cells from responding to insulin as they should. These chemicals also trigger inflammation, one of the body's ways of responding to injury. That's a good thing when you cut yourself or get the flu, but the chemicals sent out by visceral fat cause inflammation that

GET OUT THE MEASURING TAPE

What's even riskier than being overweight? Carrying excess fat around your middle. "Apple-shaped" people are at greater risk for insulin resistance, diabetes, heart disease, cancer, and other illnesses than those who are "pear-shaped" and carry more of their fat on their hips and thighs. According to the government-sponsored National Health and Nutrition Examination Survey, people with the largest waistlines have a tenfold greater risk of developing diabetes than those with the smallest. And the risk for heart disease is also greater for those with a larger waistline. Even someone at a healthy weight may be in trouble if his or her belly is too large. If you already have diabetes, your heart disease risk is more than double that of the general population, and a big belly only further adds to the risk. In addition, it can worsen your insulin resistance. How big is too big? For women, a waist measurement of more than 35 inches, and for men, a waist measurement of more than 40 inches.

To take your waist measurement, find the top of your pelvic bone on either side of your body. Starting at that point, place a paper or cloth tape measure around your bare abdomen. (And if you're a man who wears his belt *under* his belly—sorry, you can't measure there!) The tape should be snug (but not pressing into your skin) and parallel to the floor (not crooked). Exhale a little before measuring.

can target your blood vessels, triggering heart disease, and may underlie other diseases, including certain forms of cancer.

So you can see why shedding some weight is such a good idea, not just for diabetes management but for staving off other illnesses, too. This might be a little tougher for those of you with type 2 diabetes. Part of the nature of this illness is that your body is genetically programmed to lay down more intra-abdominal fat than that of a person without diabetes. It may not be fair, but it's no reason to throw in the towel. It just means that you must work a little harder at eating right and burning calories. The good news: exercise can make a big dent in visceral fat, as we'll explain in the Phase One chapter. You have so much to gain from losing!

SUGAR DOES NOT CAUSE DIABETES, BUT . . .

Diabetes is a disease of high blood sugar, so people often think that it's caused by eating too much sugar. That's not true in the case of type 1 diabetes, which is an autoimmune disease. But it's not as straightforward when it comes to type 2. Sugar *may* play a role in this disease, but it's not a direct cause-and-effect relationship. For instance, people who consume more sodas and sweetened beverages are more likely to be overweight, which is a primary trigger of type 2 diabetes. In fact, the research on sugary beverages is startling. According to the Harvard Nurses' Health Study, which tracked more than 91,000 nurses for about eight years, women who drank one or more regular (not diet) sodas per day had an 83 percent higher risk of developing diabetes than those who drank no more than one per month. Even worse than soda was fruit punch, a sugary drink containing very little fruit juice. Drinking one or more glasses daily doubled the diabetes risk compared to drinking one or less per month.

It's not just sugary drinks that are the problem; unhealthy diets in general can set you up for type 2 diabetes. Take, for instance, the British Whitehall study, which, for eleven years, tracked 7,339 men and women who, at the start of the study, did not have diabetes. Those whose diets included a lot of white bread, potato chips, burgers, and soda were 50 percent more likely to develop type 2 diabetes than those who ate very little of these foods and instead followed a diet that included a lot of whole grains and salads.

It's true that in these studies the people who consumed an unhealthy diet or drank soda were more likely to be overweight, but experts say that the weight differences alone were not enough to account for the dramatically increased risk of diabetes. They speculate that foods that shoot glucose into the bloodstream quickly, such as sugary sodas, candy, potatoes, white bread, and other foods made with refined flour, simply cause the pancreas to wear out over time. This, in turn, causes the blood sugar to rise, triggering the glucose toxicity described on page 16. Clearly, limiting your intake of sugar and refined carbohydrates is a way to avoid packing on extra pounds. Keeping a lid on these foods, as you'll start doing in Phase One, will also help slow the progression of both type 1 and type 2 diabetes and help prevent the complications described later on in this chapter. In Phase Two, you'll be working on replacing refined-flour products with whole grains and other high-fiber foods.

Pre-Diabetes

The diabetes epidemic pales in comparison to the number of people with pre-diabetes—now estimated at 57 million Americans. It strikes one in four Americans over age 20. If you're one of them, then your blood sugar is high enough to be abnormal, but not high enough to reach the diabetic range (see page 8 for the numbers). If you were diagnosed using a fasting blood sugar test, your condition can also be called impaired fasting glucose; if an oral glucose tolerance test (OGTT) detected your condition, your doctor might refer to it as impaired glucose tolerance. Both mean you have pre-diabetes. Some people will have abnormal results on both tests. Researchers are finding that the OGTT appears to catch more cases than the fasting glucose test. And they're noticing that people who test positive on both tests have a higher likelihood of developing type 2 diabetes compared to those who test positive with just one test.

Pre-diabetes is really "pre–type 2 diabetes"; it is not a precursor to type 1, which is an autoimmune disorder. Pre-diabetes is, in essence, a milder form of type 2 diabetes: your cells are insulin resistant, but you're still producing enough insulin to partially overcome the problem. Pre-diabetes progresses to diabetes when the pancreas can no longer release enough insulin and blood sugar soars to diabetic levels.

The term pre-diabetes is still controversial because the condition does not always progress to diabetes. While most people who have type 2 diabetes started out with pre-diabetes, not everyone who has pre-diabetes will go on to develop diabetes; estimates range from 33 percent to 70 percent. Fortunately, about a third of people with pre-diabetes are able to reverse their condition, winding up with normal blood sugar.

However, if you don't get rid of your pre-diabetes—even if it never turns into diabetes—you still have a serious condition that can set you up for many of the same complications of diabetes, such as heart disease, retinopathy, and neuropathy. Your heart disease risk is particularly high if you have some of the other conditions that often tag along with pre-diabetes, such as high blood pressure, insulin resistance, a big belly, high triglycerides, and low HDL ("good") cholesterol. If you have three or more of these conditions, you have metabolic syndrome or insulin resistance syndrome. Metabolic syndrome often goes hand in hand with pre-diabetes. It's estimated that a whopping 40 percent of middle-aged Americans have metabolic syndrome, which not only makes heart disease and diabetes more likely to occur, but also increases the risk of cancer.

Scary stuff, but pre-diabetes and metabolic syndrome are very treatable with a good diet, regular exercise, and weight loss. (Exercise alone can increase insulin sensitivity and shave off belly fat—more on this in the Phase One chapter.) A landmark study called the Diabetes Prevention Program (DPP) found that losing 5 to 7 percent of body weight by cutting calories and stepping up exercise prevents or delays the shift to diabetes. If you or anyone in your family has pre-diabetes or metabolic syndrome, following the plan in this book may completely reverse both conditions.

Diabetes During Pregnancy

When you're pregnant, the last thing you want is to develop a condition that could threaten you or your baby, but out-of-control blood sugar can do just that. Whether you develop diabetes for the first time while pregnant (what's called gestational diabetes mellitus, or GDM) or you had diabetes prior to becoming pregnant, you're putting you and your baby at risk if you don't get your blood sugar into the best possible range. Somewhere around 4 to 7 percent of all pregnant women—that's between 135,000 and 200,000 women—in the United States develop gestational diabetes each year. Another 0.3 to 0.5 percent have type 1 or type 2 going into pregnancy. Although this number is smaller than that for gestational diabetes, more women than ever are entering pregnancy with diabetes, mirroring the rise in type 2 cases over the past decade.

Gestational diabetes usually strikes in the second half of pregnancy, but this isn't always the case. Most obstetricians screen for gestational diabetes around the twenty-second week of pregnancy by giving their patients a version of the oral glucose tolerance test described on page 8. Gestational diabetes is sometimes thought of as a unique kind of diabetes, but it's really a form of type 2. Women who get GDM have the same risk factors as those with type 2 diabetes—genetics and obesity—and are pushed over the edge into diabetes by hormonal shifts during pregnancy that trigger insulin resistance. Gestational diabetes often goes away after delivery, but once you develop the condition, you're at an increased risk for a recurrence during later pregnancies and for the development of type 2 diabetes later in life.

Both GDM and preexisting diabetes can affect the fetus, although birth defects, such as congenital heart disease or problems in the brain and spinal cord (such as spina bifida), are much more likely to happen when the diabetes is preexisting. That's because these conditions occur earlier in pregnancy. Preexisting diabetes also heightens the likelihood of miscarriage or stillbirth. Fortunately, the risk of developing any of these conditions is strikingly reduced in women who have good blood sugar control. Interestingly, prevention depends in large part on having good blood sugar levels for several months *prior* to becoming pregnant, not just controlling it during pregnancy. It's critical for a woman with diabetes to work with her doctor, diabetes educator, and dietitian well before becoming pregnant. It's also essential to take a multivitamin supplement daily if you even think you may become pregnant. According to a Centers for Disease Control and Prevention study, women with diabetes who took a multivitamin during the time of conception greatly reduced the risk of birth defects. Most of the credit goes to folic acid, a B vitamin that helps prevent neural tube defects.

Another risk of a diabetic pregnancy is macrosomia, meaning "big body." This can happen with both gestational and preexisting diabetes. It's basically a case of overfeeding the fetus: if a woman's diabetes is not well controlled, excessive amounts of glucose pass through the placenta and into the fetus's circulation. Now the fetus's pancreas has to ramp up its own insulin production to bring down the excess sugar. Too much sugar means too many calories, so the fetus grows abnormally large, with excessive body fat. These hefty babies can have a rough vaginal birth, which can damage their shoulders as they try to squeeze through. Sometimes they just can't make it, so the delivery winds up being a cesarean section. After birth, even though the excess glucose infusion from the mother has stopped, the baby continues making extra insulin for a while. This can cause hypoglycemia—very low blood sugar—which can lead to neurological damage. These babies are also at higher than normal risk of developing breathing problems and of becoming obese and getting type 2 diabetes later in life.

Remember, diabetes-related effects on the baby can almost always be prevented by good blood sugar control during pregnancy. So if there's ever a case to be made for good diabetes management—pronto—it's when you have diabetes and are thinking of becoming pregnant or you get pregnant and develop gestational diabetes. Your blood sugar level needs to get into the normal range as quickly as possible.

Although the diet and exercise goals in this program are appropriate for many pregnant women with preexisting diabetes or those who develop gestational diabetes, this book shouldn't be used as a guide for treatment during pregnancy. That's because each woman's situation is different, and she may require unique dietary and activity recommendations. A pregnant woman with diabetes needs the care of a team dedicated to the management of a high-risk pregnancy, and with such a team approach, the pregnancy usually ends happily with the birth of a healthy baby. After delivery, a woman who had gestational diabetes can apply the principles of *The Best Life Guide to Managing Diabetes and Pre-Diabetes* to help control her diabetes if it persists or to prevent its recurrence if it has gone away.

COMPLICATIONS OF DIABETES AND PRE-DIABETES

You might think you have just one disease: diabetes. But if it's not managed properly, you could wind up with a whole host of other problems. Pre-diabetes can also trigger a number of chronic illnesses. We're not saying this to panic you but to give you a heads-up on just how serious diabetes and pre-diabetes can be. As we emphasize over and over throughout this book, with proper care, you don't have to develop these other problems. If you already have some of the complications of diabetes, good management can slow down their progression or even reverse them to some degree. Below, we run through the basics of the complications of diabetes. In Chapter Five, we'll give some additional information, including which tests can help you track and avoid these problems.

How do diabetes and pre-diabetes set off so many other diseases? One trigger is the excess abdominal fat that often accompanies those two conditions. Another cause is blood sugar itself. At this writing the prevailing theory is that excess glucose in your bloodstream fastens onto proteins all over the body and damages them. These glucose-damaged proteins are called advanced glycation end products, or AGEs. (Glycation is the term for glucose attaching to protein.) Everyone gets some AGE damage as he or she ages, but people with out-of-control diabetes get it earlier and at a higher rate. The accumulation of AGEs in tissues causes many of the complications of diabetes. For instance, AGEs cause inflammation that can trigger clogged arteries, resulting in heart disease and erectile dysfunction. They can also damage the eyes, kidneys, and nerves. Lowering blood sugar reduces AGE damage, and medications that prevent AGE formation are being studied as a way to stop or slow the development of diabetic complications.

Take a deep breath; the complications of diabetes are pretty sobering. Here's the important thing to remember, though: if you follow this program, which means eating healthfully, exercising, and taking your medications properly, you will dramatically reduce the likelihood of developing any of these problems, and you'll help slow their progress if you already have one or more of them.

Heart Disease, Peripheral Vascular Disease, and Stroke

Heart disease, peripheral vascular disease, and stroke are all caused by clogged arteries, which are the blood vessels carrying oxygen to the heart, legs, feet, brain, and other areas of the body. Having diabetes puts you at double the risk (or more) for developing these conditions. In fact, heart disease is the main killer of people with diabetes, and they get it earlier in life than those without high blood sugar. And pre-diabetes heightens the risk of heart disease and stroke by 50 percent. A large-scale European study called DECODE (Diabetes Epidemiology: Collaborative Analysis of Diagnostic Criteria in Europe) found that testing positive for pre-diabetes through an OGTT makes it even more likely that heart disease will ensue than if you simply tested positive via a fasting blood sugar test. If you regularly have your blood cholesterol and blood pressure checked, you should be able to pick up any early warning signs for these conditions (more on this in Chapter Five, "Drugs Used to Treat Diabetes and Prevent Complications").

The type of heart disease that's most common in diabetes is the one in which arteries leading to the heart become narrowed or completely blocked with cholesterol-laden plaque. You might feel this as angina (chest pain) or shortness of breath when you try to exert yourself. A heart attack occurs when one of the arteries becomes completely blocked.

Peripheral vascular disease results from the same process, but it occurs in areas other than the heart, mainly the legs and feet. You might feel pain in the calf (claudication) because the leg is deprived of blood and oxygen. In severe cases, poor blood flow to the lower extremities can result in tissue death that may require amputation of the affected limb.

Strokes happen when blood flow to the brain is interrupted by a clot that blocks an artery. Or an artery with a weakened wall, such as an aneurysm, may simply burst. A TIA, or transient ischemic attack, results from temporary interruption of blood flow in the brain. In this case, the person recovers brain function. If blood flow is cut off too long, permanent damage will occur.

Kidney Disease (Nephropathy)

Remember those AGEs? Well, the theory is that they damage the kidneys to the point where they can no longer filter your blood. High blood pressure is also a major cause of kidney disease, and diabetes and high blood pressure together are really rough on the kidneys. When enough kidney cells are damaged, kidney failure ensues and blood must be artificially filtered with a dialysis machine. The bad news: diabetes is the leading cause of kidney failure and even pre-diabetes is thought to harm the kidneys. The good news: keeping blood sugar levels and blood pressure as close to normal as possible can prevent most cases of kidney damage. There are tests to give you advance warning of kidney problems; we'll tell you about them in Chapter Five.

Eye Disease (Retinopathy)

The most dangerous eye disease caused by diabetes is retinopathy, damage to the retina, the light-sensitive membrane at the back of the eye. This can cause vision loss and, in severe cases, blindness. Again, AGEs are probably the culprit. Pre-diabetes can also cause retinopathy: in the Diabetes Prevention Program discussed on page 20, 8 percent of people with pre-diabetes developed the condition. In addition, having diabetes puts you at greater risk for developing cataracts and weakened eye muscles, which can cause double vision. Widely fluctuating blood sugar levels often cause blurred or changing vision, but this usually goes away when the blood sugar level becomes stable. Regular visits to an ophthalmologist (eye doctor) are a must for anyone suffering from diabetes or pre-diabetes.

Nerve Damage (Neuropathy)

Neuropathy is the term for a broad range of problems that can come from diabetes-related nerve damage. The most common form is peripheral neuropathy (peripheral nerves allow you to feel something as rough or smooth, cold or hot, sharp or dull). If you have significant peripheral neuropathy, that sensation will be diminished. The symptoms usually affect the feet. You may have a "pins and needles" sensation, a burning pain, or numbness. If your feet are numb, you can develop an ulcer without even realizing it, and this can lead to infection of the underlying bones. An increasing number of studies indicate that pre-diabetes also causes peripheral neuropathy. Doctors have long struggled to understand why about 10 percent of people already have neuropathy when they are first diagnosed with diabetes. It's most likely that the nerves were damaged during the pre-diabetes phase.

Autonomic neuropathy affects the autonomic nervous system, which controls your blood pressure, heart rate, and breathing and much of your intestinal function. This can cause severe acid reflux because the stomach isn't emptying properly, chronic diarrhea, and an inability to sense pain properly when there is ongoing damage to the heart or other internal organs, such as the gallbladder. Someone with diabetes is at increased risk of having a "silent" heart attack because the neuropathy numbs the angina pain.

It's easier to reverse neuropathy in its early stages, but the longer you have it, the harder it is to beat. So ideally, you want to prevent it from the get-go with good diabetes management. And if you already have symptoms, a program like the one in this book can prevent further damage.

Sexual Problems

Erectile dysfunction is very common in men with diabetes and pre-diabetes and results mostly from poor blood flow to the penis. High blood pressure and elevated cholesterol, which many people with diabetes have, may be additional culprits. There may also be damage to the nerves that affect erections caused by neuropathy. Men with diabetes also have a higher likelihood of a low testosterone level, which may contribute to poor erections and a loss of interest in sex. We talk about this in detail on pages 243 to 246.

Cut Complication Risk—Dramatically

Fortunately, these spin-off diseases of diabetes and pre-diabetes can be prevented. The theory that good control of blood sugar can dramatically lower your risk of developing these conditions got a big boost in the 1990s from the Diabetes Control and Complications Trial, or DCCT. In this study, 1,400 people with type 1 diabetes (all taking insulin, of course) were divided into two groups receiving either conventional or intensive treatment. When the study began in the early 1980s, conventional treatment meant keeping blood sugar levels just low enough to prevent symptoms such as blurred vision and frequent urination. As long as the person felt okay, it was considered perfectly acceptable to consistently have blood sugar levels in the 200s, which is now considered too high. That's because home blood sugar monitors weren't widely available (when they first hit the market, they were very expensive and not very easy to use). So people with diabetes had to err on the high side in order to prevent hypoglycemia or low blood sugar (see page 70). The intensive treatment group tried to get their blood sugar levels as close to normal as possible through more regular testing with their newly acquired home blood sugar monitors, tests at the doctor's office, and more frequent insulin administration. The study lasted for 10 years.

The results, reported in 1993, were striking. In the intensively managed patients, the frequency of kidney disease was reduced by more than 50 percent. Damage to the nerves and eyes was reduced by 60 percent or more. Even those people who suffered from established complications of diabetes slowed the progression of their problems. From that point on, a relaxed attitude about blood sugar levels was no longer acceptable.

Studies published over the next several years confirmed the same overall encouraging results for people with type 2 diabetes. The United Kingdom Prospective Diabetes Study (UKPDS) included more than 5,000 people with newly diagnosed type 2 diabetes treated with either insulin or oral medications and followed for about eleven years on average. With a fall in average hemoglobin A1c (see page 31 for an explanation of A1c) from about 8 to 7, kidney disease was reduced by 33 percent, and eye disease dropped by 21 percent. Several studies that followed these landmark trials have confirmed the benefit of good diabetes control in terms of preventing or reducing the progression of kidney, eye, and nerve disease, the so-called microvascular complications of diabetes.

Unfortunately, good control of blood sugar is not enough to stave off all the complications of diabetes. The biggies—especially for those with type 2—are heart disease and other macrovascular complications, like stroke and peripheral vascular disease. Although intensively treated patients in the UKPDS had a 14 percent reduction in cardiovascular disease, the results were not as impressive as they were for the microvascular complications like retinal or kidney disease. One important study, the ACCORD (Action to Control Cardiovascular Risk in Diabetes) trial, published in 2008, even suggested that lowering blood sugar levels too much might *increase* mortality from heart disease and other causes. This is puzzling, because nearly all the other studies have shown that lower is better. One important point is that people in the ACCORD trial were chosen because they had known heart disease or a very high risk for it, and the results may not hold for the average person with diabetes. Also, this is the only study to date that has shown an increased risk from lower day-to-day blood sugar levels. In fact, two other large studies published in 2008 showed no such increase in heart disease risk among those who had better blood sugar control. Placing too much emphasis on just one study can lead to a roller-coaster ride of medical recommendations. So far we think it's better to shoot for lower blood sugar levels as long as you don't have too many episodes of hypoglycemia.

Here's the bottom line: in order to reduce macrovascular problems, including heart disease and stroke, it's important to keep your body weight, blood pressure, and LDL ("bad") cholesterol in the normal range, get enough exercise, and, if you smoke, it's essential to quit. And of course, it's important to control blood sugar. Remember, though, that insulin resistance causes vascular inflammation and blocked arteries even without high blood sugar, so becoming less insulin resistant by maintaining a healthy body weight is your goal.

MANAGING DIABETES AND PRE-DIABETES

It might be tempting to imagine that simply popping some pills or injecting insulin will take care of your problem. But diabetes and pre-diabetes are diseases for which medication alone isn't enough. In fact, many people with these conditions could be treated *without* medication if they would make the changes in diet and exercise that we recommend in this book. Even for those who must be on medication, lifestyle makes a big difference in the prognosis down the road.

If one leg of a three-legged stool is missing, the stool topples over. The same holds true for the management of your diabetes: it needs to be supported by a good diet, enough exercise, and proper medications. Addressing all three is the only way to achieve the best possible blood sugar control, stave off complications, and increase the chances that you'll live your best possible life. If you already have some complications, this program can help prevent them from progressing any further and, in some cases, can reverse the damage.

In addition, we think you'll be very happy with the side benefits. You may look and feel dramatically different, especially if you lose weight—and you can lose a lot of weight on this program. You'll also become more fit and have lots more energy. You may lower your blood sugar level to a point where you will need less medication—always a big bonus.

Admittedly, there's a lot to do. Right from the start, you'll be eating the appropriate amounts of carbs and getting more exercise. If you have diabetes, you'll be monitoring blood sugar. You'll check in with your doctor to see if these new habits warrant any shifts in your medications. *This is very important*—the changes you're making on this plan may lower your blood sugar so that your old dose of medicine is too high.

The truth is that managing your disease can be very challenging, and that's why we've broken it down into three phases, so you work up gradually to the best way of eating and exercising. Even with this approach, you're bound to feel overwhelmed sometimes. But hang in there, because the longer you do it, the easier it gets. When you regularly carve out space in your schedule for exercise, it's easier to get to the gym or take that power walk. After you've measured your cereal a few times, you no longer have to do it; eyeballing works fine. The more you use your blood sugar monitor, the easier it becomes, as does injecting insulin if that's how you're treated. When you're lighter and fitter, you can fly through tasks that were once fatiguing and difficult. When your blood sugar is under control, you will have far more energy. So be patient, work through the learning curve, and life will get easier.

Treating Diabetes and Pre-Diabetes with Drugs

Even with good diet and exercise habits, most people with diabetes still require medications. Nearly all medications for diabetes do one of two things: either they increase the amount of insulin in your body, thus overcoming insulin deficiency, or they improve how your body responds to insulin, helping to correct insulin resistance. If you have pre-diabetes, you probably won't need medication, though studies have shown that medications that improve insulin resistance may delay the onset of diabetes in those with pre-diabetes. If you have type 1 diabetes, the drug choice is pretty simple: insulin. On occasion, you may benefit from other medications as well, especially to combat insulin resistance if you are overweight. If you have type 2 diabetes, a dizzying array of treatment options opens up. In the best-case scenario, you won't need any medication, at least for a while; diet and exercise may do the trick. But as the condition progresses, these lifestyle changes may not be enough. Figuring out which medications are best for you may take a little trial and error, even with an experienced doctor. We devote a lot of time to this subject—see "Drugs Used to Treat Diabetes and Prevent Complications," beginning on page 189.

Many people with type 2 diabetes will also need insulin therapy, just like people with type 1. Let's be honest: most people find the idea of taking insulin frightening or intimidating. But here's one of the most important things we're going to say in the entire book: *there is no reason to be afraid of insulin treatment.* People are often scared of insulin because they don't like the idea of shots or because they believe that being on insulin means that their disease is more severe. As for the first issue, we don't blame people— nobody really likes to be stuck with a needle—but the injections are very easy to give and hurt very little. When it comes to the second issue, the truth is often the complete opposite of what people believe: the simple fact is that someone who is on pills but has a high blood sugar level has a much more serious condition than someone who is on insulin and has good blood sugar control. Even though most people are hesitant at the beginning, what we usually hear from someone who has started insulin is "I can't believe I was afraid of this!" or "I wish I had started insulin a long time ago. I feel so much better now!"

Monitoring Your Progress

If you improve your diet and exercise habits, how will you know whether your efforts are paying off? Two important tools—one for home use, the other from your doctor—will let you know how your blood sugar is responding. As for keeping an eye on all the complications of diabetes, such as kidney and heart disease, there are tests for these conditions as well. We'll look at those in Chapter Five.

BLOOD SUGAR MONITOR

This is the device you use to prick your finger and get a blood sugar reading (discussed in detail in the Phase One chapter). Finger-stick measurements provide an instant snapshot of your blood sugar at precisely that moment. You'll find out the effects of the chicken sandwich you had for lunch, the after-dinner walk, or the overnight fast. It's critical to log this information so you can discover patterns, such as "My blood sugar is usually high in the morning before breakfast" or "I go too low after I take my power walk." The Best Life Diabetes Management Log on page 335 is an ideal way to record this information. You'll find out everything you need to know about testing and logging, a must on this program, in the Phase One chapter.

HEMOGLOBIN A1c (A1c)

This test is usually done at the doctor's office, although home kits are now available. While finger-stick blood testing reveals the blood sugar reading at that moment in time, the A1c test gives you a sense of how your blood sugars have been behaving over the past two to three months.

You might wonder what hemoglobin, which transports oxygen in red blood cells, has to do with your blood sugar. Here's the link: Glucose in the blood makes its way into red blood cells, where it reacts with hemoglobin to form a new chemical combination called hemoglobin A1c. The higher your blood sugar, the more A1c is made. The A1c hangs around for as long as the red blood cells live (about four months), so when you measure the A1c in your blood, you get an average of how much is in all your cells. Because some cells are new and some cells are up to four months old, the average is something like two months. Therefore, the A1c test will tell you, on average, how high your blood sugar has been for the two or three months prior to the test. A normal A1c is under about 6 (meaning that just 6 percent of the hemoglobin in your body is in the form of hemoglobin A1c). The higher it goes, the higher your average blood sugar levels have been (see "A1c's Got Your Number," page 32).

As valuable as it is, the A1c test has its limitations. It tells you how your blood sugar has been doing on average, but it can't tell you how you got to that average. Let's say your A1c is 6.5, which is considered excellent control, corresponding to an average blood sugar reading of about 140. Was your blood sugar humming along in a nice tight range of 90 to 190 to get there? Or, were you swinging from dangerous lows in the 30s to dangerous highs in the upper 200s? The home blood glucose monitor completes the picture by letting you know your blood sugar range on an

A1c'S GOT YOUR NUMBER

Because the A1c test reflects your average blood sugar levels over the past two to three months, it's an excellent indicator of how well you're managing your diabetes. You should know your A1c and how it's been changing over time. You'll still need your finger-stick numbers to complete the picture, as these tell you how much you're fluctuating and if there's a daily pattern to your numbers.

Note that a lower A1c is *usually* better, but only if you get there without having frequent or severe low-blood-sugar reactions. Remember, the lower your A1c, the lower your average sugar and the more likely you are to have episodes of hypoglycemia. An A1c of 6.5 may be a terrific result for someone who very rarely goes too low, but someone who has a lot of problems with low blood sugar levels may have to shoot for a higher value in order to be safe.

Here's what the A1c numbers mean:

6.0 and under: Normal. People without diabetes are under 6, but only a small percentage of people with diabetes consistently get into this zone.

6.5: Excellent overall control.

Under 7: Good control.

Between 7 and 8: Fair control. In most cases, you can probably do better.

Over 8: Poor control, and the higher you go, the worse off you are. Someone with a hemoglobin A1c of 11, for example, would regularly have glucose levels over 300, and his or her average glucose levels would be running more than 100 points higher than ideal.

DIAGNOSING DIABETES WITH THE HEMOGLOBIN A1c:

Currently, A1c is used to track the progression of your disease, but in 2009, a group of leading diabetes experts proposed using it to diagnose diabetes as well. Here's what they are recommending:

6.0 and under: Normal.

From 6.0 to 6.5: Values in this range indicate a "heightened risk of diabetes," roughly, though not exactly, corresponding to the current definition of pre-diabetes. The risk of developing diabetes and cardiovascular disease goes up as the A1c rises through this range.

6.5 and over: This would mean a diagnosis of diabetes, and ongoing control would be as outlined above.

ongoing basis. In addition, there are some conditions, such as sickle-cell disease and other hemoglobin disorders, where the hemoglobin A1c test is not reliable.

Some people find it confusing to keep the two numbers straight—blood sugar numbers, where normal is around 100, and A1c numbers, where normal is around 6. Because a given A1c represents the average blood sugar level over time, you can convert the A1c to that blood sugar level, called the estimated average glucose or eAG, by using a simple calculation described in the "What's Your eAG?" box. Some doctors and diabetes researchers have proposed that A1c values be converted to eAG so that people can compare their finger-stick glucose values with their average glucose levels over the past few weeks. The eAG value may become the

---

WHAT'S YOUR eAG?

The estimated average glucose, or eAG, translates your A1c value into a much more familiar number: an average blood sugar reading. For example, as you can see from the table below, an A1c of 6.5 means that if you took many blood sugar readings at all different times throughout the day, the average of all the readings—the eAG—would be about 140. You can calculate your own eAG by multiplying your A1c by 28.7 and then subtracting 46.7 (the formula is 28.7 × A1c − 46.7 = eAG). Below are the eAGs corresponding to various A1c values:

A1c %	eAG (mg/dL)
6	126
6.5	140
7	154
7.5	169
8	183
8.5	197
9	212
9.5	226
10	240

standard over the next several years, but for now most people still refer to the A1c, and that's what we'll do in this book.

LIVING YOUR BEST LIFE WITH DIABETES AND PRE-DIABETES

We've given you the straight facts about the damaging effects of diabetes not to scare you or make you felt guilty but rather to empower you. The ability to prevent diabetes-related problems is almost completely in your hands, and we hope this will motivate you to make the habit changes laid out in the rest of this book.

But there's something else we want for you: to enjoy your life. There's a balance you'll have to strike between discipline and reward, between sacrifice and pleasure. When we talk about the management of any medical problem, including diabetes, we quote mortality statistics and research studies. But managing your disease shouldn't be just about staying alive; it should be about living life and enjoying it. It wouldn't be reasonable for you—or us—to expect that you'll never indulge in an ice cream sundae or just laze around the house one day. We will have failed miserably if you follow this program to a T but walk around feeling deprived. Our diet plan allows for treats that should satisfy cravings, and we're flexible enough with our exercise plan that if you want a little break, it's okay. The overall goal is not for you to simply "eat right" or "exercise enough." The goal is for you to feel well and be healthy, and we think this program will help you do that without making it seem like an impossible task. Sure, it's going to take some effort to manage your diabetes, but we hope you'll find parts of it interesting and, yes, even enjoyable. (For instance, we bet that you'll love many of our recipes and that many of you are going to find physical activity rewarding.) We want you to be healthy and take pleasure in your life—your *Best Life*!

2

PHASE ONE: TAKING CONTROL OVER YOUR BLOOD SUGAR

WE'LL SAY IT AGAIN: the way your diabetes or pre-diabetes plays out is largely in your hands. You might be feeling a little frightened by both the diagnosis and the responsibility; try to turn that fear into a determination to get your diet and exercise habits on track. Right now, you may be very motivated to do what it takes to lower your blood sugar level; hold on to this motivation as you begin to make some important lifestyle changes.

In Phase One of the plan, you won't have to drastically change everything you eat, nor will you have to spend hours each day at the gym. Instead, this phase focuses on making a few simple, but critical, habit changes that will help you drop pounds (if you need to) and improve your blood sugar levels. Your main focus in this phase will be eating appropriate amounts of carbohydrates; you don't have to worry about changing much else about your diet. As for exercise, you'll challenge yourself to increase your activity gradually. Meanwhile, you'll be using a blood glucose monitor to check your sugar at appropriate points in the day and recording these numbers alongside your meals and exercise. This log will clue you in to any necessary adjustments to your diet, medication, or exercise. If you have pre-diabetes you will not be monitoring your blood sugar, but all other aspects of the program apply to you. Further fine-tuning of your diet and exercise routine will come later. We know there is no single perfect diet or workout that fits everyone; throughout all the three phases of this book, we'll help you develop a plan that works for *you*.

There's one other critical component we haven't mentioned yet: emotions. It's natural to become anxious, upset, and stressed out when you are first diagnosed with diabetes or pre-diabetes. If you're an emotional eater, you may be tempted to turn to food to cope with this new stressor. But as those of you who've taken a few turns on the weight-loss roller coaster know very well, emotional eating only perpetuates the vicious cycle. You may feel soothed for a little while after eating, but then the guilt and stress from overdoing it set in, which will likely drive you to seek comfort, once again, from food. And so on. In addition, having diabetes increases the likelihood of having depression. In Phase Three, we'll be addressing the emotional side of managing diabetes and pre-diabetes and offer advice on maintaining your motivation. Phase Three is eight weeks away, but if you'd like some help on the emotional issues now, just read ahead, starting on page 154.

All the diet, exercise, and other goals in this phase and throughout the rest of the program apply whether you have type 1 diabetes, type 2 diabetes, or pre-diabetes. (The only exception: you don't have to test and log blood sugar if you have pre-diabetes unless your doctor suggests it, as might be the case if your blood sugar takes a steep climb.) For instance, the meal plans will benefit you no matter where you fall on the diabetes spectrum. Although they're optional, we encourage you to give them a try—they are a delicious way to learn how to put all our diet prescriptions into action.

Note that even though the meals and recipes from this book can be enjoyed by the whole family, and there are a number of family-oriented exercise ideas, this program is not for children. It's also not for pregnant women. That's because children—especially those with type 1 diabetes—and pregnant women have special needs that go beyond the scope of this program. Pregnant women should team up with their ob/gyn and, perhaps, a registered dietitian or certified diabetes educator to manage the disease. And if your child has diabetes, you should work with his or her doctor and turn to the following resources for more help and information:

the Juvenile Diabetics Research Foundation International (www.jdrf.org), a leading organization in the fight against diabetes in children and adolescents; the American Diabetes Association (www.diabetes.org), which offers tips and information on research; the National Diabetes Education Program (www.ndep.nih.gov), which offers information and news on diabetes research; and *487 Really Cool Tips for Kids with Diabetes* and *Getting a Grip on Diabetes*, both by Spike Nasmyth Loy and Bo Nasmyth Loy, which will help you and your child meet the challenges of the disease.

For now, let's start at the beginning. If you make the Phase One habit changes listed below, you'll be well on your way toward managing diabetes.

PHASE ONE

TIME FRAME: About four weeks.

WEIGH IN: Weigh yourself on the day you start Phase One, then no more than once a week. Or don't weigh yourself at all until four weeks into the program. It's your choice.

FOCUS: Monitoring and recording your blood sugar level, medications, and activity (if you have diabetes), eating appropriate amounts of carbohydrates, increasing your physical activity.

OBJECTIVES:

- If you have diabetes, regularly test your blood sugar and keep a blood sugar/drug/food/exercise log.

- Eat appropriate amounts of carbohydrates.

- Eat three meals and two snacks each day, three snacks if you're taking in 2,250 calories daily.

- Eat a Best Life Breakfast.

- Eat lightly—or not at all—during the two hours before bedtime.

- Eliminate sweetened beverages and alcohol.

- Drink six glasses of water daily.

- Increase your activity.

JUDGING YOUR SUCCESS: Compared to when you began, your blood sugar is closer to, or in, the acceptable range, you're eating a more appropriate amount of carbohydrates, and you're getting more exercise.

PHASE ONE OBJECTIVES

Test It, Log It

(If you have pre-diabetes, you can skip this monitoring section unless your doctor has suggested you test at home.)

Our goal for you: blood sugar in the normal range, consistently, every time you check—or at the very least, blood sugar readings in the acceptable range (see "Target Blood Glucose Level" page 40). Knowing how your blood sugar responds to different medications and doses, to meals, to exercise, to an overnight fast, and to the length of time between meals will help you craft a plan that is right for you.

You'll find all this out with the help of your new best friend: a blood glucose monitor (also called a glucose meter), an electronic device that reads your blood sugar level. The numbers flashing on the screen of this little device let you know how well you're managing your disease. Using the monitor is a critical component of this program. We'll help you set up a testing schedule of the best times of the day to check your sugar. Already using a monitor? Look at the testing suggestions anyway; you may find a better approach. If you've been erratic about using the monitor, we hope to make a good case for picking it up again more regularly. Of course, you must discuss the schedule with your doctor and make sure it doesn't need to be tweaked for your particular issues.

As we've said, testing with a blood glucose monitor lets you know how that morning bowl of oatmeal, that long walk, or your medication is affecting your blood sugar. It's what clinicians call pattern management: managing your diabetes by discovering your own unique blood sugar patterns and adjusting your diet, medications, and activity accordingly. For instance, you might be one of those people who have a high blood sugar level upon waking but not after meals. Figuring out your pattern will help you and your doctor determine the type and dose of medication you'll need.

We're going to make it easy for you to detect your blood sugar patterns with the Best Life Diabetes Management Log on page 335, which you can copy to keep track of blood sugar, meals, exercise, and doses and timing of your medication. You can also log your blood sugar numbers, meals, and exercise online if you join www.thebestlife.com/diabetes. This Web site also offers carbohydrate-controlled meal plans and lots of other resources for people with diabetes.

By entering meals into your log, you'll soon discover which are kindest to your blood sugar. For example, one of the goals of Phase One is to eat a Best Life Breakfast every day. Check out the meal plans starting on page 250—you have quite a choice of breakfasts: eggs, cereal, peanut butter and toast, and much more. What they all have in common: the same amount of carbohydrates. Say you pick the oatmeal-based breakfast on Day 1, and two hours after eating, your blood sugar is near normal, but the waffle-based breakfast on Day 8 left your blood sugar too high. A number of factors influence blood sugar levels, so you can try those breakfasts again. If you get a similar result each time, it means the oatmeal breakfast is a keeper, and from now on you'll skip the waffles. Pretty soon, you'll have a great collection of blood-sugar-friendly meals that work for you. On www.the bestlife.com/diabetes, you can save your favorite meals and create daily meal plans around them.

Monitoring your blood sugar doesn't just help you pick the best meals, it also lets you know whether you're taking the right amount of medication to prevent a large spike in blood sugar after eating. And monitoring before bedtime and first thing in the morning will help you know if your meds are keeping your blood sugar in a good range overnight.

Your blood sugar monitor will also clue you in to the effects of exercise. Does your blood sugar go up or down after a short walk, a long walk, an aerobics class, a jog, or any other form of exercise? Do you need to adjust your medicine to safely cover exercise? That's what your trusty monitor will reveal. On this plan, you'll be moving your body more, and that may mean you need less medication, whether you're taking insulin or any other diabetes drug. For some of you, the combination of diet and exercise could mean a dramatic decrease in medication or even that you can stop taking medication. However, your body's ability to make insulin tends to decrease as time passes, so even with the best diet and exercise regimen, your blood sugar levels may eventually rise again and you may need to increase or restart medications in order to keep them normal.

By helping you keep your blood sugar in line, your monitor can help you ward off diabetes-associated conditions such as heart disease and neuropathy. That's what a 2009 study at the German Diabetes Center in Düsseldorf, Germany, found. Researchers tracked 3,268 people with type 2 diabetes for 6½ years from the time of diagnosis. They found that those using glucose monitors had half the number of heart attacks and 37 percent fewer strokes than people not using the device.

Target Blood Glucose Level

These are the numbers to shoot for. "Ideal" is what blood sugar readings look like in people without diabetes. You may be able to achieve these. If not, your levels should fall into the acceptable range.

TIME	IDEAL (NORMAL RANGE), mg/dL	ACCEPTABLE RANGE, mg/dL
Before meals	70–100	70–130
Two hours after the start of a meal	Less than 140	Less than 180

GLUCOSE MONITORS (OR METERS)

Having to prick your finger to test your blood sugar level isn't on the top of many people's wish list, but believe it or not, you should actually feel pretty lucky. Until the 1980s, home monitors were not widely available and you had to see your doctor or go to the hospital to find out your blood sugar level. The monitors have gotten much easier to use and faster as time has passed, and new monitors require very little blood. These devices have revolutionized diabetes management. For example, people used to be terrified of insulin because they thought they might have a hypoglycemic reaction. Without home blood sugar monitoring, it was nearly impossible to determine an insulin dose that was safe but would also help keep the blood sugar level near normal. Now you can get immediate feedback on the effects of insulin, oral diabetes drugs, diet, and exercise on your blood sugar level. That feedback will help you shape the best possible treatment plan. And once you get the technique down, it isn't painful—we promise!

There are basically two types of monitors: the most common one, by far, is simply called a glucose monitor or glucose meter. It involves pricking a finger with a tiny needle called a lancet and placing a drop of blood on a test strip. The monitor reads the strip for your blood glucose level. They're quick—you'll know your number within seconds. The other option, relatively new and rapidly improving, is a continuous glucose monitor, or CGM, which we describe in detail beginning on page 228.

The Holy Grail of glucose monitoring would be a system that will let you know your blood sugar without breaking your skin at all, called a noninvasive glucose monitor. Some devices have been developed and even sold in the United States and elsewhere, but there are really no versions available right now that are as reliable as the standard meters or the CGMs. Some of the ads you see on TV that say "no finger sticks" are really talking about getting blood by pricking yourself somewhere else, such as the forearm (see page 42). Be sure you know what you're getting! Many companies are working hard to develop systems that will allow for noninvasive testing, because they know that millions of people around the world with diabetes will rush to their doors the minute something reliable and economical becomes available.

BUYING AND USING A GLUCOSE MONITOR

Cost. Glucose monitors themselves are not very expensive; they typically retail for between $50 and $100, and you can usually get coupons that offer a substantial discount. Sometimes you can even get a monitor free from your doctor or diabetes educator or the manufacturer. The real expense is the test strips. At full retail, these typically go for about $0.75 per strip. Even if you're monitoring just once a day, that's $22.50 per month or $270.00 per year. Because most people benefit from frequent monitoring, at least at some point during their diabetes management, the real cost of monitoring may be substantial. We know many patients who test five or six times per day or even more; that adds up to a lot of money. For many people, the single most important question is whether their insurance plan will cover the cost of a particular meter and strips. If your insurance will pay all or a portion of the cost of a certain brand, it's probably reasonable to go with that brand. Sometimes insurance companies or diabetes suppliers have contracts with brands that aren't as desirable because the meters require a larger drop of blood (meaning you have to stick yourself more deeply), aren't as user-friendly, or don't offer high-tech bells and whistles such as the ability to download the information to a computer. In this case you can either try to persuade your insurer or the supplier to give you a better model or pay for it yourself.

Check out a meter's features and tools before you make the purchase. Some meters have large displays or audio readouts for those who are visually impaired. Some meters are unusually small and light. Some meters just seem easier for some people to use. Be sure to talk to your doctor, pharmacist, or diabetes educator about your preferences. In most cases, however, what matters more than the brand of meter or the features it offers is that you use the proper testing technique and record the information consistently and in a useful manner.

Working the Device. Even just a few years ago, a large drop of blood was required to test your blood sugar. Happily, that's no longer true. Most of the current meters use very little blood, and it makes sense to choose one that requires only a very small amount so that the needle stick doesn't have to be painful. Note that meters that require only small amounts of blood often allow you to collect the sample from spots other than your fingertips; this is often called alternative-site testing and may be helpful if your fingertips are getting sore from frequent testing. The forearm is often recommended, but it's frequently more difficult to get blood from this area because there is not as much blood flowing near the surface of the skin as there is in the fingertips, and many people have a lot of hair, which prevents the drop from staying in place until it's drawn up into the strip. A lancet device that applies a small amount of suction after the needle stick (for example, the Vaculance) sometimes makes testing on the forearm easier.

Still, the finger is usually your best bet. If you do it right, you'll feel just a little pressure but no pain. Here's the technique: Place your hand on a firm surface such as a tabletop with your palm facing up. This will prevent you from unconsciously pulling away as you are about to stick your finger. Dial the lancet device—a penlike instrument containing a lancet, a sharp, disposable needle—to the lowest level (with the least penetration). Push the lancet device firmly into your finger, stretching the skin tight like a drum. This will allow it to pierce your skin without going very deep, and the pressure will push up a drop of blood. Many people have told us that this method causes them almost no pain. If the lowest setting doesn't pierce the skin, try the next to lowest, and so on.

Logging Results. You've taken a reading, but the job's only half done. Recording this information is essential. You can write it down in the Best Life Diabetes Management Log (page 335), or you can rely on your meter to store the information. Nearly all glucose meters store readings, and most come with software that lets you download the readings into your computer. The software will let your print out the readings and analyze them in various ways. The computer readings *look* good, with the blood sugar number and the date and time, but they often miss the boat on recording meals. For instance, if you eat breakfast, lunch, or another meal outside the window of time programmed for that meal, your meter might indicate that the test was taken after the meal when it was actually done before you ate.

Some of the newer meters let you enter whether a test is before or after a meal, and may let you choose from a list of common foods or enter grams of carbohydrate. These are fantastic if you are very detail-oriented and use them with great care, especially if you are on an insulin pump or are taking multiple injections of insulin daily. Some people have glucose meters that provide information directly to their insulin pumps, facilitating proper insulin dosing. We'll talk about this a bit more in the section on insulin treatment of type 1 diabetes beginning on page 219.

In our experience, a simple meter and a handwritten record work best for most people. You'll find the Best Life Diabetes Management Log a useful tool that will help you and your doctor or certified diabetes educator spot important trends and patterns. Because most physicians don't have time to wade through the diet and exercise details, we've also provided a Doctor's Log on page 339 to take to your doctor's appointments. See page 336 for tips on using the log.

WHEN TO MONITOR

Don't worry, you won't have to stick your finger all day. Though all readings are helpful, certain readings—such as those taken in the morning, before meals, two hours after meals, and before bedtime—provide particularly valuable clues as to whether your overall diabetes management is working well. You and your doctor may come up with a testing schedule; if not, here is a common approach that will provide plenty of information without your having to test your sugar constantly.

Common Monitoring Pattern

DAY 1

- Check your fasting sugar first thing in the morning, before breakfast or any activity.
- Check again 2 hours after breakfast (start counting the time at the beginning of the meal).

DAY 2

- Check right before lunch.
- Check again 2 hours after lunch.

DAY 3

- Check right before dinner.
- Check again 2 hours after dinner.

DAY 4 AND AFTER

- Repeat the above cycle, choosing a different meal each day.
- If there are several hours between the after-dinner test and when you go to bed, do a pre-bedtime test some days.

■ On a few occasions, set an alarm clock and do a test in the middle of the night (2 or 3 A.M. for most people); this is especially valuable if you wake up with a high blood sugar level or do not sleep well.

You'll record that information in both the Best Life Diabetes Management Log and the Doctor's Log. Here's an example from a 66-year-old patient, Jackie, who was diagnosed with type 2 diabetes about three weeks before completing this Doctor's Log. She was taking the oral medication metformin but had not started seriously watching her carbohydrate intake and was not yet exercising.

DATE	BEFORE BREAKFAST	2 HOURS AFTER BREAKFAST	BEFORE LUNCH	2 HOURS AFTER LUNCH	BEFORE DINNER	2 HOURS AFTER DINNER	BEDTIME	OVERNIGHT (2 A.M. TO 3 A.M.)
Feb 1	96	223						
Feb 2			105	98				
Feb 3					104	160		106
Feb 4	110	215						
Feb 5			92	117				
Feb 6					134	174		
Feb 7	87	193					162	
Feb 8			95	104				
Feb 9					86	163		

In this example, Jackie tested before and after meals in a repeating 1–2–3 day cycle and did one extra test at 3 A.M. and one extra test at bedtime during the nine days. You can see that her sugars soar after breakfast and she tends to be high after dinner but has no problem with lunch.

Jackie's log is just one example of how testing about twice a day can give very useful information. Those who have very stable and well-controlled blood sugar levels may not need to test more than two or three times a week; people who are wearing insulin pumps or taking meal-related insulin often test themselves many times a day. Your doctor or diabetes educator may have specific information that he or she would like to gather and may ask you to test according to a particular schedule. We're not trying to recommend a one-size-fits-all schedule for testing; we want to help you understand how best to use the test information. Once you do, you can develop a schedule most appropriate for you.

Interpreting Highs and Lows

What's going on when you experience a blood sugar swing? Here are some common causes. There may be other triggers as well, and we'll go into more detail about that in Chapter Five "Drugs Used to Treat Diabetes and Prevent Complications."

WHEN YOUR BLOOD SUGAR IS . . .	IT COULD MEAN . . .
High upon waking	Your liver is releasing too much sugar at night, or you had a middle-of-the-night low and your body is overcompensating (the Somogyi phenomenon). Or a rise in the hormone cortisol occurring in the early morning hours is causing the sugar to rise (the dawn phenomenon).
Much higher after breakfast	You've consumed too many carbs at breakfast, a common occurrence with typical American breakfasts (such as cereal with milk), or you've had a carryover from the high cortisol levels that cause the dawn phenomenon (see above).
High all the time	Your blood sugar is out of control; you need to see your doctor right away and adjust your medication and diet.
Low in the middle of the night or upon waking	You are taking too much long-acting medication, or your liver may not be making enough sugar during periods of fasting, such as overnight.
Higher after exercise	The adrenaline that your body makes during exercise is causing your sugar to rise. Usually this is temporary, and overall, exercise lowers blood sugars.
Lower during or after exercise	You are taking too much medication or not consuming enough carbohydrates prior to exercising. Remember: if you are getting a lot of low readings, ask your doctor about reducing your medication rather than just taking in more food, to avoid packing on extra pounds.

WHEN TO STEP UP THE MONITORING

Normally, you can follow the sample testing schedule in the "Common Monitoring Pattern" section on page 44 or develop one with your doctor. This should give you a good idea about your personal blood sugar pattern. However, there are certain situations when you'll need to take more regular readings. These include:

- When you are first diagnosed. You'll benefit from frequent testing for the first several weeks or until you see your blood sugar levels stabilize.

- When you make any changes to your exercise frequency or intensity.

- When you make any changes to your diet, such as cutting calories or adjusting carbohydrate, protein, or fat intake.

- When your doctor changes your medication or dosage.

- When your blood sugar levels were well controlled but now have gone off course.

- When you become ill with a cold or flu or other condition, especially one that makes you sick to your stomach or prevents you from keeping down fluids.

Controlling Your Carbs

YOUR DAILY CARBOHYDRATE ALLOWANCE

If you like your morning bowl of cereal, you're a fruit lover, or sandwiches are a staple of your diet, you'll be very happy with this plan. Yes, we've limited carbohydrates to help stabilize blood sugar, but there are still enough to make eating enjoyable. There is no one-size-fits-all carb prescription; some people can handle more at a meal than others. In the charts and meal plans in this book, we offer a model that should be easy on your blood sugar while providing the vitamins, minerals, and phytonutrients (beneficial plant compounds) unique to carbohydrate-rich foods.

How many carbs you're allowed each day is tied to your daily calorie needs, which, in turn, are based on genetics, whether you need to lose weight, and how much exercise you're getting. Obviously, the more calories you burn through physical activity and the faster your inherent metabolism, the more calories you can consume and still stay at a healthy weight or lose weight.

We've created a few handy charts to help you get a handle on carbs. Don't worry—you won't have to do much calculating or difficult math to figure it all out. In fact, all you'll have to do is learn how many servings of various carbohydrate-rich foods, such as fruit, vegetables, starchy foods, milk, or yogurt, to eat each day. Here's how to get started.

Step One: Pick a calorie level from the "Find Your Daily Calorie Level" table, on page 53. The descriptions of the people best suited for each calorie level are very general; for example, we're estimating that a woman at Activity Level 3 looking to lose weight should consume 1,700 calories per day, but at that level you might need to adjust your calorie intake up or down. If after a week or so you're hungry nearly all the time, you can bump up to the next calorie level. If you're feeling pretty satisfied but not losing weight, you should go down a calorie level (and make sure you're getting enough exercise!). As you can see, 1,500 calories per day is the lowest-calorie plan we offer; any lower, and not only do you risk falling short on key nutrients, but you'll also be so hungry that you won't be following the plan for long!

Step Two: Become familiar with carbohydrate servings. Use the "Daily Servings" table on page 53 to get a sense of how many servings from the different high-carbohydrate food groups you get daily. As you can see, on the 1,500- and 1,700-calorie plans, you get four grain/starchy vegetable servings daily, two fruits, etc. The "What's a Carbohydrate Serving?" lists (page 59) will tell you what a serving size looks like.

Step Three: Limit the amount of high-carb foods you consume at each meal. Turn to the "High-Carbohydrate Foods at Each Meal" table on page 54 to see how best to divvy up your high-carb foods among breakfast, lunch, dinner, snacks, and treats. Try out our model—it makes for an even distribution of carbohydrates throughout the day, and it's practical.

You'll have a milk/yogurt serving at breakfast, which is when most people have dairy products, and there's enough starch at lunch for a sandwich. Look at the meal plans, which start on page 250, to see how these servings translate into real breakfasts, lunches, dinners, and snacks.

Step Four: Test your blood sugar more often and check in with your doctor. (See "Common Monitoring Pattern" on page 44.) The way of eating that we're recommending on these pages is not low-carb, but at 38 to 42 percent of total calories from carbohydrates it might be lower in carbs than your current diet, especially if you're cutting calories and eating less food overall. When your carbohydrate intake drops, so can your blood sugar level—that's the point—but it may warrant a lower dose of medication. If you were on a low-carbohydrate diet and are now eating more carbs, you should still monitor more and check in with your doctor, as your medication may still need to be changed.

TRACKING CARBOHYDRATES IN FOODS: "SIZE UP SERVINGS" METHOD

Once you know how many servings of carbohydrates you can consume each day and what constitutes a serving, you'll be able to put that knowledge into practice on your plate. Over the next few weeks, you are going to become a serving size expert. You'll be able to eyeball your plate at a restaurant and say, "That's a cup of rice—three servings." You'll be able to pour a nearly perfect amount of cereal into your bowl. But before that happens, you'll have to do a little measuring.

Dealing with serving sizes is much simpler than counting carbohydrate grams. Just think how much easier it is to plan your dinner around one grain/starchy vegetable serving (for instance, a small dinner roll) and three vegetable servings (such as 1½ cups of sautéed broccoli) than trying to figure out how much bread and broccoli will amount to 45 grams of carbohydrate.

Some food manufacturers make it really easy for you by posting food group information along with other nutritional information right on the package. ("Diet exchanges" and "food exchanges" are terms used for the food group classification system we're using in this book.)

The "Size Up Servings" approach will work for most meals, but there will still be times when you'll have to deal with carbohydrate grams, as you'll see below. Those of you on short-acting insulin may have to be more precise about carbohydrate grams (for details, see pages 219 to 230).

MEASURING UP

While the "Size Up Servings" method will rarely give you the *exact* carbohydrate gram count of a meal, if you know your stuff, you'll get close enough to make a big difference in your diabetes management. To become savvy about servings, you have to do a little homework. Instead of pen and paper, your tools are measuring cups and spoons and bowls, plates, cups, and mugs.

You won't have to carry around measuring cups and spoons forever! But over the next few weeks, measure, at least once, all the high-carbohydrate foods you eat; it's especially important to measure foods you eat regularly.

Measuring your food is an essential step for weight loss and diabetes management, and you will probably be surprised by how much you've been putting on your plate!

WHAT YOU'LL NEED

A set of measuring spoons

A set of measuring cups

WHAT YOU'LL DO

1. Measure out the correct portion of the carbohydrate-containing food you want to eat. Sometimes you can go straight off the "What's a Carbohydrate Serving?" lists on page 59. Say you're having blueberries as part of a snack. Just measure out a serving—⅔ cup—into your bowl. For packaged foods, you'll have to rely on the nutrition label to help you out. For instance, cold cereals are all over the map; a cup of granola has 61 grams of carbohydrate, while a cup of whole wheat flakes has 23 grams of carbohydrate. Looking at the "What's a Carbohydrate Serving?" lists, you see that a grain/starchy vegetable serving contains 15 grams of carbohydrate. You're allowed 1½ serv-

ings from that food group for breakfast no matter what daily calorie level you're on—that's 22 to 23 grams of carbohydrate. You can enjoy a cup of wheat flakes or about a ⅓ cup of granola.

It's worth memorizing the carb counts of serving sizes; fortunately, there are just a few numbers to remember:

15 grams for each serving of fruit, grain, and starchy vegetable

12 grams for each milk/yogurt serving

10 grams for dessert if you're on the 1,700-calorie-per-day plan; 15 grams on the 2,000- or 2,250-calorie plan

5 grams for each serving of nonstarchy vegetable

Using these numbers and the nutrition labels on prepared foods, you can figure out how much of a chocolate bar you get for 10 grams of carbohydrate, and you can tell if a slice of bread exceeds the 15-gram carbohydrate limit.

Carrying around the "What's a Carbohydrate Serving?" lists with you at all times isn't a bad idea; you can make a copy from the book or print out a version on www.thebestlife.com/diabetes.

2. Use the same bowls, plates, and glasses for all your meals and snacks. Measure your oatmeal or cereal into the same-size bowl each time and pour your milk or soy milk into the same glass. If you take food to work, portion it out in the same-size containers.

3. At restaurants, use these rules of thumb:

1 pancake is about the size of a CD.

A medium apple is about the size of a tennis ball.

2 tablespoons raisins or chopped dried fruit is about the size of a small egg.

For cooked rice, pasta, or other grains or flaky cereal or cut-up fruit:

¼ cup is about the size of a golf ball.

¾ cup is about the size of a tennis ball.

1 cup is about the size of a woman's fist.

4. With dishes such as casseroles, soups, and stews, do your best to estimate carb servings from various food groups. This is much easier if you're the chef: just take note of the total amount of high-carb ingredients, measure the finished product, then measure your portion. For instance, let's say the high-carb ingredients in a chicken and bean chili are 1 cup of beans, 1 cup of canned tomatoes, and 1 cup chopped onion. With the chicken, oil, some water, and spices the entire recipe comes to 6 cups. Your portion was 2 cups, or ⅓ of the recipe, so you had ⅓ cup beans (1 grain/starchy vegetable serving), ⅓ cup tomatoes (close enough to 1 nonstarchy vegetable serving), and ⅓ cup onions (1 nonstarchy vegetable serving).

If it's commercially prepared, or if you're at a restaurant that posts nutrition information for its menu items, take note of the serving size, then look at the number of total carbohydrates and calories per serving on the nutrition label/information. Dish out a portion that stays within your carbohydrate limit for that meal. For instance, say you have a can of chicken, vegetable, and barley soup. Looking at the label, you see that a cup has 15 grams of carbohydrate and 125 calories. From "High-Carbohydrate Foods at Each Meal," you know you're allowed 425 calories for lunch and 48 grams of carbohydrate. Have two cups of the soup, and you've hit 30 grams of carbohydrate. That leaves room for a fruit for dessert at about 15 to 18 grams of carbohydrate.

If you're at a dinner party or restaurant that does not post nutritional information, it's safest to order foods that aren't mixed dishes if at all possible. But if you really have a hankering for lasagna or eggplant Parmesan (which, by the way, should be very occasional splurges because they're high in calories and saturated fat) or you have no other options, you'll have to size up the inches or estimate cups. We have measurements for these types of foods in the "Mixed Dishes" section of the "What's a Carbohydrate Serving?" lists.

Find Your Daily Calorie Level

There's a lot of trial and error involved in finding a daily calorie level. Use this table as a starting point, but you may find that you need to move up or down a calorie level.

IF YOU'RE...	YOUR DAILY CALORIES MIGHT BE...
A woman who is sedentary or at Activity Level 1 and wants to lose weight	1,500
A woman at Activity Level 2 or 3 who wants to lose weight or a man or woman who is sedentary or at Activity Level 1 maintaining your weight	1,700
A man at Activity Level 2 or 3 or a woman at Activity Level 3 or 4 who wants to lose weight, or a woman at Activity Level 4 or a man at Activity Level 2 or 3 who is maintaining weight.	2,000
A man at Activity Level 4 who wants to lose or maintain weight; or a woman at Activity Level 4 who wants to maintain weight or at Level 5 who wants to lose weight. NOTE: A man at Level 5 will probably need more calories, even if trying to lose weight. See suggestions on page 56–58 and 252–253.	2,250

Daily Servings

The chart on the next page outlines a healthful, balanced diet based on the six food groups. A treat/dessert is also included for all calorie levels except for the lowest level (1,500); there's no room for empty calories at this level. During Phase One, you need to focus only on carbohydrate-rich foods; that's why the high-protein foods and fats are grayed out. All you need to know for now is that you should have some protein and fat at every meal; they help reduce the rise in blood sugar triggered by the carb-rich foods. Then you can turn to the "What's a Carbohydrate Serving?" lists on page 59 to become familiar with serving sizes. As for how to distribute high-carb foods in meals, check out "High-Carbohydrate Foods at Each Meal" on page 54. A note for high-level exercisers: you'll need more carbohydrates than are in the plan; see "More Carbohydrates for the High-Level Exerciser" on page 56.

Daily Calories

	1,500	1,700	2,000	2,250
DAILY CARBO-HYDRATE GRAMS	144 g	154 g	191 g	212 g
DAILY SERVINGS OF HIGH-CARBOHYDRATE FOODS				
GRAINS/STARCHY VEGETABLES	4	4	5	6
MILK/YOGURT (FAT-FREE OR 1 %)	2	2	3	3 1/2
FRUIT	2	2	2	2
NONSTARCHY VEGETABLES	6	6	7	7
DESSERT CARBOHYDRATE ALLOWANCE	—	A 100-calorie treat with no more than 10 grams of carbohydrate	A 150-calorie treat with no more than 15 grams of carbohydrate	A 150-calorie treat with no more than 15 grams of carbohydrate
THE REST OF THE DIET				
PROTEIN-RICH FOODS	7	7 1/2	8	9
HEALTHY FATS	6	7	8	9

High-Carbohydrate Foods at Each Meal

The way carbohydrate-rich foods are distributed on the following page ensures that no single meal will send you into carbohydrate overload. (For serving sizes of food listed, go to the "What's a Carbohydrate Serving?" table on page 59.) You'll notice that even though some meals have the same number of servings of high-carb foods, they may differ in calories. For instance, at all daily calorie levels, lunches have the same number of grain/starchy vegetable servings and the same number of vegetable and fruit servings. But the extra calories on the higher calorie plans come from protein-rich foods or healthy fats. More on protein and fat in Phase Two; for now, just include some in each meal.

DAILY CALORIES:	1,500	1,700	2,000	2,250
BREAKFAST				
TOTAL CALORIES	325	325	400	400
TOTAL CARBOHYDRATE GRAMS	34	34	40	40
HIGH-CARBOHYDRATE SERVINGS	1 milk/yogurt 1 1/2 grain/starchy vegetables	1 milk/yogurt 1 1/2 grain/starchy vegetables	1 1/2 milk/yogurts 1 1/2 grain/starchy vegetables	1 1/2 milk/yogurts 1 1/2 grain/starchy vegetables
LUNCH				
TOTAL CALORIES	425	425	500	550
TOTAL CARBOHYDRATE GRAMS	48	48	48	48
HIGH-CARBOHYDRATE SERVINGS	1 1/2 grain/starchy vegetables 2 nonstarchy vegetables 1 fruit	1 1/2 grain/starchy vegetables 2 nonstarchy vegetables 1 fruit	1 1/2 grain/starchy vegetables 2 nonstarchy vegetables 1 fruit	1 1/2 grain/starchy vegetables 2 nonstarchy vegetables 1 fruit
DINNER				
TOTAL CALORIES	500	500	550	550
TOTAL CARBOHYDRATE GRAMS	45	45	52	52
HIGH-CARBOHYDRATE SERVINGS	1 grain/starchy vegetable 1 fruit 3 nonstarchy vegetables	1 grain/starchy vegetable 1 fruit 3 nonstarchy vegetables	1 1/2 grain/starchy vegetables 1 fruit 3 nonstarchy vegetables	1 1/2 grain/starchy vegetables 1 fruit 3 nonstarchy vegetables
SNACK NO. 1				
TOTAL CALORIES	175	175	200	200
TOTAL CARBOHYDRATE GRAMS	12	12	18	18

(continued on next page)

DAILY CALORIES:	1,500	1,700	2,000	2,250
HIGH-CARBOHYDRATE SERVINGS	1 milk/yogurt	1 milk/yogurt	1½ milk/yogurts	1½ milk/yogurts

SNACK NO. 2

	1,500	1,700	2,000	2,250
TOTAL CALORIES	75	175	200	200
TOTAL CARBOHYDRATE GRAMS	5	5	18	18
HIGH-CARBOHYDRATE SERVINGS	1 nonstarchy vegetable	1 nonstarchy vegetable	2 nonstarchy vegetables ½ grain/starchy vegetable	2 nonstarchy vegetables ½ grain/starchy vegetable

SNACK NO. 3

	1,500	1,700	2,000	2,250
TOTAL CALORIES	—	—	—	200
TOTAL CARBOHYDRATE GRAMS				21
HIGH-CARBOHYDRATE SERVINGS				1 grain/starchy vegetable ½ milk/yogurt

TREAT

	1,500	1,700	2,000	2,250
TOTAL CALORIES	—	100	150	150
TOTAL CARBOHYDRATE GRAMS		10	15	15

High-carbohydrate servings: Treats can be based on fruit, grains (such as a cookie), dairy products, or vegetables. The only "must" here is that you stay within the calorie and carbohydrate limit. Check out the list of treats in the "What's a Carbohydrate Serving?" lists on page 59.

MORE CARBOHYDRATES FOR THE HIGH-LEVEL EXERCISER

If you're a competitive athlete or working out at Activity Level 4 or higher (see "The Best Life Activity Scale" starting on page 83), you may need more carbohydrates, and if you're working out hard enough, even our highest daily calorie level—2,250—won't be enough. You'll need extra carbohydrates to replenish glycogen, the storage form of glucose used as fuel by muscles. Long, strenuous workouts and athletic events such as marathons deplete your glycogen stores, whether or not you have diabetes. But if you have type 1 or type 2 diabetes and are taking insulin or have type 2 and are taking any other drug that lowers blood sugar, there's another reason to add carbs to our plan: to guard against exercise-induced hypoglycemia (see "Hypoglycemia," on page 70).

Having diabetes can throw off the way the body regulates insulin and other hormones during exercise. That, in turn, can cause blood sugar to go either too high or too low. But that doesn't mean you can't exercise or even become an athlete. It just means that you have to make sure to get the right combination of medications, carbohydrates, and calories to keep your blood sugar in a safe zone while exercising. This is particularly critical if you're taking insulin and/or oral medications that raise insulin levels, because if you have too much insulin in your system and not enough carbohydrates, your blood sugar level will fall. The fall could be anything from a slight dip that makes you feel a little more fatigued than usual to a serious hypoglycemic plunge. Getting enough carbohydrates is just half your glucose-stabilizing strategy; most likely you will, in consultation with your doctor, also decrease your dose of insulin or insulin-raising medication before exercising (see "Exercise and Your Medications," page 99).

There isn't a one-size-fits-all carbohydrate prescription for high-level exercisers. To figure out how many grams of carbohydrates you should tack onto the basic plan outlined in this book, first look at your particular blood sugar patterns. In general, what is your blood sugar level going into a workout? What tends to happen to your blood sugar level during a workout, a long run, or another athletic event? What's your blood sugar right after the event? An hour later? Many hours later? For this, you'll need to take blood sugar readings and record them, along with your carbohydrate intake, in the Best Life Diabetes Management Log (page 335). "Some of my clients test blood sugar three times prior to an event so they know the direction their blood sugar is heading. For instance, if blood sugar is trending downward, then they'll cut insulin back or possibly increase their preexercise carb intake," says Susan Weiner, M.S., R.D., a certified diabetes educator and exercise physiologist in private practice in New York. "And," she says, "they check during and afterwards. Because blood sugar response to exercise is so individual—for instance, some people's sugar falls during exercise, for some it's two hours later, for others it could be ten hours after the marathon—you must get to know your unique pattern."

That pattern dictates your carbohydrate needs. If you're taking insulin and/or drugs that lower your blood sugar level, these general guidelines are a good jumping-off point:

1. Add 15 to 30 grams of carbohydrate to each breakfast, lunch, and dinner. As you'll see from the "What's a Carbohydrate Serving?" lists on page 59 a grain/starchy vegetable serving has 15 grams of carbohydrate and 80 calories; a fruit serving has 15 grams of carbohydrate and about 60 calories. So if you use a starch or fruit serving to bolster your carbohydrate intake, you'll be adding 60 to 80 calories per meal. At the high end, adding two grain/starchy vegetable servings to each main meal will tack on another 480 calories each day. Add that to the 2,250-calorie plan, and you're up to 2,730 calories per day. That still may not be enough if you're a competitive althlete or if you're putting in a lot of hours a week exercising. If your weight is dropping too low, add even more carbohydrate-rich foods to meals, or add snacks, as described on pages 252 to 253.

2. Reach for carbohydrates before and/or during and/or after exercise. (We explain this in more detail in "Timing Meals to Exercise" on page 97.) The rule of thumb is that you need 15 grams of carbohydrate for each 30 minutes of intense exercise. But your needs may be different; see what your blood sugar monitor tells you. If your blood sugar level is under 100 before working out, you'll need the 15 grams of carbohydrate before exercising. You can use the snacks outlined in the "High-Carbohydrate Foods at Each Meal" chart on page 54 to bolster carbs during exercise. Or, if you can afford the calories, add on more snacks. Good choices: peanut butter on low-fat whole grain crackers, dry cereal with dried fruit, energy bars, and unsalted nuts with raisins. You should always have glucose gels, juices, or sports drinks handy in case of a low-blood-sugar response.

One more bit of advice: Keep in close touch with your doctor when you make any changes to your exercise patterns. This may require a shift in medications.

WHAT'S A CARBOHYDRATE SERVING?

In the lists below, you'll find familiar high-carbohydrate foods. This is your bible of serving sizes—get to know it *very* well. Make a copy if you'd like, and keep it with you for reference. You'll find more foods in the "Carbohydrate Counts" tables starting on page 343.

Grains/Starchy Vegetables:

15 grams of carbohydrate and approximately 80 calories per serving

Many foods on the following list have a wide range of carbohydrates; for instance, a slice of bread can contain 8 to 21 grams of carbohydrate. So, if there's a nutrition label on your food, check it. If you'd like, jot down the carbohydrate count of your staple items next to the foods below. Use a pencil; manufacturers change formulations all the time!

You might notice that we're not asking you to switch to eating more whole grains at this point; for instance, we simply list bread, 1 slice, instead of whole wheat bread. Whole grains are more healthful, and if you're already eating them, keep doing so. But if you don't already eat them much, now's not the time to make that shift. Your priority in Phase One is to learn appropriate serving sizes. In Phase Two, we'll help you make the switch to whole grains.

GRAIN-BASED CARBOHYDRATES

One serving equals:

Bagel: ¼ large bagel or ½ medium

Barley: 1½ tablespoons dry or ⅓ cup cooked

Bread: 1 medium slice

Cereal, flake type: about ¾ cup (this varies; check the label and choose one with at least 4 grams of fiber per 100 calories)

Couscous: 1½ tablespoons dry or ⅓ cup cooked

Crackers: 80 calories' worth (and no more than 2 grams of fat)

English muffin: ½

Flatout Healthy Grain Multi-Grain flatbread: 1 (100 calories and 17 grams of carbohydrate per serving)

Granola, low-fat: ¼ cup

Grits: 2 tablespoons dry or ½ cup cooked

Muesli: ¼ cup

Muffin: ¼ large muffin or ½ of a 2.75-inch × 2-inch-diameter muffin

Oatmeal, plain (or other unsweetened hot cereal): ¼ cup raw or ½ cup cooked (steel cut: ⅛ cup raw; ¾ cup cooked)

Pancakes: Two 4-inch diameter

Pasta: ¼ cup or ¾ ounce dry or ⅓ cup cooked

Pita bread: ½ of a 6-inch round

Polenta: 2½ tablespoons dry or ⅓ cup cooked

Popcorn: 3 cups (air-popped or no more than 3 grams of fat)

Pretzels, hard: ¾ ounce

Rice: 1 tablespoon plus 2 teaspoons dry or ⅓ cup cooked

Rice cakes: Two 4-inch cakes or 8 minis

Roll: 1 small (29-grams or 1-ounce) dinner roll or ½ of a 65-gram (2.3-ounce) hamburger roll

Tortilla: One 7-inch

Tortilla chips, baked: ¾ ounce

Waffles: One 4½-inch square

STARCHY VEGETABLES

One serving equals:

Beans (such as black beans, pinto beans, white beans, garbanzos, lentils, etc.): 1 tablespoon plus 2 teaspoons dry or ⅓ cup cooked or canned

Corn: ½ cup or one 5-inch ear

Peas: ⅔ cup

Potato: heaping ½ cup cooked (no fat added), or half of a medium baked potato

Squash (butternut, acorn, or other winter squash): 1 cup cooked

Sweet potato: ½ cup cooked or ½ medium potato

Fruit:

15 grams of carbohydrate and approximately 60 calories per serving

Instead of fruit juice, go for whole fruit, which is more filling, lower in sugar, and higher in nutrients.

One serving equals:

Apple: 1 small

Applesauce, unsweetened: ½ cup

Apricots: 4 fresh or 8 dried halves

Banana: ½

Blueberries: ⅔ cup

Cantaloupe: ⅓ melon or 1 cup cubed

Cherries: 14

Dates: 3

Figs: 2 medium or 1½ dried

Grapefruit: ½ large

Grapes: ½ cup

Juice (100%): ½ cup

Kiwi: 1½

Orange: 1 medium

Mango: ½ mango or ½ cup slices

Peach: 1

Pineapple: ¾ cup cubed or ⅓ cup plus 1 tablespoon canned pineapple, juice pack

Plums: 2

Raisins: 2 tablespoons

Raspberries: 1 cup

Strawberries: 1¼ cups

Nonstarchy Vegetables:

5 grams of carbohydrate and approximately 25 calories per serving

General rule: One serving equals 3 cups lettuce or spinach, 1 cup chopped raw vegetable, ½ cup cooked vegetable. Note: ⅓ cup or less of lettuce is a free food; no need to count it.

One serving equals:

Artichoke hearts: ⅓ cup

Asparagus: 8 medium spears (4½ ounces raw)

Bean sprouts: ¾ cup

Beets: Two 2-inch diameter raw or ½ cup cooked

Broccoli: 1 cup raw or ½ cup cooked

Cabbage: 1¼ cups raw shredded or ¾ cup cooked

Carrot: 1 medium (about 5½ inches long), ⅓ cup chopped, ½ cup grated, or ½ cup chopped, cooked

Cauliflower: 1 cup raw or cooked

Celery: 4 medium stalks or 1½ cups chopped

Cucumber: 1½ cups sliced

Eggplant: 1 cup raw or ⅔ cup cooked

Greens (collard, kale, spinach, turnip greens, etc.): ¾ cup cooked

Onion: ⅓ cup chopped raw or ¼ cup cooked

Salad greens (arugula, mixed greens, romaine, etc.): 3 cups

String beans: ⅔ cup raw or ½ cup, cooked

Tomato: 1 medium or ¾ cup chopped, ½ cup canned, or 1 cup cherry tomatoes

Tomato juice: ½ cup

Tomato sauce (plain): ⅓ cup

Water chestnuts: 5

Milk and Yogurt:

12 grams of carbohydrate and approximately 100 calories per serving

Make fat-free or 1% milk or yogurt your mainstays. Yogurts sweetened with sugar or other caloric sweeteners are very high in carbohydrates so it's best to avoid them.

Cheese has virtually no carbohydrates, so it's considered a high-protein food (the protein foods list is in Phase Two).

One serving equals:

Milk, fat-free or 1%: 1 cup

Soy milk: 1 cup (no more than 100 calories) calcium-enriched, at least 25 percent of the daily value for calcium, such as most Silk varieties

Yogurt, low-fat or nonfat plain: 6 ounces or ⅔ cup

Mixed Dishes:

Counting the carbohydrate grams in your seving of boxed frozen pizza or from a can of chili is easy—all you need to do is measure your portion and compare it to the serving on the nutrition facts panel. But how do you calculate the carbs in your aunt Sofia's lasagna, or in the mushroom barley soup at your local lunch spot? You can guesstimate; the numbers below are bound to be somewhat imprecise, but they are better than nothing.

Lasagna, vegetable, meatless: ⅛ piece of 7 × 12-inch lasagna, 45 grams of carbohydrate

Lo mein with shrimp: 1 cup, 35 grams of carbohydrate

Macaroni/pasta salad: ½ cup, 20 grams of carbohydrate

Pizza, thin crust, cheese only or cheese and vegetable(s) topping: 1 slice of 14-inch pie, 17 grams of carbohydrate (check pizza restaurants' Web sites for exact carbs and other nutrition information per slice and read food labels on frozen pizza brands for accurate nutrition information)

Stew, beef with vegetables and potatoes: 1 cup, 16 grams of carbohydrate

Sushi with fish and vegetables rolled in seaweed: 1 roll cut into 6 pieces, 43 grams of carbohydrate

Tuna casserole in white sauce: 1 cup, 25 grams of carbohydrate

SOUPS

(choose brands with 500 mg sodium or less per serving)

Chicken noodle soup: 1 cup, 11 grams of carbohydrate

Lentil soup: 1 cup, 25 grams of carbohydrate

Mushroom barley soup: 1 cup, 15 grams of carbohydrate

Tomato soup: 1 cup, 17 grams of carbohydrate

Treats/Desserts:

On the 1,700-calorie-per-day plan, you get a treat with approximately 100 calories and 10 grams of carbohydrate; on the 2,000- and 2,250-calorie plans your treat is about 150 calories and 15 grams of carbohydrate. The examples below lead off with the treat for the 1,700-calorie plan, followed by the version for the higher calorie levels.

One serving equals:

Chocolate: 0.7 oz (20 grams) such as 2 Hershey's Extra Dark

Pure Dark tasting squares, any flavor with the exception of Pomegranate (2,000 and 2,250 calories per day: have one ounce, such as 3 Hershey's squares.)

Chocolate-covered raisins: 1 tablespoon, such as Raisinets, with 7 unsalted almonds
(2,000 and 2,250 calories per day: have 1 tablespoon plus one teaspoon of the chocolate-covered raisins with 11 unsalted almonds.)

Pudding, no sugar added: 4 ounces (about 90–100 calories, 9–11 grams of carbohydrates), such as a number of Kozy Shack flavors including chocolate and rice (check other flavors as carbohydrate contents vary)
(2,000 and 2,250 calories per day: along with the pudding, have a heaping tablespoon of cashew pieces or slivered almonds.)

Cookies or biscotti with no more than 10 grams carbohydrates and no more than 1.5 grams saturated fat (if chocolate chip, can have up to 2 grams saturated fat because the type of sat fat in chocolate does not clog arteries)
(2,000 and 2,250 calories per day: Cookies or biscotti with 15 grams carbohydrates and no more than 1.5 grams saturated fat (up to 2 grams sat fat if chocolate chip for same reasons cited above)

Graham crackers: 30 calories, 5 grams of carbohydrates, such as half a rectangle spread with 2 teaspoons creamy peanut butter, such as Smart Balance
(2,000 and 2,250 calories per day: have an entire rectangle spread with 2½ teaspoons peanut butter.)

Popcorn, air-popped, no salt, no butter added: 1⅔ cups drizzled with 1 teaspoon melted healthy spread, such as Bestlife Buttery Spread (2,000 and 2,250 calories per day: have 2¼ cups popcorn with 2 teaspoons melted spread and 1 tablespoon grated Parmesan cheese.)

Skinny Cow Mini Fudge Pop: 1 pop paired with 3½ unsalted walnut halves
(2,000 and 2,250 calories per day: have 1 pop paired with 7 walnut halves.)

Tortilla chips (⅓ ounce, or about 5 chips) dipped in 3 tablespoons guacamole
(2,000 and 2,250 calories per day: Have ½ ounce (about 8 chips) dipped in 4 tablespoons (¼ cup) guacamole

Free Foods:

These foods have only ½ gram of carbohydrate and are low in calories. If you have no more than three servings total per day, these foods are free (more than three, and the carbs start adding up and will affect your blood sugar).

- Cucumber: ⅓ cup

- Gum, sugar-free: 1 stick

- Salad greens (romaine, mixed greens, etc.): ⅓ cup

Eat Three Square Meals and Snack as Needed

Eating is one of life's great pleasures; that doesn't have to change when you have diabetes. You'll have to think about what goes into your mouth a little more than most people, but you'll be healthier for it. You may see your mood and energy levels improve on the Best Life plan because you'll be eating regularly throughout the day, not skipping meals, and using snacks in between meals to keep your blood sugar level, and your appetite, in check.

That doesn't mean you'll have to be a slave to the clock. It used to be that having diabetes meant leading a regimented life: you had to eat breakfast, lunch, dinner, and any snacks at the same time each day or risk dangerously high or low blood sugar levels because there were no instruments to check blood sugar levels at home. Also, the older oral medications were more apt to send blood sugar plunging (hypoglycemia); many of the ones in current use are much safer. And the newer forms of insulin can help you better match your own body's glucose patterns. So, nowadays, you make the meds fit your schedule and lifestyle, instead of the other way around.

Still, sticking with a fairly regular eating schedule has advantages for your blood sugar and your waistline. If you eat every three to four hours, you won't get too hungry, making it easier to control your calorie and carbohydrate intake at your next meal. Skipping meals and letting your hunger build can make you feel weak and irritable and sets you up for overdoing the calories—and often the carbohydrates. That's a problem especially if you're on a stable dose of long-acting insulin alone or in combination with oral medications; you may not have enough insulin to bring down your blood sugar after a high-carbohydrate meal. While waiting too long between meals could set you up for some serious overeating, not waiting long enough is also a problem. Eating before feeling a tug of hunger interferes with the cues that help you eat when you need to and stop when you're full. In Phase Two, you'll be tracking your hunger with a 10-point hunger scale.

For now you need to commit to eating breakfast, lunch, and dinner, and a few snacks. Eat one of the breakfasts on the meal plan (starting on page 250); that's a must in Phase One. You can continue following the meal plan for the rest of the meals or choose your own lunch, dinner, and snacks. Meanwhile, monitor your blood sugar so you can start figuring out what types of meals put you into the best blood sugar zone.

SMART SNACKING, BETTER BLOOD SUGAR LEVELS

Snacking used to be essential in diabetes management because of the between-meal hypoglycemia risk posed by older medicines. Despite the improved medicines, hypoglycemia is still a very common problem in people with diabetes. Snacking can help reduce occurrences of this condition by ensuring controlled intake of carbohydrates throughout the day. For some people, snacks are particularly useful at helping prevent exercise-induced hypoglycemia or low blood sugar that strikes in the middle of the night.

The right snacks can also help keep your blood sugar level from going too high. If you move 10 grams of carbohydrate from your usual breakfast into a midmorning snack, you might solve that high post-breakfast blood sugar problem. That could mean that you'll need less medication to cover meals. Our breakfasts—both in the meal plan and as outlined in the chart on page 55—are low enough in carbs to combat most post-breakfast blood sugar spikes so you won't need to subtract 10 grams of carbs.

Not to mention, smart snacking can also help you lose weight. For instance, if you're cutting calories, you may feel hungry in between meals. A 100- to 200-calorie snack may be just the thing to ward off hunger so that you don't overeat when mealtime does come around. Just make sure that you don't get into the dangerous grazing-all-day pattern, which makes it hard to control calorie intake.

Our meal plans offer two snacks a day on the 1,500-, 1,700-, and 2,000-calorie-per-day plans and three snacks if you're taking in 2,250 calories. One snack is always high in calcium, so that, along with the high-calcium breakfasts, you're automatically covered for at least 600 milligrams of calcium per day. That goes a long way to meeting your daily calcium needs—see page 145 for advice on supplementing with calcium.

Eat a Best Life Breakfast

Everything you've heard about the importance of breakfast is even truer for you. Eating the right type of breakfast will not only help control your blood sugar but will help slim you down and reduce your risk of heart disease and possibly cancer and other chronic diseases. One of your Phase One goals is to eat any of the breakfasts on our meal plan, which starts on page 259. Why are we such sticklers about breakfast? Because morning is the time when many people experience the highest blood sugar levels, and the right type of breakfast can help. Coffee and a doughnut won't cut it, but one of our egg wraps or a hot whole grain cereal–based breakfast might mean the difference between a normal and high blood sugar level two hours later. Because many people have a higher blood sugar level in the morning, we've made breakfast lower in carbs than lunch and dinner. All our breakfasts offer 1½ starch servings and 1 dairy serving and differ a little in the amount of protein-rich foods and healthful fats.

And don't forget about this other breakfast benefit: in our experience (and research studies have also proved this), breakfast eaters are slimmer, so that morning meal might be a real boon to those of you trying to lose weight.

Experiment with the Best Life Breakfasts, and stick to those that give you the best blood sugar readings two hours later. There are lots of delicious choices starting on page 259 to make it easy for you breakfast skippers to come back to the table.

Stop Eating Two Hours before Bedtime, if Possible

It's 10 P.M., dinner's long over, and you're back in the kitchen opening cupboards or munching chips in front of the TV. If this sounds familiar, adapting this one change can make a big difference in your waistline. Why does so much overeating occur during those last few hours of the evening? Maybe you didn't eat enough calories during the day and are truly hungry. Or maybe you didn't get enough sleep and are tired (or even worse, you're tired in the kitchen!), and eating, especially high-carbohydrate foods, is the body's attempt to perk itself up. Or maybe you're using food to soothe you, calm you, numb you, or any of the other reasons so many people become emotional eaters.

Of course, salad or roasted broccoli isn't what people usually eat at night—they're reaching for cookies, crackers, chips, ice cream, and other high-carbohydrate foods. These are foods that not only send blood sugar soaring immediately but easily pack on the pounds over the long haul, increasing insulin resistance and heart disease risk.

For some, the two-hour cutoff is not a good idea. Those of you who have low blood sugar before you go to bed or have a history of low-blood-sugar reactions in the middle of the night may need a snack to help offset these blood sugar dives.

Before writing off the low evening blood sugar level as inevitable, check with your doctor to make sure it's not a medication issue. For instance, you may be taking too much short-acting insulin (called regular insulin, brand names Novolin R or Humulin R) at bedtime or a fast-acting insulin analog, such as Humalog, NovoLog, or Apidra (see page 209). Too much of these medications taken before bed without eating can be dangerous. Certain oral medications such as the sulfonylureas (see page 194) can also lower blood sugar overnight, especially if taken late in the day.

HYPOGLYCEMIA

Jitteriness, tremors, sweating, anxiety, lightheadedness—the symptoms of hypoglycemia can be frightening. Hypoglycemia is, simply, abnormally low blood sugar levels. It's not really defined by a number, though a sugar level under 65 is usually too low and much lower is almost always a concern. It's often caused by a mismatch between your insulin dose (or other medications that cause insulin levels to rise) and meals or exercise. In other words, you have too much insulin in your system and are putting away so much blood sugar that the level falls too low.

When symptoms strike, check your blood sugar level if possible. If you can't because your meter isn't around or the symptoms are coming on too quickly, just go ahead and treat it (see below for details) immediately to prevent your blood glucose from going even lower and possibly causing you to lose consciousness.

Unfortunately, some people can't tell if their blood sugar level is dropping too low; they have what is called hypoglycemic unawareness. This is especially common in people who have advanced neuropathy or have had so many hypoglycemic episodes that they've lost the ability to sense that low blood sugar is coming on. Hypoglycemia is a real challenge for these people, and they must test more frequently than most in order to avoid having their blood sugar level go too low.

When you feel the effect of low blood sugar, eat a 15-gram portion of sugar or sugar-containing food. The ideal choice is glucose tablets or a glucose gel, both available at any pharmacy. They're portioned to make it easy to grab 15 grams' worth and don't have to be refrigerated. Keep them in places where you might need them in a hurry, such as next to your bed or couch, at your desk, or in your car. If neither of these is available, the next best choice is four to five pieces of hard candy or ½ cup of fruit juice. After taking the glucose or other sugar-rich food, wait fifteen minutes and check your blood sugar level again. If it's not rising, you can repeat the process. Avoid the temptation to eat more than one 15-gram portion of glucose or sugar-containing food during that initial fifteen-minute period. It can be hard, especially when you feel so bad as a result of the low blood sugar, but eating too much too quickly will simply drive your sugar very high once you've recovered. After your blood sugar level begins to rise, eat a small snack that includes some longer-lasting carbohydrates, healthy fat, and protein, such as a whole-grain cracker topped with a little mayonnaise and a slice of chicken or spread with nut butter. This will help prevent your blood sugar level from falling once the glucose or sugar is used up.

Treating hypoglycemia promptly is crucial, but just as essential is figuring out why it's happening and then making the necessary changes to your diet, medication, or exercise to prevent further episodes. An occasional, mild low-blood-sugar reaction is not a problem, and, in fact, most people with diabetes will experience these from time to time. However, if you are having frequent or severe episodes of hypoglycemia— more than one every two weeks or even a single episode that leads to the loss of consciousness—it means that your diet, exercise, and medication are out of balance. It may be that an amount of medication that was just right when you were not exercising is too much once you start or that the medication dose is too high now that you are watching your serving sizes or losing weight. Or it might be that the low-sugar reactions occur only on days when you do a particularly strenuous activity (lots more on this starting on page 99). There are many possible explanations, so if it's not clear what's going on, talk to your doctor.

There's another case to be made for a healthful bedtime snack: it can actually help lower your morning blood sugar level. Here's why: in some people, the liver produces too much glucose during the night; the glucose goes to the bloodstream, causing high blood sugar upon waking. A night-time snack sends sugar into the blood, which sends a signal to the liver that there is enough sugar in the body. So if you have high sugar upon waking, slot in one of your daily snacks shortly before hitting the pillow and see if your A.M. readings drop.

If you need a snack during the two-hour window before bed, *eat the type of snack recommended on your plan.* You're allowed two snacks (three if you're on 2,250 calories per day), so simply save one for before bedtime; you won't be adding any extra calories and you'll be sticking to a safe carbohydrate level. Experiment with your snacks to see which one helps stabilize your blood sugar level best.

Eliminate Sweetened Beverages

When looking for reasons for the spike in overweight and obesity in this country, experts point to our increasingly sedentary lifestyles, the gigan-tic portions on our plates, and sweetened beverages: sodas, juice drinks, and other sugary drinks. In fact, some experts had suggested that a single ingredient in these beverages, high fructose corn syrup (HFCS), was a major contributor to the obesity epidemic because the increased use of the sweetener paralleled the rise in obesity and because of the appetite-stimulating effects of *pure* fructose (see page 75). But structurally, HFCS is very similar to regular table sugar—it's 55 percent fructose and 45 percent glucose while sugar is a 50/50 split of these two compounds. And recent research shows that your body treats HFCS and sugar the same way; both have similar effects on appetite, insulin, and blood sugar. The real problem boils down to calories—and although HFCS is no more caloric than sugar, it is more widely used in food products because it's cheaper, so we're consuming more of it than any other sweetener. If manufacturers used sugar in place of HFCS, we'd simply be overdoing calories from that instead.

And we are certainly overdoing calories, particularly from beverages, in a big way. In 1965 about 12 percent of calories came from beverages; in 1977 about 14 percent. Today, about 21 percent of daily calories are sipped away, translating to 222 more calories per day from beverages than in the 1960s. For some people simply ending their soda habit can bring them down to a healthy weight.

But when you have diabetes, it's more than just a weight issue. Down a 12-ounce can of soda, and you've consumed about 40 grams of carbohydrate (10 teaspoons of sugar), which will send your blood sugar level soaring. The bottom line: if you've been drinking sodas, they have to go, right now. If you need to lean on diet soda for a while, that's okay, but aim to whittle down that habit, too (for all the reasons mentioned in "The Skinny on Other Sweeteners," page 74).

During the next four weeks, you should also stop drinking other sweet drinks, such as fruit juice, fruit drinks, energy drinks, sport drinks, and sweetened iced tea (unsweetened is fine). You'll be rewarded by better blood sugar readings and a drop in numbers on the scale. Later on, after your blood sugar is under good control, if you really miss sweet beverages, you can experiment with reintroducing them in small quantities of about 4 ounces. But that's for Phase Two.

What to drink instead? Any of the following is fine:

Water

Sparkling water (plain or calorie-free flavored)

Unsweetened iced tea

Hot tea*

Coffee*

---

* Caffeine can raise the blood sugar level in some people, so if your blood sugar level rises consistently after drinking tea or coffee, switch to decaf. (More on this on page 174.) You can put a teaspoon of sugar or honey (4 grams of carbohydrate) into these beverages, but you must count it toward your treat serving. If you are allowed 15 grams of carbohydrate for your treat and you use a teaspoon of sugar in your tea, you have 11 grams of carbohydrate left for dessert. If you're on the 1,500-calorie-per-day plan, you don't have a treat, so just subtract the sugar or honey carb grams from the meal's total carbohydrate grams. To minimize blood sugar spikes, have the sweetened hot drink with a meal instead of by itself.

In addition to these beverages, soy milk and fat-free or 1% milk are part of your plan. You get 2 milk or soy milk servings on 1,500 and 1,700 calories per day, 3 servings on 2,000, and 3½ servings on 2,250. The protein in these beverages helps reduce the rise in blood sugar.

Eliminate Alcohol

We'd like you to hold off on drinking any alcohol during Phase One; you can bring it back in Phase Two if you choose. Here's why: while you're learning to make the best food choices, alcohol can detract from your goals because it adds extra calories and no nutrients to your diet, making weight loss, a goal for many of you, that much harder. Alcohol has 7 calories per gram, while protein and carbohydrates have only 4 calories per gram (fat has 9 calories per gram). A 5-ounce glass of wine has 100 calories, a 12-ounce glass of beer has 148 calories, and a 4½-ounce piña colada has 262 calories. Another reason alcohol and weight loss don't mix is because alcohol is quickly absorbed into your bloodstream and can slow down your metabolism. In addition, drinking can impair your judgment about what you eat while stimulating your appetite; a double whammy you don't need while trying to control blood sugar and lose weight!

THE SKINNY ON OTHER SWEETENERS

You already know that regular sodas and sugary drinks are linked to obesity, but you may be wondering about diet soda or foods sweetened with artificial sweeteners, sugar alcohols, or other sweeteners.

NO-CALORIE SWEETENERS

While the calorie-free sweeteners, such as sucralose (Splenda), aspartame (Equal or NutraSweet), saccharin (Sweet 'N Low), acesulfame K (Sunett or Sweet One), and stevia (TruVia and PureVia), don't raise blood sugar or contribute extra calories to your diet, they do have other issues, like safety. All the sweeteners mentioned above (except stevia) are approved by the Food and Drug Administration (FDA), the U.S. government's agency that handles food safety issues. But a major consumer watchdog organization, the Center for Science in the Public Interest (CSPI), has given the nod only to sucralose (Splenda), saying the research isn't clear enough on the safety of the others at this point.

Sugar substitutes are certainly marketed as weight-loss aids, but the research into their effectiveness is mixed. A few studies indicate that switching to diet drinks can help you drop some pounds. But still, diet soda drinkers are typically heavier than the general population. That could be because they were overweight to begin with and turned to diet sodas to help them shed pounds. Or, as some researchers have suggested, because they taste sweeter than sugar, artificial sweeteners train your taste buds to prefer very sweet foods. This, in turn, drives you to eat more sweets—and calories. And of course, there's that little rationalization you may do with yourself: "Well, I saved calories on diet soda so I can have an extra slice of pizza."

SUGAR ALCOHOLS

Sugar alcohols are not calorie-free (they have about half the calories of sugar), but because they are chemically different from sugar, they are allowed to use the "sugar-free" claim. The ones that commonly show up on ingredient lists are xylitol, mannitol, lactitol, and erythritol. The pros: they have a minimal impact on blood sugar, they don't cause dental caries, and CSPI considers them safe. The catch: consumed in excess, they cause bloating and gas because they aren't completely absorbed into your system. (Erythritol seems to have the fewest gastrointestinal side effects and is the lowest in calories.)

FRUCTOSE

Fructose—the same sugar that occurs naturally in foods like fruit and corn—is starting to appear in energy drinks and bars and some foods marketed to people with diabetes. Not to be confused with high fructose corn syrup, which is 55 percent fructose and 45 percent glucose, this is pure fructose (a popular brand is "crystalline fructose," which has been processed to look and feel like table sugar). Fructose has been touted as a good choice for people with diabetes for two reasons: it has a much lower glycemic index than sugar or honey, meaning it has a blunted impact on blood sugar (more on the glycemic index starting on page 124). It's also sweeter, so you need about 20 percent less to achieve the same taste, thereby saving calories.

But research is showing that its risks outweigh its benefits. For instance, a groundbreaking University of California–Davis study tracked overweight and obese people who took in 25 percent of their daily calories from either a fructose- or a glucose-sweetened drink. Ten weeks later, both groups gained an average of 3 1/2 pounds, but only the fructose group was hit with a host of diabetes-promoting side effects, such as an increase in insulin resistance, levels of artery-clogging LDL cholesterol, and dangerous intra-abdominal fat (whereas glucose consumers gained the less risky subcutaneous fat). Ideally, the study would have pitted fructose against the two most common sweeteners—table sugar and high fructose corn syrup—but still, the results don't bode well for this sweetener and your health. And don't worry about the fructose in fruit—you're not getting a concentrated source because fruit is fairly low in calories and it contains a mix of fructose and glucose.

The bottom line: if you're taking in more than 1,500 calories per day, you can afford a 100- to 150-calorie treat made with real sugar, high fructose corn syrup, honey, maple sugar, or other caloric sweeteners (see guidelines on page 56 for calories and carbs in treats). If having a diet drink or other treat sweetened with no-cal or low-cal sweeteners (ideally Splenda or sugar alcohols) a few times a week helps your weight loss efforts—and doesn't instill cravings for sweets—then go ahead. And do your best to avoid foods sweetened with pure fructose.

Although research suggests that alcohol can provide some heart-healthy benefits, it's important to note that similar benefits can be gained by eating a diet low in saturated fat and rich in fruits and vegetables as well as by following a regular exercise program. Plus, research is building an ever-stronger case that drinking increases cancer risk. Breast cancer may be most affected by alcohol; the risk appears to increase even at one drink per day for women. If you don't already drink, there's no reason to start for your health's sake. But if you do drink, the general recommendation for most healthy people, including people with diabetes, is to keep consumption to one daily drink for women, and two for men. That advice may change soon for women with a personal or family history of breast cancer.

We're assuming that you'll stop drinking during the course of Phase One. If you do decide to drink before the start of Phase Two, read up on alcohol's effect on your blood sugar level on page 138, before you do.

For now, taking a break from alcohol will allow you to see clearly how to best fit the pieces of a healthy diet into place. Later, you can reassess how much alcohol means to you and use your treat calories to add it back to your diet in Phase Two if you choose.

Drink Enough Water

If excessive thirst and urination were the symptoms that tipped you off to your diabetes, then you know what it's like to be dehydrated; those symptoms are a result of persistently high blood sugar, over 300. Once blood sugar is in better control, you must guard against the garden-variety reasons for being dehydrated: sweating a little more now that you've stepped up the exercise, and, simply not drinking enough water the rest of the time.

With all the other adjustments you're making in Phase One—monitoring your blood sugar, reining in the carbs, and getting more exercise—do you really have to worry about water? Yes, because if you're well-hydrated, it will make the rest of this program easier.

For starters, staying hydrated will help you lose weight. Nutritionists and trainers always notice that their clients seem to lose weight more easily if they drink enough water, and now researchers from the University Medicine Berlin in Germany may have discovered why. Their studies show that drinking two cups of water raises metabolic rate (the rate at which your body burns calories) by about 30 percent. This effect peaks in about thirty minutes and disappears completely in about an hour. Researchers estimate that if you drink about six cups of water daily, you could, theoretically, burn an extra 48 calories a day, which could translate into a 5-pound weight loss for the year.

Other ways water may lower the number on your scale: it might help you eat a little less. We often mistake thirst for hunger; instead of filling up a glass with water, we turn to food. So stave off thirst, and you may shave off some calories. And going into your workout well-hydrated gives you more energy and endurance. You'll get the most out of your hour at the gym or your walk, burning more calories and increasing fitness.

So starting today, drink 6 glasses (48 ounces) of water daily. Drink these in addition to any other beverages. Plain water is best; keep a glass at your desk and by your bedside. Bottled water is especially convenient when you're on the run; Nestlé Pure Life Purified Water carries the Best Life Seal of Approval because it's a nationally available, reputable brand that uses less plastic. Sparkling water, water with a little squirt of juice (no more than 2 tablespoons), or flavored unsweetened water is also okay.

Move Your Body, Lower Your Blood Sugar

Exercise is not optional if you want the best possible control over blood sugar. Nor is it optional if you want a higher quality of life.

Exercise can work wonders on type 2 diabetes; in combination with proper diet (and usually weight loss), it can reduce your need for medication, sometimes drastically. In some cases your blood sugar levels will return to normal and you can go off the meds completely! (However, as we've explained, diabetes is a progressive disease. Even after your blood sugar level returns to normal, you must continue to monitor it and see your doctor regularly. Even with the best diet and exercise regimen, high blood sugar levels can return.) The combination of exercise and weight loss can completely reverse pre-diabetes. Because type 1 diabetes results from making little or no insulin, exercise alone isn't going to reverse the disease. But it can mean better blood sugar control and creates the same long-term protection against heart disease and other chronic conditions as it does for people with type 2 diabetes (and everyone else).

As compelling as the diabetes and exercise research is, about a third of people with type 2 diabetes don't exercise regularly, according to the latest figures from the U.S. government's National Health Examination Survey. The American Diabetic Association recommends 150 minutes of aerobic exercise per week, plus strength training. If you haven't put on a pair of sneakers in years, exercise might be a scary thought. But maybe you've taken a swim, and surely you've taken a walk. We've helped many people with diabetes become more fit by simply encouraging them to walk more. After taking that first step (literally), they have the confidence to work up to higher levels of fitness. That's what we have in mind for you. No matter what your level of fitness, we're going to help you gradually build up to the highest level that you can realistically sustain, given your time constraints and any physical limitations. The twelve-week fitness plan starting on page 355 lets you start at your current level and build from there.

The good news is that all types of exercise work. Both aerobic exercise (brisk walking, cycling, and other activities that get your heart rate up) and resistance training (lifting weights or using weight machines) help lower your blood sugar. And the combination, according to a study at the University of Ottawa Heart Research Institute in Canada, is even more effective than either one alone. We'll explain all the ins and outs of both types of exercise later in this chapter.

Need a little more motivation to lace up your athletic shoes? Take a moment to consider the amazing effects of exercise on your disease as well as on your weight-loss efforts and your overall health. For instance, exercise reduces the insulin resistance that usually accompanies type 2 diabetes and pre-diabetes. The insulin becomes more effective and allows more glucose from your blood into your muscle cells to use as fuel when you work out.

Plus, there's a bonus: The blood sugar–lowering effect lingers from twenty-four to seventy-two hours after exercising! Muscles continue soaking up glucose, turning it into stored glycogen. You'll use that glycogen to fuel future workouts and for other times when the body needs energy. The liver is also more insulin-sensitive after a workout, so it will have less of a tendency to release too much glucose into the blood.

Meanwhile, exercise whittles your waistline, further increasing insulin sensitivity. In a French study at the Hôpital Saint-Louis in Paris, people with type 2 diabetes who exercised for about 55 minutes three times a week (twice on an exercise bike, once doing another aerobic activity) burned off a whopping 48 percent of their visceral fat, the type of belly fat deep in the abdomen that, in excess, is actually a cause of pre-diabetes and type 2 diabetes. And once you have these conditions, visceral fat adds fuel to the fire, making you more resistant to insulin and increasing your triglyceride levels. Dropping some of this fat sent insulin sensitivity shooting up 42 percent in the French exercisers, and of course their fitness levels improved. A bonus: they also lost 18 percent of the belly fat lying right beneath the skin (subcutaneous fat). And get this: it all happened in just two months— without their dieting!

Increased insulin sensitivity is just one way exercise literally helps save your life when you have diabetes. "Why You Have to Move" (page 80) gives a more complete description of the benefits of exercise.

But before you step up your physical activity, you *must* talk to your doctor, even if you're already exercising. Increasing exercise may lower your blood sugar and, therefore, your medication dose—both great things. But if you start exercising on your old dose of medication, hypoglycemia could result. For some, the gradual increase in activity that we're recommending in Phase One might not, in itself, cause much of a blood sugar dip. But if you're also taking in fewer carbohydrates as a result of the Phase One diet guidelines, the combo could drive down your blood sugar to a level that merits a medication tweak. In any case, it's very important that you use your blood glucose meter more often during this time. Aside from the blood sugar issues, if you have high blood pressure, you must get your doctor's okay before doing any resistance training (weight lifting or using resistance training machines). In some cases, this type of exercise can increase high blood pressure.

SAFE MOVES

Steve, age 47, has a dozen marathons under his belt. He has had type 1 diabetes for twenty years. Shelley, age 62, was 50 pounds overweight when she was first diagnosed with type 2 diabetes. She went from sedentary (Activity Level 0) to a solid Activity Level 4 in six months, lost 30 pounds, and was able to stop one of her diabetes medications. Having diabetes, even long-standing type 1, does *not* mean you can't exercise or even become a serious athlete. It *does* mean that you must work with your doctor to adjust your medication and, if you have any complications from diabetes, work around them.

One of those complications is peripheral neuropathy. If you have this tingling or deadening of nerves in the feet, then exercises such as swimming or biking, which don't put as much stress on your feet as walking, jogging, and running, would probably be a good choice. Having heart disease or risk factors for it, such as high blood pressure, is another issue you might have to deal with when choosing an activity that's right for you. You may also have to take special precautions if you are sedentary or overweight. For instance, extra pounds may have triggered a condition like osteoarthritis that might make certain activities difficult or painful. Following this program should help alleviate those conditions. But no matter which of these issues you're facing, you can—and should—exercise. It's

WHY YOU HAVE TO MOVE

Exercise is just as important as diet and in some cases as important as drugs in managing diabetes. That's because exercise:

- **Lowers blood sugar and improves insulin sensitivity.** Both cardio (aerobic, such as fast walking, biking, and so on) and strength training (such as push-ups or using weight machines or free weights) lower blood sugar levels during and after exercise. A University of Ottawa review of the research found that people with type 2 diabetes who do eight weeks of aerobic exercise wind up with A1c levels—a measure of blood sugar control over the preceding two to three months—about 8 percent lower than nonexercisers (A1c of 7.65 versus 8.31). This small change can translate into a significant reduction in complications.

- **Prevents or delays type 2 diabetes.** People with pre-diabetes can lower their risk of developing type 2 diabetes by about 30 to 65 percent if they exercise. The effects of exercise are independent of weight loss; even if a person doesn't meet his or her weight-loss goals, exercise alone reduces the risks.

- **Lets you store more blood sugar.** Strength training builds muscle, and that extra muscle soaks up more blood sugar in the form of glycogen.

- **Burns more body fat.** The better trained your muscles, the better they burn fat. Losing body fat not only makes you look and feel better, but if it's belly fat you're losing, you'll also become more insulin-sensitive.

- **Keeps the weight off.** Study after study shows that exercisers are better at maintaining their weight loss than nonexercisers.

- **Dramatically reduces the risk of heart disease.** Having diabetes doubles your risk for serious cardiovascular disease and makes it two to four times more likely that you'll die from it compared to the general population. But stay active, and you'll reduce that risk by 35 to 55 percent.

- **Prevents or delays neuropathy.** Neuropathy—damage to nerves in the feet and other areas—is a common complication of diabetes and pre-diabetes. Motor neuropathy affects nerves involved in movement—walking, grasping objects, etc. In sensory neuropathy, nerves that control pain and the sensation of touching are affected (for details see page 239). Exercise may help stave off both types, according to an Italian study. Seventy-eight participants, with either type 1 or type 2 diabetes, were divided into two groups. One group got on a treadmill 4 hours a week (yes, that's a lot, but they worked up to it!); the other group didn't make any changes to their exercise habits. Four years later, none of the exercisers developed motor neuropathy, compared to 17 percent of the control group. And just 6 percent of treadmill users got sensory neuropathy compared to 30 percent of nonexercisers.

- **Prevents or delays retinopathy.** Retinopathy is damage to the blood vessels behind the retina (the light-sensitive membrane in the eye); it can cause vision loss if left untreated. In a Danish study, the risk of retinopathy fell by 42 percent in people who exercised compared to those who did not. (Exercisers were also eating a diet lower in saturated fat, but exercise was still considered largely responsible for the reduced risk.)

- **Reduces stress.** Managing any chronic disease can be stressful, and diabetes is no exception. Working out can reduce stress, anxiety, and depression.

simply more important that you ease into it instead of jumping into a level that's too strenuous.

Show your doctor the activity levels in this book and the twelve-week fitness plan on page 355, and the two of you can decide on an appropriate starting point. In some cases, your doctor may recommend a stress test before you begin. (You walk on a treadmill while having your heart monitored by an electrocardiogram [EKG]; the doctor will evaluate your heart health based on the findings.) The American Diabetes Association recommends seriously considering getting a stress test if you:

- Are over age 40, whether or not you have risk factors for cardiovascular disease (such as high blood pressure, high cholesterol, ventricle enlargement)

- Are over age 30 and you:

  - Have had type 1 or type 2 diabetes for more than ten years

  - Have high blood pressure

  - Smoke cigarettes

  - Have high levels of LDL ("bad" cholesterol) or high triglyceride levels

  - Have proliferative or preproliferative retinopathy (damage to the retina in the eye)

  - Have the kidney disease called nephropathy, including microalbuminuria (protein in the urine)

- Have any of the following conditions, regardless of age:

  - Known or suspected coronary artery disease (narrowing of the arteries leading to the heart), cerebrovascular disease (narrowing of the arteries to the brain), and/or peripheral vascular disease (narrowing of the blood vessels to the limbs and organs)

  - Autonomic neuropathy (damage to nerves that regulate blood pressure, heart rate, digestion, and other bodily functions)

  - Advanced nephropathy with kidney failure

THE BEST LIFE ACTIVITY SCALE

Ready to get moving, or at least, to consider adding more activity to your day? The Best Life Activity Scale is your starting point. First, find out where you fall on the scale. Then, read "Strategies for Increasing Your Activity," starting on page 89, for tips on getting to the next level. The twelve-week fitness plan (page 355) offers you a cardio program with optional strength training that lets you start at your currrent Activity Level and move up.

The American Diabetes Association recommends that you get at least 150 minutes per week of moderate-intensity aerobic physical activity and unless there's a medical reason not to (as in certain cases of high blood pressure), it recommends resistance training three times a week. Looking at the Activity Scale, you can see that those recommendations match up nearly perfectly with Activity Level 3.

When increasing your activity, do so safely: move up just one level from where you are now; don't skip over a level to try to get right to 150 minutes. For instance, if you're very sedentary (Level 0), transition to Level 1, don't skip to Level 2. Don't worry, you'll get there! For all the issues discussed above (heart disease, neuropathy), it's very important that you get accustomed to one level before moving on to the next.

TRACKING YOUR ACTIVITY

The Best Life Activity Scale is composed of six different levels of physical activity. Level 0 is basically just what it sounds like—doing nothing. But all the other levels include aerobic exercise and Levels 3 to 5 also include strength training.

Aerobic exercise is also called "cardio" because your heart (and lungs) are working harder than usual to get enough oxygen to fuel the workout. The more intensely you exercise the more of a workout your heart and lungs get. We'll show you how to gauge intensity using the Perceived Exertion Scale (page 93). You'll notice that we're not requiring long hours of workout time for most of the activity levels. We expect you to make the most of the minutes we do recommend by working out intensely because you'll reap greater fitness and blood sugar rewards. Of course, some of you won't be able to do that at first; you'll have to build up to it. Or you may have medical issues that won't allow you to work out vigorously. If you can do only light aerobic exercise, such as slow walking, biking, or other activities that don't raise your heart rate much, then ask your doctor if you can increase the number of minutes you exercise. More minutes partially compensates for less intensity. For instance, Activity Level 1 requires at least 90 minutes a week of aerobic activity. You might be able to do 120 minutes of slow walking or another low-aerobic activity to satisfy the requirements of Level 1.

There are two ways to track the aerobic component of the Activity Scale: steps per day (logged by a pedometer) and minutes per week. Remember: both types of exercise should be aerobic, which is defined as any activity that uses large muscle groups, can be maintained continuously, is rhythmic in nature, and elevates your heart rate and breathing. For it to count toward your weekly goal you should see an increase in breathing and heart rate not only with the workouts you do on the treadmill, bike, elliptical trainer, or in an aerobic class, but also for any walking you do.

Because it's hard to convert steps to minutes and vice versa, it's best to choose one way to track your aerobic exercise. (On www.thebestlife .com you can log both in a given day; the program converts the figures to give you one aerobic total.) Pedometers are inexpensive, offer an easy way to track your progress, and can be very motivating. Sportline, Sportbrain, Gaiam, and Nike Plus make reliable models with good tracking features. They're found in most sporting goods shops.

Aerobic exercise is not interchangeable with strength training, so log your strength-training moves separately. Strength training builds and tones muscle tissue using resistance in the form of free weights, machines, or even your own body weight. If you've never done it, don't be intimidated. Just start out with light weights, and you'll be amazed at how quickly your strength builds. Strength training starts at Level 3.

FIND YOUR LEVEL

Level 0

At Level 0, you're moving around just enough to get through your day—walking around the house or office, to and from the car, and other necessary moves—but you make no attempt to get any extra exercise. Physical activity just isn't on your radar, and it may happen only by accident—for instance, if the parking lot is very full and your car winds up far away from the store. You rarely, if ever, take a walk. Your job doesn't require physical activity, and at home at night, you're usually on the couch.

Pre-diabetes and type 2 diabetes are often caused by being overweight and inactive, so some of you may recognize yourself in this description. And you may be worried that exercise might be too strenuous for your heart or might worsen complications of diabetes, such as neuropathy. As we've discussed earlier, these are real concerns, but for most of you, consulting your physician first, starting out slowly, and building up gradually, will make exercise safe—and very beneficial—for you.

Aerobic exercise: none
or
Steps per day: 3,499 or less

Strength training: none

Level 1

At Level 1, you make an effort to get a little more exercise than just the necessary everyday moves, but the exercise you get isn't consistent or intense. You may have a job that keeps you on your feet—maybe you're a nurse, waitress, electrician, or teacher—or perhaps you just make an extra effort to move throughout the day. Maybe you often go for a stroll after dinner or ride bikes with your kids. You take the stairs when you can, and return your shopping cart to the front of the store instead of leaving it next to your car, just so you can get a few more steps in. Maybe you get off a stop or two early when you're taking public transportation and walk the rest of the way. You may be someone who hasn't participated in structured exercise since high school, or maybe you used to have a regular workout program but some change in your life, a complication of diabetes, or sustaining an injury led you to quit and you haven't picked it up again. In general, you look for creative ways to move more throughout the day.

Aerobic exercise: up to 90 minutes per week *
or
Steps per day: approximately 3,500–5,999

Strength training: none

Level 2

You're at Level 2 if you have a structured, consistent exercise schedule. It's fairly moderate, but has helped you reap some diabetes-management, cardiovascular, body-shaping, and calorie-burning benefits. You may work out in any number of ways—by yourself on a stationary bike, at home with an aerobics DVD, or with a fellow walker on the streets of your neighborhood—but you always get in at least three 30-minute sessions a week.

Aerobic exercise: three times a week, 90–150 minutes per week
or
Steps per day: approximately 6,000–9,999

Strength training: none

Level 3

You're at Level 3 if you're serious about exercise and work out at least five and possibly six days a week. On at least four of those days, you do cardiovascular exercise—usually the same workout, whether it be walking, jogging, swimming, or something like going to a spinning or aerobic dance class—for a total of at least 150 minutes a week. At least two days a week, you strength train with weights, performing at least six different exercises per session. You're so committed to activity that on the weekends you also take leisurely but long walks.

Aerobic exercise: five times a week, 150–250 minutes per week
or
Steps per day: approximately 10,000–13,999

Strength training: at least two times a week, a minimum of six exercises

* If you haven't done aerobic exercise in a while, keep the intensity moderate—under a 7 on the Perceived Exertion Scale on page 93.

Level 4

You're at Level 4 if you not only work out almost every day but also cross-train (engage in multiple aerobic activities) to get added benefits and to lower your risk of an overuse injury. For example, three days a week you run, walk, or use the elliptical trainer at the gym, and on the other two days, you do other aerobic activities, such as swimming, riding a bike, or taking an aerobics class. Altogether you rack up at least 250 minutes of aerobic exercise a week. You're also into strength training and do so consistently three days a week, performing at least eight different exercises per session. You may even use a challenging yoga or Pilates class to satisfy one of your strength-training workouts.

> **Aerobic exercise: five times a week, at least 250–360 minutes per week**
> or
> **Steps per day: approximately 14,000–17,999**
>
> **Strength training: at least three times a week, a minimum of eight exercises**

Level 5

You're at Level 5 if exercise isn't just how you stay fit and healthy, it's a way of life. You may belong to a workout group, such as a running, walking, or cycling club. Perhaps you challenge yourself by participating in races and competitions. You work out almost every day, maybe doing your main workout three times a week and cross-training three other days, for a total of six hours (360 minutes) of cardiovascular exercise a week. You've been strength training for some time now, and you're up to at least ten different exercises, a minimum of three days a week. While this level of exercise is optimal for blood sugar control and avoiding heart disease and other conditions that accompany diabetes, it's not an option for all of you. For instance, high levels of exercise can further damage the eyes if you have severe retinopathy. So, as always, check with your doctor before you get to this level.

> **Aerobic exercise: six times a week, 360 minutes or more per week**

or

Steps per day: approximately 18,000 or above

Strength training: at least three times a week, a minimum of ten exercises

GOING TO THE NEXT LEVEL

Your exercise goal for Phase One is to move up a level from where you are now on the Best Life Activity Scale. The twelve-week program in Appendix Three is one way to do it. Getting more exercise and increasing your intensity, in particular, will decrease your blood sugar levels as well as the risk of diabetic complications, such as heart disease and retinopathy. If you already have some of these complications and you're a regular exerciser, you may not be able to bump up a full level on the Activity Scale, but you could look for ways to be a little more active.

Ideally, everyone should work toward reaching Activity Level 3—the level recommended by the ADA—or higher. For many of you, that's very doable—maybe not today or next month, but perhaps in six months. If you have a physical limitation that prevents you from getting to the full-blown Level 3, you and your doctor can decide how close you can get.

Whether you ever make it to Level 3 or not, one thing is for sure: no one should be at Level 0. Being sedentary is just going to make your diabetes worse. By the end of Phase One, you should be at Level 1 or higher. It's really not that hard—it's as simple as walking down the hall to talk to your coworker instead of e-mailing her, or going out for an after-dinner walk.

The key is to stay motivated and aim high but always be safe. Move up just one level at a time, staying at that new level for at least a few weeks or months until it's no longer very challenging. And be consistent. It's better for your health to be a consistent Level 2 exerciser, faithfully completing the 90 to 150 minutes at the gym or on your walks, than going through spurts of hitting Level 3, then falling back to a Level 1. You might wind up feeling as if you've failed and getting turned off to exercise altogether. Take a realistic look at your schedule and your physical limitations, and find a level you can sustain.

STRATEGIES FOR INCREASING YOUR ACTIVITY

The tips below will help you ease into the next activity level. (For more fun exercise ideas and motivating tips, and to watch videos showing exercise routines and safe strength-training techniques, go to www.thebestlife .com.) As you read these strategies for increasing your activity, remember that you can gauge your aerobic exercise either in minutes per week or in steps per day or week. To move up to Level 3, 4, or 5, you must include strength training in your program in addition to your aerobic exercise/ steps per day, as outlined in the program on pages 355 to 358.

To Go from Level 0 to Level 1 . . .

You more than anyone else will benefit from having a pedometer, because the easiest and best way to move to Level 1 is simply to walk more. To gauge how much you're walking now and help you increase that number, use a pedometer to measure how many steps you currently take each day. For the first week, don't change your routine at all so you can get a baseline number. Then gradually increase the number of steps you take. Your initial goal should be to get up to at least 3,500 and preferably 6,000 steps a day. Walk to the store for milk. Walk your kids to school. Walk around while you talk on the phone or give a presentation. Walk up stairs instead of using elevators and escalators (and if you do take an escalator, walk up; don't just stand there while it moves you). Walk to church or other community activities (and if it's too far to walk the whole way, park a good distance away and walk the remainder). As your pedometer will show you, you'll ultimately rack up some significant mileage, and that will translate into a lower blood sugar level as well as a significant number of calories burned—and pounds lost!

Think, too, about how vigorously you move. Studies show one of the big differences between people who are overweight and people who aren't is that lean people not only fidget more, they use more energy for everyday movements. For instance, someone who's energetic jumps up and picks up something that's fallen off her desk; someone who barely moves slides his chair over to grab it. The calorie-burning difference between the two ways of moving hardly seems as if it would make one person slender and another person heavy, but multiply it by the thousands of small moves you make each day, then by weeks, months, and years, and it all adds up to a big difference.

To Go from Level 1 to Level 2 . . .

You're about to make a substantial leap that may seem difficult at first, but it's going to get easier, and you'll feel the rewards right away. You'll sleep better, feel better, and eventually even have more energy—and you might see a drop in your blood sugar readings as well. You may feel more tired than usual at first, but once the training effect kicks in and your body adapts, you'll definitely feel more lively. Choose one or more types of aerobic exercise that you like; it could be walking, jogging, aerobic dance, spinning, salsa dancing, swimming, cycling, or kickboxing. Working out on machines such as treadmills, stationary bikes, rowing machines, and elliptical trainers is a great way to go, too.

Start by putting in as much time as you can comfortably handle— 15 minutes a session, three sessions a week if you can do it, less if you can't. Each week, add 2 minutes to your workouts until you reach 30 minutes per session; you'll then be meeting the 90-minutes-a-week minimum requirement. Consider getting a workout partner, too; having someone to whom you're accountable can really help keep you on track. If you prefer to count steps to satisfy the aerobic requirement, increase your steps per day, working up to over 6,000 daily.

To Go from Level 2 to Level 3 . . .

By adding strength training to your regimen, you're not only fulfilling the ADA's guidelines, you're further improving your insulin sensitivity. You're also doing your bones a big favor; strength training can help prevent osteoporosis. At this point, you're moving up to a whole new level of commitment, so be creative about working strength training into your schedule. Some people find that they prefer to complete their strength training right after their aerobic workouts so that they can get everything out of the way in one fell swoop. Other people like to break their workouts up and do their aerobic/step component and strength training on separate days or on the same day but at separate times. One way isn't better than the other; whatever routine ensures that you're able to get everything done should be the one you choose.

To strength train, start with one to two sets of six exercises at least two days a week. Choose a selection that involves all the major muscle groups; the "Basic Eight" starting on page 179 offers ideal options. More strength-training tips, including videos, can be found on www.thebest life.com. After six weeks, increase the number of sets you do to two or three. You may want to consider working with a trainer at this point. A trainer can make sure you're doing the moves properly and also help you evaluate your current routine to make sure you're on track to meet your health and weight-loss goals. If cost is a concern, you can split the fee with a friend. Or invest in just one 2-hour session, during which your trainer can design a program for you for the next six months. Also, gradually increase your aerobic sessions by 2 minutes per week, working toward a total of at least 150 minutes per week. If you're counting steps, increase your steps per day, working up to a minimum of 10,000 to satisfy the aerobic requirement.

To Go from Level 3 to Level 4 . . .

At this stage, you should already be fairly fit, which will make advancing to the next level that much easier. Step up your strength-training regimen to include at least eight different exercises, two to three sets each, and do this for a minimum of three days a week. Also, continue to boost your aerobic workout times by 2 minutes a week and raise the frequency of your workouts to six per week. Aim for a minimum total weekly aerobic exercise time of 250 minutes. This is a good time to diversify your workouts, too. Choose a second aerobic workout you like, and alternate between that and your original workout so that you're not overworking the same muscles. Plus, by including different types of activities in your routine, you'll train more muscles and, as a result, lose more fat. If you've been running on the treadmill, try the elliptical or rowing machines. If you've been cycling, why not try an aerobic dance or salsa class? If possible, also throw in a yoga, Pilates, or stretch class during the week. If you're counting steps, increase your steps per day, working up to at least 14,000 to satisfy the aerobic requirement.

To Go from Level 4 To Level 5 . . .

You're working out so often now that it's part of your lifestyle, and you're reaping significant benefits from both weight-loss and diabetes-management standpoints. But if you can do even more, you'll be well rewarded. There's a body of new research indicating that people who do at least an hour of exercise a day make gains in everything from weight control to increased immunity to diseases.

One of the best ways to kick up your activity a degree is to test your skills. If your condition permits and your doctor approves, enter 10Ks and half marathons or maybe even full marathons. Join workout clubs; there are organizations for just about every possible activity, and these groups often train for both fun and serious competitions. To find a club, search the Web or check with local sporting goods stores, which usually can point you in the right direction. To reach Level 5, you'll be raising your total aerobic workout time to 6 hours (360 minutes) or more a week. If you're counting steps, increase your steps per day to at least 18,000 to satisfy the aerobic requirement. Increase your strength training to a minimum of ten different exercises and the number of sets you do to three, at least three days a week. Now is a good time to consider finding a training partner. You're putting a lot of hours into exercise, and having someone to talk to and encourage your effort will make the time go faster.

GET INTENSE

Of course, any kind of activity or movement you do is beneficial, as long as you're out there burning calories (and, hopefully, enjoying it!). But some studies are showing that the more intensely you work out, the better your A1c numbers and, perhaps, the smaller your waistline. In a University of Virginia study, obese women with metabolic syndrome (a precursor to type 2 diabetes) who walked or jogged at a moderate intensity two days a week and three days a week at high intensity lost 9 percent of their visceral belly fat in sixteen weeks; they also shed another 9 percent of subcutaneous belly fat. Women in that same study who worked out at low intensity didn't lose belly fat, but they did lose, on average, 5 pounds. No one in this study was dieting.

That said, it's much more important to play it safe and work out lightly or moderately until you're fit enough to increase your exercise intensity.

How do you know how intensely you're working out? Find your level on the Perceived Exertion Scale below. This tool uses your breathing to determine how hard you're working out based on a scale of 0 to 10. You breathe harder as your body requires more oxygen, and the more oxygen required, the more intensely you're working out. Ideally, you want to be between 7 and 8. Here's a look at what each number represents.

THE PERCEIVED EXERTION SCALE

0   This is the way you feel at rest. There is no fatigue, and your breathing is not elevated.

1   This is how you'd feel while working at your desk or reading. There is no fatigue, and your breathing is normal.

2   This is what you'd feel like when you're getting dressed. There is little or no feeling of fatigue, and your breathing is still normal.

3   This is how you'd feel while slowly walking across the room to turn on the TV. You may feel a little fatigued and you may be aware of your breathing, but it is still slow and natural. You might also feel this way at the beginning of your warm-up.

4   This is the way you'd feel if you were walking slowly outside. There is a slight feeling of fatigue and your breathing is slightly elevated but comfortable. You should experience this level during the initial stages of your warm-up.

5   This is how you'd feel while walking somewhere at a normal pace. You're aware of your breathing, which is now deeper, and there is a slight feeling of fatigue. You should experience this level at the end of your warm-up.

6   This is similar to how you'd feel if you were walking to an appointment that you were late for. There is a feeling of fatigue, but you know you can maintain this level of exertion. Your breathing is deep, and you're aware of it. This is how you should feel as you transition from your warm-up to your regular exercise session.

7   This is how you'd feel while exercising vigorously. There's a feeling of fatigue, but you're sure you can maintain this level for the rest of your exercise session. Your breathing is deep, and you're aware of it. You could carry on a conversation but would probably choose not to do so. You should try to maintain this level during your workouts.

8   This is how you should feel while exercising very vigorously. You're feeling fatigued, and if you asked yourself if you could continue for the remainder of your exercise session, your answer would be that you think you could but you're not sure. Your breathing is very deep, and though you could still carry on a conversation, you don't feel like it. You should try to exercise at this level only after you feel comfortable at level 7. This is the level that produces the most rapid weight loss for many people.

9   This is what you'd feel like if you were exercising very, very vigorously. You'd definitely feel fatigued, and you probably wouldn't be able to maintain this level for very long. Your breathing is very labored, and it would be very difficult to carry on a conversation. You may sometimes hit this level when trying to reach an 8 on the scale; if you hit this point, slow up a bit until you feel as if you're back down to a 7 or 8.

10 This level is all-out exercise, so difficult that you couldn't maintain it for very long. You don't want to experience level 10 because there's no way to maintain it for very long, and hence there's no benefit to it.

Be patient—learning how to use the Perceived Exertion Scale will take a bit of time, but once you get the hang of it, it will be very easy to use.

For the vast majority of people, the Perceived Exertion Scale will be the easiest and most effective way to gauge intensity during exercise.

However, in certain cases, such as if you have a heart arrhythmia or other complication that requires you to stay below a certain heart rate, your doctor may recommend instead that you figure out your target heart rate and work out within this range. Your target heart rate is best measured on a maximal treadmill test administered by a health professional, but you can also estimate it with a simple formula. (Note that this figure is accurate for only about a third of the population. That's because your heart rate doesn't always reflect your oxygen consumption or how hard you're working. Plus, other factors, such as your emotional state, caffeine consumption, or medications like beta-blockers used to treat high blood pressure or heart disease, can alter your heart rate. In these cases, your heart rate might not increase as it should with exertion or you might work out too hard or too easy even though your heart rate suggests you're working out at your target rate.)

To figure out your maximum heart rate, subtract your age from 220; if you're 40 years old, your max heart rate would be 180. You'd then use this number to find your target heart rate—simply multiply 180 by 80 percent to get 144. That means you'll want to stay near this number when you're exercising. How can you tell if you're close? You can check your pulse, although this obviously has limitations; once you stop to take your pulse, your heart rate will drop. You could also rely on the monitors on treadmills, bikes, and other cardio equipment, but these aren't always very accurate. Your final option would be to buy a heart rate monitor, such as the Polar or Timex brands, which you can find at most sporting goods stores.

A target heart rate of 80 percent of your maximum will not be safe or achievable for everyone, especially in the early stages. Your prime consideration has to be safety, and it's critical that you check with your doctor before starting your exercise program or increasing the intensity of your workouts. Your doctor may recommend a target of 60 percent of your maximum heart rate at the beginning and suggest gradually working up from there. If you develop shortness of breath, chest pain, or lightheadedness while exercising, you should stop your workout. Let your doctor know what happened; he may recommend a stress test, as discussed on page 82.

Exercise, Meals, and Medications

As beneficial as exercise is, when you have diabetes, you have to be careful; in some cases, your workout can trigger blood sugar swings in both directions. (This shouldn't be an issue if you have pre-diabetes.) The eating and medication tips in this section will help keep your blood sugar level stable throughout your workout. You'll learn what works best for you by using your blood glucose monitor. Monitoring your blood glucose frequently is going to be critically important, both when you begin your exercise regimen and when you move up on the Activity Scale later in this program. Of course, anytime you change the balance of diet, exercise, and medication, you will need to test most when the change is first made. Once things are stable, you can relax just a bit, knowing that you've increased your exercise safely.

HOW DIABETES AFFECTS YOUR WORKOUT

When you hit the treadmill, take an aerobics class, or do any other type of exercise, most of your physical reactions are the same as everyone else's. You sweat, you become a little out of breath, you eventually feel fatigued, and, if you're lucky, you get that exercise-induced endorphin high. Regular exercise will do the same great things for your body and mind, but having diabetes or pre-diabetes does change one important response to exercise—the way your body adjusts the level of glucose, which is needed to power your workout. It boils down to the way diabetes alters insulin and other hormones that control blood sugar.

Here's what's supposed to happen during exercise: At the beginning of a workout, muscles use mainly glucose, pulled from the blood, and glycogen(the stored form of glucose in muscles). As the workout progresses, the fuel shifts to a mix of glucose and fatty acids. Insulin, as you know, plays a key role in ushering glucose into muscle cells. During exercise, insulin needs to be available to help sugar get into your cells, but must also keep a low profile because a high level of insulin in the blood tells the liver not to release glucose—glucose you need to keep your energy up.

In a person without diabetes, insulin ebbs and flows as the body needs it. But when you have diabetes, several things can throw this system off. In one case, you don't make enough insulin, so you can't get enough sugar into your cells and you start feeling pretty tired on the treadmill. Or you're taking insulin or a medicine that revs up insulin production and you have too much insulin in the bloodstream, which tells the liver to stop releasing sugar just at the time you need it most. That can cause a hypoglycemic reaction.

Normally, with vigorous exercise, the body releases several other hormones. The main one is adrenaline, also called epinephrine. Adrenaline is the body's "fight-or-flight" hormone. It causes your heart rate to go up, increases blood flow to the muscles, enhances breathing, and generally prepares you for a burst of physical activity. That increased activity requires fuel, so adrenaline also causes the release of glucose into your bloodstream from the glycogen in your liver. So when you step out onto the tennis court, your blood sugar level may actually go up after you start to play.

Normally the body hums along, releasing the right amounts of insulin and adrenaline to keep the blood sugar level normal even with vigorous exercise. But if you have diabetes, you don't make adequate levels of insulin on your own, and you may not make adrenaline properly either, particularly if you have autonomic neuropathy, damage to the nerves that help regulate heart rate, blood pressure, and other internal organ functions. Too little adrenaline and/or too much insulin can plunge your blood sugar to hypoglycemic levels.

Over the long term, exercise almost always improves blood sugar levels. But during the short term, it can sometimes be hard to predict how your blood sugar level will react. The whole situation can get even a bit more complex when you are taking medicines designed to lower your blood sugar levels. That's why it's so important to monitor yourself carefully as you increase your exercise routine.

TIMING MEALS TO EXERCISE

To sustain a workout, you need to have enough energy, which comes from calories, primarily from glucose, along with some fat. For people who don't have diabetes, it's pretty simple: if they eat enough food that day, they have the energy to work out. Going into a workout fueled but not full (which makes it uncomfortable to work out) is optimal. This is also true for you, but you're grappling with another issue too: making sure your blood sugar level remains in a good zone. Depending on what you eat and what type of medicine you're taking, if you're not careful, exercise can send your blood sugar level either soaring or plunging.

Test your blood sugar level before working out; don't work out if it's under 100 or over 300. Here are the strategies that will help you stay safe during your workout:

- If you're under 100, have a snack that provides 15 grams of carbohydrate (see the meal plans page 251). Retest in 15 minutes to see if your blood sugar level is 100 or above. If so, it's safe to start exercising. Remember, though, that the exercise itself will tend to lower your blood sugar level and there is the possibility that it will fall again even though you've brought it up with the snack. Stopping for a quick test during your workout will help ensure you don't go too low again. If your glucose level has fallen again, stop exercising for that session, eat a 15-gram carbohydrate snack, and retest in 15 minutes. You'll need to repeat the snacks every 15 minutes or so until your glucose level rises, and if you've needed more than one 15-gram snack or if your blood sugar level fell very low, you'll need to eat a bigger meal so that it doesn't fall again over the next couple of hours.

- If your blood sugar level is above 300, wait until it falls into a better range before starting to exercise. When your blood sugar level is high, it may mean that you've overdone the carbohydrates at a previous meal or snack, that you're getting sick, or something else is going on. If your blood sugar level is high enough, it may be sending you to the bathroom to urinate more frequently, and, as a result, you could become dehydrated. Starting to exercise when you are dehydrated can be downright dangerous: it saps energy and endurance and in severe cases can cause heatstroke. As we said earlier, sometimes your blood sugar level may go higher during exercise itself, even if it tends to fall later. All in all, it's probably just safer to wait until things are back to normal.

- If you have type 1 diabetes, you need to be even more careful if you have a high sugar reading. If you have a glucose value of 300 or higher before exercise, or anytime you have persistently high blood sugars, you should check your urine for ketones using a test strip. Ketones are chemicals that appear in the blood and urine when you are developing ketoacidosis, a condition in which there is plenty of glucose in your blood but your cells are literally starving because the glucose can't get inside them. Ketoacidosis can be serious and even life-threatening but in the early stages can be corrected by drinking enough fluid and taking the correct amount of insulin. If the test is positive, you need to postpone your workout, drink plenty of fluids, monitor your blood sugar level, and probably take extra insulin. A small amount of ketones in the urine may not be serious, but if your blood sugar level remains high or the ketones stay positive, you should contact your doctor immediately.

EXERCISE AND YOUR MEDICATIONS

If you've begun to make the changes we've recommended in Phase One, you're exercising more than you did before and probably eating fewer carbs. Both of these changes will lower your blood sugar level, and your diabetes medication may need adjustment. Hypoglycemia from too much medication is especially common with exercise. Some medicines pose more of a problem than others. We want to emphasize that you must not adjust your medications without talking to your doctor, but we also want you to be clued in to the effects of exercise on the drugs you're taking. We've already discussed what to do if you have a low or high blood sugar prior to exercise (page 98). If you are taking diabetes medication and are having low blood-sugar reactions during or after exercise, understanding the effects of the various drugs may help you pinpoint the cause. You can then discuss with your doctor what changes might need to be made. Here is an overview of how various medications impact blood sugar levels during exercise (for a comprehensive look at diabetes medications, turn to Chapter Five):

Medications Other Than Insulin

Diabetes drugs can be categorized in terms of how they help lower blood sugar. Some drugs increase the amount of insulin in the body. These carry the greatest risk of low blood sugar reactions during exercise. Some drugs improve the way your body reacts to insulin. Taken alone, these drugs carry much less risk, though given in combination with medications that increase insulin, they may make hypoglycemia worse. In the lists below, brand names are given in parentheses.

Medications That Increase Insulin Production by the Pancreas

ORAL MEDICATIONS

Sulfonylureas (pages 194 to 195): glyburide (Micronase, DiaBeta, Glynase), glipizide (Glucotrol), glimepiride (Amaryl), and others

Meglitinides (pages 195 to 196): repaglinide (Prandin) and nateglinide (Starlix)

Sitagliptin (Januvia) and saxagliptin (Onglyza) (pages 201 to 202)

MEDICATIONS GIVEN BY INJECTION

Exenatide (Byetta), liraglutide (Victoza), and pramlintide (Symlin) (pages 202 to 203)

These medications raise the amount of insulin in your body. They do so by causing your pancreas to make more of your own naturally occurring insulin. If too much insulin is made, a hypoglycemic reaction will occur. The risk is greatest with the sulfonylurea medications, which are long-lasting and are very powerful at releasing the body's insulin. The meglitinides work in similar ways but are shorter-acting and not as potent. Januvia and Onglyza carry the least risk of a low-blood-sugar reaction among these medicines. Byetta and Victoza are given by injection, increase the amount of insulin made by the body, and affect other hormones that also regulate blood sugar. Symlin doesn't raise insulin, but we mention it here because its other actions are similar to Byetta. Both Byetta and Symlin lessen appetite, which might cause you to eat less than you need to fuel a workout. If you are having frequent exercise-related hypoglycemia on any of these medications, you may need a reduction in dose or a change in the drug, you may need to eat some extra carbs prior to exercising, or you may need to change the timing of your workout.

Medications That Reduce Insulin Resistance

Metformin (Glucophage, Glucophage XR, Glumetza, Fortamet, Riomet) (pages 196 to 199)

Thiazolidinediones (TZDs): pioglitazone (Actos) and rosiglitazone (Avandia) (pages 199 to 200)

These drugs help lower blood sugar not by increasing insulin, but by helping the body react better to the insulin already present. Metformin works primarily by reducing glucose production by the liver, but it doesn't usually shut off the production completely, so you can still meet your fuel needs. The TZD medicines Actos and Avandia improve how your muscle cells react to insulin. All these drugs are much less likely to cause hypoglycemia because when your blood sugar starts to go low, your pancreas automatically reduces the amount of insulin that it is making. You're responding better to the insulin, but the amount in your blood is not usually enough to cause hypoglycemia.

Medications That Slow the Digestion of Starch

Acarbose (Precose) and miglitol (Glyset) (pages 204 to 205)

Precose and Glyset are medications that slow down the rate at which your digestive system breaks down the starch in foods into sugars. These drugs are unusual in that they don't depend on insulin for their action. They help keep blood sugar low by slowing the rate at which you absorb the glucose that comes from starchy foods, such as breads, potatoes, rice, and pasta. They don't usually cause hypoglycemia when used alone, and probably won't need to be adjusted for exercise in most cases. However, these drugs also slow the rate at which your body breaks down sucrose—table sugar or cane sugar—to glucose. This means that you'll recover less quickly from a low-blood-sugar reaction if you drink orange juice or eat hard candy. Therefore, if you are taking either Precose or Glyset, you should always have glucose tablets or glucose gel available for the treatment of hypoglycemia, including with exercise, as glucose is absorbed directly by the body without having to be broken down in the intestine.

Insulin

All forms of insulin carry the risk of hypoglycemia. The risk with exercise comes down to timing. Insulins differ in terms of how long they last and when they reach their maximum effect, as described on pages 207 to 216. The most common forms of insulin are:

Very-fast-acting: NovoLog, Humalog, and Apidra

Fast-acting: regular insulin (Novolin R and Humulin R)

Intermediate-acting: NPH insulin (Novolin N or Humulin N) or Lente insulin (Novolin L or Humulin L)

Very-long-acting: Lantus and Levemir

The very-long-acting insulins Lantus and Levemir have little or no "peak" in their activity. They provide a relatively steady amount of insulin action over many hours and are rarely a problem with exercise. All other insulins rise to a point of maximum or peak activity, after which their action begins to decline.

The fast and very-fast-acting insulins, which peak between one and three hours after injection and are usually taken with meals, rapidly lower blood sugar. The same dose of insulin that lowers your blood sugar to just the right level after meals could cause your sugar to dip too low during exercise, especially if you are exercising during the period of maximum blood sugar lowering action. In general, you should not exercise during the peak time periods after injecting the insulin because this is when there is the greatest likelihood of hypoglycemia.

If you become hypoglycemic during exercise, it probably means that the last dose of insulin you took was too high. So next time you exercise, you should probably decrease your insulin dose. For example, let's say you took eight units of insulin before lunch, then hit the gym after work and experienced hypoglycemia. Talk to your doctor about how much to reduce that prelunch insulin dose and see if that helps the next time you work out.

If you are taking an intermediate-acting insulin, now you're contending with a five- to seven-hour peak. For example, let's say you're taking NPH at breakfast and at dinner, and you experience a low-blood-sugar reaction during afternoon exercise. That's probably because you took too much insulin in the morning. Work with your doctor on reducing that morning dose on exercise days. And while you may need to lower your evening dose right after having the hypoglycemic reaction, this should *not* be the way you deal with this problem in the future. It's all about preventing the hypoglycemia to begin with by hitting on the right A.M. dose.

JUDGING YOUR SUCCESS

We'd like you to spend a minimum of four weeks in Phase One. Once the four weeks are up, ask yourself the nine questions below to determine if you're ready to move on to Phase Two. If you can answer yes or usually to each of the first seven questions, you're ready for Phase Two. If you're answering no or not usually, then it's best to remain in Phase One for a few more weeks. (Remember, if you're making substantial lifestyle changes, it may take a little longer for them to stick.) Although a yes or usually isn't required of the final two questions to move on, you have a greater chance of success if you're consistently achieving these two goals as well. If you're not, you can still continue on to the next phase as long as you make a commitment to keep working on them.

1. If you have diabetes, is your blood sugar under better control, meaning when you test, is it more often in the good zone?

2. If you have diabetes, are you monitoring and logging your blood sugar regularly?

3. Are you familiar with carbohydrate servings of foods you regularly eat?

4. Are you eating appropriate amounts of carbohydrate-rich foods at most meals?

5. Are you eating three meals and the number of snacks recommended for your calorie level?

6. Did you increase your activity level?

7. Are you comfortable enough with the lifestyle changes you've made in Phase One, and are you prepared to take on new challenges?

8. Are you drinking six 8-ounce glasses of water daily?

9. Have you eliminated alcohol and soda?

3

PHASE TWO: FINE-TUNING YOUR DIET

HOPEFULLY, ALL THE BLOOD sugar monitoring, carbohydrate watching, and exercise you've been doing has started to pay off in the form of better blood sugar levels, a heightened sense of well-being, and perhaps even weight loss.

As you've become more accomplished at managing your diabetes, there's still more you can do to tighten your control over your blood sugar levels. In Phase Two, you'll try to bump up to the next level on the Activity Scale (it's optional but encouraged). You'll be putting the right amount and type of high-protein foods and fats on your plate. You'll be improving the *quality* of your carbohydrates, eating more of the ones that are easy on the blood sugar, while continuing to work on the Phase One goal of eating the right amount of carbs. If you've been a fan of fat-filled baked goods, such as doughnuts and cookies, and fried foods, you'll be reining in your consumption of these notoriously fattening foods. If you need to lose weight, the pounds should drop off even faster in this phase, not only because of the food choices you'll be making but also because you'll be using an excellent weight-control tool: the Hunger Scale (see page 137). If you decide to step up your exercise, you'll shed even more weight. We'll also help you pick a multivitamin/mineral tablet and discuss the pros and cons of other nutritional supplements.

Meanwhile, you'll continue to do most everything you've been doing in Phase One, including monitoring your blood sugar, watching your carbohydrates, eating regularly, eating lightly (or not at all) before bedtime, cutting out soda, drinking your six cups of water every day, and meeting your activity level. You can relax the alcohol restriction in this phase; we'll offer some guidance on how, and whether it's a good idea, later in this chapter.

PHASE TWO

TIME FRAME: At least four weeks.

WEIGH IN: Weigh yourself once a week.

FOCUS: Improve your blood sugar levels by putting the best mix of carbohydrates, protein, and fat on your plate, losing more weight (if you need to) by listening to your body's hunger and satiety cues, and, if possible, getting more exercise and taking the right supplements.

OBJECTIVES:

- Continue all your Phase One goals:
  - If you have diabetes, regularly test your blood sugar and keep a blood sugar/drug/food/exercise log.
  - Eat appropriate amounts of carbohydrates.
  - Eat three meals and two snacks each day, three snacks if you're taking in 2,250 calories daily.
  - Eat a Best Life Breakfast.
  - Eat lightly—or not at all—during the two hours before bedtime.
  - Eliminate sweetened beverages.
  - Drink six glasses of water daily.
- Increase your activity (optional).
- Incorporate lean protein into your diet.

- Switch to healthy fats.

- Eat healthier, high-carbohydrate foods.

- Cut out fried foods.

- Understand your body's natural hunger and fullness cues, and use the Hunger Scale to eat reasonable portions and cut back on emotional eating.

- Take a multivitamin and calcium or omega-3 supplements if needed.

JUDGING YOUR SUCCESS: The majority of your blood sugar readings should be in the ideal or acceptable range; you're losing weight if you need to; the mix of carbohydrates, protein, and fat should be well balanced; you've cut back on overeating; and you're getting more exercise.

PHASE TWO OBJECTIVES

Go Up One Level on the Activity Scale

Because of the tremendous importance of exercise in diabetes management, we're going to encourage you to move up a level on the Activity Scale, or you can keep progressing with the cardio and strength-training program provided on page 357. After Phase One you should be fitter and stronger, and your body should be more used to exercise. If your exercise routine has become easy, you're definitely ready to make this move, but if you're still very challenged by your current activity level, you might want to stay where you are for a few more weeks.

Unless physical limitations or health issues are standing in the way, you should be at least at Activity Level 1, and by the end of this phase at Activity Level 2 and preferably higher. Find the time, push yourself a little, and you'll be well rewarded in so many ways: better blood sugar, more energy, accelerated weight loss, and possibly less medication.

The Rest of Your Plate: Protein and Fat

We spent a lot of time discussing carbohydrates in Phase One, so let's turn now to the other components of your meals: protein and fat. Protein holds an almost magical place in the weight loss world—high-protein diets gained the public's attention years ago and have managed to maintain their popularity. Fat, on the other hand, is widely considered a diet downer; something to be feared and avoided, and that apprehension has spawned a huge market for low-fat and fat-free foods. If you've put protein on a pedestal and/or have become a fat-phobe, we hope to change those views. We've included moderate amounts of both healthy fat and lean protein in Phase Two, levels designed to help you on both the blood sugar and weight-loss fronts. Plus, we've factored in taste and the pleasure of eating. We want you to enjoy your food—whether it's a diet of your design based on our guidelines, or if you're eating straight off the meal plans in this book.

PROTEIN

Have you ever had toast and coffee for breakfast, or a Danish, and felt hungry an hour later? On the flip side, ever notice how much longer you can go on an egg-based breakfast or if you spread a little peanut butter on that slice of toast? If you have, you've experienced the staying power of protein, and research confirms that there is something uniquely hunger-quelling about the macronutrient. Don't get us wrong: fat and carbohydrates (especially certain types, which we'll get into later) help make a meal filling and satisfying. But a slew of studies show that protein's the most satiating of the three major macronutrients.

In a University of Washington/Oregon Health and Science study, people who switched from eating 15 percent of their total calories from protein to eating 30 percent of their calories from protein (and 20 percent from fat and 50 percent from carbs) spontaneously reduced their calorie intake by an average of 441 per day and lost, on average, 11 pounds, most of it body fat, in twelve weeks.

Your protein goal on the Best Life plan will be 24 percent, well within the 10 to 35 percent range recommended by the National Academy of Sciences. At this level, you'll be consuming more than average Americans, who get 13 to 16 percent of their calories from protein.

We've found that this protein level helps manage diabetes in a few ways. First, it will help take the edge off hunger and can speed up your weight loss, which, in turn can lower your blood sugar level. Plus, protein has a few other tricks up its sleeve. Pairing protein-rich foods with carbohydrates slows the rise in blood sugar. For instance, topping your pasta and tomato sauce with grilled chicken causes your blood sugar level to take longer to peak than if you'd skipped the chicken, because protein stimulates insulin release (in those of you who still produce insulin). In addition, protein causes your stomach to empty more slowly, so when the chicken and pasta hit your stomach, they stick around a little longer. This in turn delays the starch from reaching your gut, where it's turned into glucose before entering your bloodstream. This delayed gastric emptying helps prevent sharp spikes in blood sugar. That's the reason we encourage you to have your daily treat immediately after a meal instead of by itself. Including protein (and, as you'll soon find out, fat) in your meals will cause a more gradual and smaller rise in your blood sugar levels.

Healthy Protein Picks

You can have it all—beef, poultry, seafood, and tofu; both animal and vegetable sources of protein are fair game on this plan—but you should avoid or limit your consumption of fatty meats and processed and cured meats, such as salami and bacon. Our recommendations:

- Have fish at least twice a week. Make at least one of those servings a fattier fish, such as bluefish, salmon, sardines, or trout, which are rich in beneficial omega-3 fatty acids but low in mercury, a contaminant that has health risks.

- Vary your seafood picks. Lobster, crab, scallops, mussels, clams, squid, and octopus are all low in saturated fat; so is shrimp, although it's high in cholesterol. But for most people, saturated fat is a much more potent cholesterol-raiser than dietary cholesterol.

- Remove skin from poultry. Skinless light (breast) and dark (drumstick and thigh) meat chicken and turkey are both fine.

- Try vegetarian sources of protein. Tofu and tempeh (fermented tofu), made with soy, and seitan (wheat protein) are virtually carb-free and can be substituted for animal protein. (Check tempeh labels carefully; some include wheat and are higher in carbohydrates. That's okay, just count those carb grams toward your grains/starchy vegetable servings.) Another great alternative are foods that have the taste and texture of meat or poultry but are made from plant-based protein, such as the gardein line, found in the deli and frozen food sections of natural food stores and some mainstream supermarkets. Tofu stars in recipes on pages 291, 300, 324, and a number of our other recipes offer a vegetarian alternative. Protein-rich beans are also high in carbohydrates, so on this program they're a much encouraged high-carbohydrate choice—not a protein option.

- Limit red meat to no more than twice a week, and stick with lean cuts, such as flank steak, sirloin, top loin or tenderloin, top round or eye of round, and ground beef that's at least 90% lean. Buffalo rib eye, shoulder, top round, and sirloin are lean cuts, as are lamb arm chop, leg shank, leg sirloin, leg top round, and loin chop. For pork, stick with center loin chop, lean ham, loin rib chop, shoulder blade steak, sirloin roast, tenderloin, top loin chop, and top loin roast.

- Have cured or processed meats, such as pepperoni and bacon, no more than twice a week. Less frequently is even better. This also applies to lean processed meats, such as turkey breast, because they're so high in sodium and most are preserved with nitrites and nitrates, which are linked to cancer. However, eating nitrite- and nitrate-free versions, such as Applegate Farms and Hormel Natural Choice, three times a week should be fine. Ideally, a serving should have no more than 300 milligrams of sodium per 2 ounces, but that's hard to find. Just make sure to limit the sodium at the rest of your meals.

No matter which protein source you choose, aim to have some protein at each meal and snack. In the meal plans, high-protein foods, such as chicken, fish, and lean beef are fairly evenly distributed between lunch and dinner. Milk, soy milk, tofu, and eggs are the main protein sources at breakfast. Even if you're not following our meal plans, it's worth glancing through them to see how much and what type of protein-rich foods we recommend. Checking out our meals can spark ideas for your own eating plan. (And there are lots more meals on www.thebestlife.com/diabetes.)

WHAT'S A PROTEIN SERVING?

High-Protein Foods:

Make the protein sources on the following pages your mainstays. They're all low in saturated fat, which raises LDL or "bad" cholesterol. If you want to indulge in the occasional fatty steak or full-fat cheese, keep the portion small (4 ounces for the steak, 2 ounces for the cheese), and remember that "occasional" means no more than once a week!

Some general guidelines:

- Have 2 to 6 servings at a given meal. A serving looks small— just 1 ounce of lean meat or 2 ounces of tofu—but remember, you get 7 to 9 servings of high-protein foods daily. (It varies with total daily calorie level, as you can see on the chart on page 114.) For instance, at a meal you could have 3 ounces of lean roast beef in a sandwich (3 servings), or 6 ounces of tofu in a stir-fry (3 servings), or 6 ounces of broiled fish (6 servings). While you can have a high-protein food, such as eggs or scrambled tofu, at breakfast, you don't have to. Milk, yogurt, or soy milk has enough protein to balance out the meal.

- Size it up. Three ounces of meat, poultry, or fish is roughly the size of a deck of cards, 1 ounce of cheese is about a 1-inch cube, and 6 ounces of tofu is about the size of a tennis ball (about ¾ cup).

- Limit cheese to 2 ounces, even reduced-fat versions. As you'll see from the list on the following page, only low-fat cheese makes the cut; full-fat cheeses are too high in saturated fat. But at 3 grams of saturated fat per ounce, even reduced-fat cheese is a higher source of this fat than the other picks on the list. (Technically, cheese is a dairy food, but on this plan it's considered a high-protein food because cheese is virtually carbohydrate-free, while milk and yogurt are major sources of carbohydrates.)

■ Count peanut butter as *both* protein and fat. Peanut butter is fairly high in protein, but the bulk of the calories come from fat, so it straddles the high-protein and high-fat groups. In order to get the 7 grams of protein in an ounce of animal protein, you have to eat 2 tablespoons of peanut butter, but it costs you calorie-wise: those two tablespoons have three times as many calories as an ounce of lean animal protein. Despite the calories, peanut butter is a very nutritious food, so go ahead and eat it, and don't worry that it's lower in protein than animal sources. As long as you're getting more concentrated sources of protein at other meals, you'll be fine. Here's how to handle it: Count each tablespoon as one high-protein serving and one fat serving (fat servings are explained later in this chapter). So, if your peanut butter and jelly sandwich has 2 tablespoons peanut butter, check off 2 protein servings and 2 fat servings.

Protein-Rich Foods:

About 7 grams of protein and 65 calories per serving

One serving equals:

Beef, lean (such as sirloin, tenderloin, trimmed of fat): 1 ounce cooked

Beef, ground 95% or more lean: 1½ ounces cooked

Cheese, reduced-fat hard (such as reduced-fat cheddar, jack, or Swiss): 1 ounce (check label for no more than 3 grams of saturated fat per ounce)

Chicken/turkey, skinless broiled: 1½ ounces or ¼ cup diced

Chicken/turkey, skinless, stewed: 1 ounce or 3 tablespoons diced

Edamame: ⅓ cup (also counts as half of a grain/starchy vegetable serving)

Egg: 1 large

Eggs, liquid (such as Better'n Eggs): ½ cup

Fish, white-fleshed (such as grouper, flounder, or snapper): 2 ounces cooked

Fish, oily (such as salmon, trout, or bluefish): 1 ounce cooked

Peanut butter (such as Smart Balance): 1 tablespoon (also uses up 1 fat serving)

Pork tenderloin: 1 ounce cooked

Salmon, canned, packed in water, drained: 2 ounces

Seitan (wheat protein): 2 ounces

Shellfish (clams, mussels, oysters, scallops, shrimp): 1½ ounces cooked

Tempeh (fermented soy): 1¼ ounces

Turkey bacon: 1½ medium slices or ½ ounce cooked, from 1 ounce raw (high in sodium so eat only occasionally)

Tofu: 2 to 4 ounces (check label as calories vary)

Tuna, canned, light, packed in water, drained: 2 ounces

THE PROBLEM WITH RED MEAT

You'll notice that we've recommended a lot more seafood and poultry options than red meat, and you'll see this in our meal plans, too. Red meat has a lot of strikes against it. For starters, it's high in iron. Though we need iron for healthy red blood cells, in excess it becomes an oxidant, causing damage to cells (the type of damage countered by antioxidants in foods). Then there's the way meat is cooked—Americans love meat barbecued or grilled at high temperatures, which causes the formation of two types of carcinogens: heterocyclic amines and polycyclic aromatic hydrocarbons (PAHs). And fatty cuts of meat are loaded with saturated fat, which is linked to heart disease, diabetes, and breast and colon cancer.

So if you like red meat and processed meat products, you can enjoy them once a week and eat healthier sources of protein, such as skinless poultry, fish, and tofu the rest of the time.

Vegetable burger, soy-based: ½ patty (check label as products differ; ideally, the entire burger should have at least 12 grams of protein and no more than 9 grams of carbohydrate, which you must count toward your grain/starchy vegetable servings)

Daily Servings

You saw this chart in Phase One, but now the protein and fat servings are not grayed out. That's because in this phase, you'll be concentrating on these two food groups, incorporating the right amounts and making the healthiest choices. With protein-rich foods and fats, you don't have to worry about exactly how many servings you have at each meal. Just try to meet the daily goal and to make sure you consume fat and some protein-rich food at each meal. At breakfast, you may not need a protein-rich food; the protein in your dairy serving might be enough. High-level exercisers: you may need more carbohydrates. See page 56 for your prescription.

Daily calories

	1,500	1,700	2,000	2,250
DAILY CARBO-HYDRATE GRAMS	144 g	154 g	191 g	212 g
DAILY SERVINGS OF EACH FOOD GROUP				
GRAINS/STARCHY VEGETABLES	4	4	5	6
MILK/YOGURT (FAT-FREE OR 1 %)	2	2	3	3½
FRUIT	2	2	2	2
NONSTARCHY VEGETABLES	6	6	7	7
DESSERT CARBOHYDRATE ALLOWANCE	—	A 100-calorie treat with no no more than 10 grams of carbohydrate	A 150-calorie treat with no no more than 15 grams of carbohydrate	A 150-calorie treat with no no more than 15 grams of carbohydrate
PROTEIN-RICH FOODS	7	7½	8	9
HEALTHY FATS	6	7	8	9

FAT

If you've struggled with your weight, you've probably struggled to control the amount of fat in your diet. How many times were you afraid to pour olive oil onto a salad or have a scoop of regular ice cream? (Or hated yourself when you had those foods?) The fear of fat has derailed more than one dieter because fat-free foods just aren't satisfying. And when a meal isn't satisfying, you go back to the fridge, the cupboards, and the vending machine for more food.

Including a little bit of fat in your meals and snacks will help you feel satisfied, and it will do so on two levels: in your mouth and in your stomach. Fat makes things taste good; using fat wisely can transform boring but healthful foods into dishes you actually crave. You might dutifully chomp through five cups of raw spinach, but you'd actually look forward to that spinach sautéed in olive oil with a little garlic and pine nuts. Fat also slows the rate at which your stomach empties, keeping you feeling full longer.

Just as too *little* fat is no good, neither is too *much*. Very-high-fat diets, where more than 45 percent of the calories consumed are from fat, can also be dangerous to your waistline. At 9 calories per gram, fat has more than double the 4 calories per gram of protein and carbohydrates. Translated to real food, that's why 14 grams of olive oil (1 tablespoon) has 120 calories while 14 grams of sugar (a heaping tablespoon) has 54 calories, and 14 grams of cooked rice (a heaping tablespoon) has just 18 calories. You can see why it's so easy to quickly run up a big calorie tab when you eat foods high in fat. That's one of the reasons we'll be asking you to completely avoid fried foods in Phase Two; if you've been eating them, this change alone will help you drop some weight.

Finding the Ideal Fat Zone

What we've found works best for most people is a Mediterranean-style diet of about 35 to 40 percent of your calories coming from fat. The principles of a Mediterranean-style diet—olive oil as the staple fat, the abundant use of fruits, vegetables, nuts, fish, and other lean protein sources, and whole grains—are easy to adapt. For instance, instead of fried fish and French fries, you can brush the fish with a mix of olive oil, lemon juice, and garlic, broil it, and serve it with a side of potatoes roasted in olive oil and rosemary.

Countless research studies show that a Mediterranean diet lowers heart disease risk. But recent studies are showing that it's also a great way to lose weight and that it may help prevent type 2 diabetes. For instance, a Harvard Medical School study, in conjunction with Israeli medical institutes, compared a Mediterranean diet (35 percent calories from fat) to a lower-fat plan (30 percent calories from fat) and an Atkins-type low-carbohydrate, high-protein diet. Researchers checked in on the 322 participants at six months, one year, and two years. Most everyone lost weight, but those on the Mediterranean and low-carb diets lost a lot more than the low-fat group. Women did especially well on the Mediterranean plan, keeping off, on average, 14 pounds over the two years compared with 5 pounds on the low-carb diet and virtually nothing on the low-fat diet. Men did a little better on the low-carb plan, maintaining, on average, an 11-pound loss compared to 9 pounds on the Mediterranean diet and nearly 8 pounds on the low-fat diet.

Obviously, weight loss is important, but what's more impressive is the effect this style of eating had on the blood sugar levels of the 36 subjects with type 2 diabetes. A year into the study, their average blood sugar level fell an impressive 23 points (mg/dL) on the Mediterranean diet, 18 points (not bad) on the low-carb diet, and just 3 points on the low-fat diet. Two years later, the average blood sugar level was even better on the Mediterranean plan—33 points down from the start of the study. Meanwhile, blood sugar returned to baseline levels for those on the low-carb diet and actually went up 12 points on the low-fat diet.

So if a low-fat diet just doesn't do it for you, you'll be very happy with this plan. At about 40 percent of daily calories from fat, it's along the lines of the Mediterranean diet. From our experience, that's the sweet spot: the meals are tasty and satisfying and conducive to weight loss, and we've kept saturated fat low enough (less than 8 percent of total calories) to help ward off heart disease.

Healthy Versus Unhealthy Fat

Everyone has to watch their intake of unhealthy fats, but if you have diabetes, you have to be extra vigilant. As you'll learn shortly, unhealthy fats can worsen insulin resistance and make your already heightened risk for heart disease that much greater. It's not the total fat consumption that matters so much; it's the *type* of fat consumed that affects your health. Your mission: to bring in more healthy fats and root out the unhealthy ones. We're not necessarily suggesting that you add *more* fat to your diet, although if you've been on a very-low-fat diet and aren't enjoying it, that may be a good idea. The goal here is to *replace* the unhealthy fatty foods with foods containing healthy fats.

If ordering a side of guacamole with your chicken fajita, snacking on a handful of mixed nuts, and sautéing your favorite vegetables in olive oil and garlic all sound appealing to you, you're already a fan of healthy fat. The reason these foods—avocados, nuts, and olive oil—are considered healthy fats is because of the type of fatty acids they contain. These and other foods we think of as fat—oils, butter, margarine, the fat surrounding a steak or under the skin of a chicken—are actually composed of different types of fatty acids. And it's the fatty acids that are either good or bad for your body.

The four types of fatty acids are polyunsaturated, monounsaturated, saturated, and trans. Though most foods contain a mix, usually one type of fatty acid predominates. For instance, olive oil contains 73 percent monounsaturated fat; the rest is polyunsaturated and saturated fat.

The different types of fatty acids have different effects on your health; here's the scoop.

Healthy Fats: Polyunsaturated and Monounsaturated (Both Called Unsaturated Fatty Acids)

These are the fats you should be including in your diet because they are linked to disease prevention. Monounsaturated fats are healthiest, so aim to get the most of these, while polyunsaturated fats are next in line.

Monounsaturated fatty acids are considered healthy because they don't raise LDL (the "bad" cholesterol that contributes to clogged arteries and heart disease) and they do raise HDL (the "good" form that actually removes cholesterol from your body). Plus, they've been linked to greater insulin sensitivity. Nearly all the monounsaturated fat in our diet comes from oleic acid.

Sources: Olive oil and canola oil are loaded with monounsaturated fats, so make these your staple oils. Other mono-rich foods include avocados, almonds, cashews, peanuts, and sesame seeds.

Polyunsaturated fatty acids, which fall into the healthy fat category because they do not raise LDL, include two types:

Omega-3 fatty acids offer a host of health benefits, including reducing inflammation, which, in turn, helps prevent and may even treat diseases such as rheumatoid arthritis and heart disease. These fats also help prevent blood clots and lower blood pressure, can improve mood, and may increase IQ in children. The health effects are so great that there's a case to be made for taking omega-3 supplements in addition to what you get from your diet. You can find supplementation advice on page 147. The three main types of omega-3s are:

▷ **Alpha-linolenic acid** (ALA) is the omega-3 fatty acid that's found in plants. ALA is critical to our survival; it's one of the two "essential" fatty acids that the body cannot make, so we must get it from foods (linoleic is the other essential fatty acid, see page opposite).

Sources: Have one of the following every day: flaxseeds or flaxseed oil, canola oil, walnuts, and foods enriched with omega-3s, such as these products sporting the Best Life Seal of Approval: Barilla PLUS pasta, Flatout Flatbread, Silk DHA Omega-3 & Calcium Soymilk (contains both ALA and DHA), Smart Balance milk (all four types), Smart Balance Peanut Butter.

▷ **Eicosapentaenoic acid** (EPA) and **docohexaenoic acid** (DHA) are the omega-3s found primarily in fish; there are also small amounts in meat from grass-fed animals. These seem to have more potent and direct benefits to the heart, brain, and joints than ALA and are what make up most omega-3 supplements.

Sources: Have one of the following fatty fish at least two times a week: bluefish, salmon, sardines, trout, and tuna. Fresh and white albacore canned tuna come from large fish that tend to be high in mercury, so have them no more than once a week. Chunk light canned tuna is low in mercury, so it's okay to have it a few times a week. (The rest of the fish listed are low in mercury.) If you don't like fish or are allergic to it, you should take an omega-3 supplement; even if you do eat fish, there's a case for supplementing (see page 147).

Omega-6 fatty acids have also been linked to heart disease prevention. Some argue that because omega-6s can be converted into substances that encourage inflammation, they may actually be bad for the heart and other tissues. However, a 2009 review by the American Heart Association found that most of the evidence points to a heart-protective effect. The most common omega-6 in our diet is linoleic acid, which, like ALA, is an essential fatty acid. Most people get more than their share of omega-6s because these are the predominant fats in many processed foods, such as frozen foods, baked goods, and salad dressings, as well as restaurant fare. There are also omega-6 fatty acids in olive and canola oils, which should become your staple oils for home use.

Sources: Corn, sesame, sunflower (not "high-oleic sunflower oil," which is high in monounsaturated fat), soybean, and walnut oils.

Unhealthy Fats

Cut back on foods high in saturated fat, and make it a point to avoid sources of trans fat altogether.

Saturated fatty acids are considered unhealthy fats because when eaten in excess, they raise LDL ("bad" cholesterol) and have been linked to an increased risk for heart disease and breast, colon, prostate, and pancreatic cancer. To make matters worse, a high intake of saturated fat appears to increase insulin resistance.

Sources: You can't avoid saturated fat completely because it's in many healthy foods, including olive oil, but you can limit the loaded sources, such as butter, cream, full-fat cheese, whole milk, fatty meats, and chicken skin. A few plant foods, such as palm and coconut oil, are also high in saturated fat. Fortunately, the type of saturated fatty acid in the cocoa butter in chocolate (stearic acid) does *not* raise LDL. Sometimes you luck out!

NUT NUTRITION

If you've peeked at the meal plans on page 251, you've noticed that we're generous with nuts as well as seeds. Nuts and seeds top hot cereal, are used to coat vegetables and fish, are blended into smoothies, and are eaten as snacks. They're an ideal food for people with diabetes: rich in vitamins, minerals, and phytonutrients; low in carbohydrates; moderate in protein; and high in healthy fats.

Nuts weigh in at about 150 to 200 calories per ounce. Yes, that's high, but we recommend only about 1 to 2 ounces daily. In fact, people who eat nuts are thinner than those who don't. "One reason is that nuts are very filling. Studies show that after eating nuts, people compensate for about 65 to 75 percent of their energy by eating less of other foods," says Richard D. Mattes, MPH, PhD, RD, professor of foods and nutrition at Purdue University. "Eaten in moderation, nuts pose limited risk for weight gain."

A number of other studies show that nut eaters have a lower risk of heart disease; the unsaturated fat and blood pressure–lowering compounds in nuts get much of the credit. Nuts may also help prevent type 2 diabetes, if the Harvard University Nurses' Health Study is any indication. Researchers tracked 83,818 women for sixteen years and found that those eating the most nuts—5 or more ounces per week—had a 24 percent lower risk of developing type 2 diabetes than those who ate nuts less than once a week. Women eating 5 or more ounces of peanut butter weekly had a similar reduction in the risk of developing type 2 diabetes. It is also clear that adding nuts to a meal can slow down the subsequent rise in blood sugar.

Trans fatty acids are the most unhealthy fats of all. Not only do they raise LDL, but they also lower HDL ("good" cholesterol). These fats appear to promote visceral fat, the deep belly fat that surrounds the organs, which can trigger heart disease and insulin resistance. Although trans fat exists in small quantities naturally in fatty meats and high-fat dairy foods, the major source is man-made partially hydrogenated vegetable oil, a solid fat that is used in some commercial baked goods and makes foods more shelf-stable.

Sources: Foods made with partially hydrogenated oil, including some cookies, cakes, crackers, pie crusts, and other baked goods, frozen foods, and margarine. (Fortunately, now there are brands of margarine or spreads such as Bestlife Buttery Spread, that have no partially hydrogenated oil.) Check out "Don't Get Tricked by Trans" on page 122 for how to spot products with trans fat.

WHAT'S A FAT SERVING?

Fats:

About 5 grams of fat and 45 calories per serving

Most of the fats in your diet should be unsaturated. That means you should be limiting your intake of saturated fats and completely avoiding foods containing trans fat.

HIGH IN UNSATURATED FATTY ACIDS (MONOS AND POLYS):

Almond butter: 1 tablespoon

Avocado: 2 tablespoons mashed or ⅙ Hass avocado

Margarine/spread: 1 to 2 teaspoons (check labels as calories vary, and buy brands with no partially hydrogenated oil, such as Bestlife Buttery Spread)

Margarine/spread, light: 1 tablespoon (with no partially hydrogenated oil)

Mayonnaise, regular: 1 teaspoon

Mayonnaise, light: 1 tablespoon

Nuts and seeds, any kind: 1 tablespoon

Oil (such as olive oil or canola oil): 1 teaspoon

Olives: 1 ounce, about 5 to 8 or ¼ cup chopped

Salad dressing, regular: 2 teaspoons to 1 tablespoon (check labels)

Salad dressing, reduced-fat: 1 to 2 tablespoons (check labels)

Tahini (sesame seed butter): 2 teaspoons

DON'T GET TRICKED BY TRANS

"0 grams trans fat!" boasts the label of many margarines, crackers, and other packaged foods. But is it really free of this artery-clogging fat? Turn the package around, and indeed, you'll see a "0 g" after "trans fat" on the nutrition facts panel. But that still doesn't mean the product is truly trans fat–free. Due to a legal loophole in food labeling, a product can state "0 g trans fat" and still contain nearly half a gram (up to 0.49 grams) per serving. Even 1 or 2 grams daily can harm your health, and you can see how quickly a few half grams can add up.

Fortunately, the ingredients list doesn't lie; if it contains any type of partially hydrogenated oil, the product has trans fat. Because you can't tell from the label exactly how much a product may contain, it's best to opt for a brand that contains no partially hydrogenated oil.

And remember, just because a product has no partially hydrogenated oil or trans fat doesn't mean it's healthy. Some manufacturers are simply replacing that type of oil with palm oil, which is high in saturated fat. Or they're using "hydrogenated" or "fully hydrogenated" oil, which does not contain trans fat but, depending on the oil, could be high in *saturated* fat. So compare labels of similar products and choose those that are not only free of partially hydrogenated oil but also lower in saturated fat (and sodium, while you're at it).

HIGH IN SATURATED FATTY ACIDS

Bacon: 1 slice

Butter: 1 teaspoon

Cream cheese: 1 tablespoon

Cream cheese, reduced-fat: 1½ tablespoons

Half-and-half: 2 tablespoons

Sour cream, regular: 2 tablespoons

Sour cream, reduced-fat: 3 tablespoons

Whipped cream: 1 tablespoon unwhipped; 4 tablespoons whipped

Whipped cream, pressurized container: 5 tablespoons

BAD FATS—BAD FOR THE BRAIN?

The dangers of unhealthy fats go beyond damage to your heart and waistline. Women with diabetes who ate the most saturated and trans fats in midlife entered their seventies with less brainpower than women who ate less of these fats and more polyunsaturated fat, according to Harvard Medical School's Nurses' Health Study. A series of six tests measuring thinking ability revealed that those whose diets included the most unhealthy fats experienced mental declines along the order of someone seven years older. The study also found that substituting more polyunsaturated fat for saturated fat improved women's mental prowess.

Start the Switch to Healthier Carbohydrates

In Phase One you did the hard work: you figured out your daily and per-meal carbohydrate limit and learned what a serving of a high-carbohydrate food looks like. Now it's time to focus on the quality of your carbohydrates, not just the quantity. Better-quality carbohydrates mean not only better blood sugar levels but a better chance of staving off heart disease and other chronic illnesses.

In Phase Two you'll be concentrating on just one carbohydrate group: grains/starchy vegetables. For now, eat whatever type of fruits and nonstarchy vegetables you please within your daily limit, and keep working your way down to fat-free or 1% milk and low-fat yogurt.

Your carbohydrate goals in this phase are to:

1. Make at least half of your grains whole grains. Whenever possible, choose minimally processed whole grains, such as steel-cut oats, quick-cooking or regular instead of instant oatmeal, or brown rice instead of white.

2. Eat legumes (beans, such as black beans, garbanzo beans, kidney beans, and lentils) at least twice a week.

3. Limit starches that are high in fat such as most cookies, cakes, and other baked goods; relegate them to your daily treat calories. (See chart page 114.)

4. Accumulate a group of "safe carbs," starches that produce the smallest rise in your blood sugar. This is somewhat individual, as we'll explain later on.

When you look at the carbohydrate goals above—whole grains, legumes, lower-fat starches—it's easy to see where we're going with this. These foods are more nutritious than white bread and doughnuts. But for people with diabetes, these high-quality carbohydrates have an added importance: Whole grains (for the most part) and legumes elicit a less drastic rise in blood sugar than their refined-flour counterparts, and they're associated with a lower risk of heart disease. Lower-fat starches also do their part to stave off heart disease because they help you cut back on the artery-clogging saturated and trans fats found in so many fried and baked goods.

THE GLYCEMIC INDEX

Though all carbohydrate-containing foods increase blood sugar, they don't do it at the same rate. For instance, a 1-ounce slice of white bread makes its way into your bloodstream much more quickly than the same amount of pasta. Obviously, when you have diabetes, you want the slowest and smallest possible rise in blood sugar after a meal. Choosing the right carbohydrates can help you achieve this.

Why do some carbs spike blood sugar quickly while others take their time? The type of grain and the way a food is processed makes a big difference when that food hits your gut. It's all about structure—for instance, the difference between soft white bread (elicits a quick rise in blood sugar) and chewy pasta (slow rise). Enzymes in your upper intestines attack sugars and starches and break them into smaller sugar units. But the fiber, fat, and other elements of food act as obstacles and barriers to the enzymes, delaying digestion and, in turn, the time it takes to turn food into blood sugar.

A few thousand high-carbohydrate foods have been ranked on a scale from 1 to 100 according to how quickly they raise blood sugar; this ranking is called the glycemic index. This was done by giving people a fixed amount—usually 50 grams—of a carbohydrate-containing food, such as carrots or an English muffin, and watching how high their blood sugar rose over the course of two hours. That increase was compared to the effects of eating plain glucose, which has a GI of 100. The glycemic index was developed to help people with diabetes choose foods that would cause a slower and smaller rise in blood sugar. The idea is that if you choose low-GI foods (see "A Sampling of the Glycemic Index," page 134, for what constitutes low-, medium-, and high-GI food), then your blood sugar will be better controlled.

But what works in the lab doesn't necessarily work at your dinner table. In the lab, people walk in with an empty stomach after fasting overnight and eat *just* the English muffin or *just* carrots and nothing else. But when you combine those foods with others, as you'd do in a meal, you change their glycemic index (see "Lower the GI in Your Kitchen," page 126).

Another problem: not everyone has the same blood sugar reaction to foods, which means a low-GI food might actually be a medium-GI food for you when you eat it. It's also not a foolproof guide to picking healthful foods: because fat suppresses the rise in blood sugar, high-fat foods have a lower GI than low-fat versions. So a slice of frosted cake, which is absolutely loaded with unhealthy fat, might have a lower glycemic index than a slice of whole wheat bread.

Even with these caveats, eating a low-GI diet in which most of your carbohydrates have a low or medium GI is proving to be good for your blood sugar and other aspects of your health. After reviewing the literature, University of Sydney researchers concluded that there is a small but potentially important blood sugar–lowering benefit to a low-GI diet for people with diabetes. On average, A1c, a measure of average blood sugar level, was reduced by 0.5 percent. "That doesn't sound like much, but this level of reduction might well translate into meaningful reductions in risk for several complications of diabetes, including vascular disease and heart attacks," notes Bernard Venn, PhD, Lecturer and Researcher, Department of Nutrition, University of Otaga, New Zealand. The results of the review also indicated that low-GI diets reduce blood sugar levels and hyperglycemic (high-blood-sugar) episodes without increasing the risk of hypoglycemia (low blood sugar).

Another blood-sugar bonus is the second-meal effect. Eating a low-GI breakfast, for example, has a carryover effect, so that the next meal, even if eaten four hours later, will have a lower impact on blood sugar than it normally would.

The benefits don't end there. Following a low-GI diet may also help you drop some pounds because it's more satisfying for the calories consumed, and it has been linked to lower cholesterol levels, a lower risk of heart disease, and improved endurance during exercise.

If you can get your family to eat a low-GI diet along with you, all the better. The long-running Nurses' Health Study found that women eating a low-GI diet cut the risk of developing type 2 diabetes by nearly 60 percent, and a recent update on that study found that eating this way can even help protect those carrying a gene that puts them at high risk for the disease.

Our take on the glycemic index: eating strictly by the GI numbers is too fraught with limitations to be the major tool for picking the best carbs, but it can still be helpful. (You can take a look at the "Carbohydrate Counts" table on page 343 to pick out the low- and medium-GI foods you like; we listed only the healthful ones.) But eating by the principles of the glycemic index and choosing the types of foods that are kinder to your blood sugar is the driving force behind our carbohydrate goals for you. That's what this next section is about.

LOWER THE GI IN YOUR KITCHEN

You can lower the GI of some foods by cooking, cooling, and reheating as explained on page 132. You can also:

- **Add some fat.** Fat slows stomach emptying, delaying the process of converting food to blood sugar. This isn't a license to slather on the butter, however! Instead, use moderate portions of healthful fats. Adding peanut butter, nuts, avocados, or olive oil is a smart way to help tame the carbohydrates in a meal.

- **Toss it with lemon juice or vinegar.** These acidic condiments have been shown to reduce the GI of a mixed meal. For example, the vinaigrette from the salad will help blunt the rise in blood sugar from the side of rice on your plate. Marinating a potato salad in a vinegar or lemon juice dressing will do the same (plus, if you cool the salad overnight, you drive down the glycemic index even further as explained under "Resistant Starch" on page 132).

CARBS THAT PUT UP A FIGHT

There are a few broad classes of carbs that have a low GI. Instead of taking a glycemic index chart to the supermarket, you can simply pick foods that fall under one of the categories below. For instance, knowing that stone-ground whole wheat has lower glycemic index, you can pick this type of bread instead of bread made with regular whole wheat flour.

All the foods listed below are highly nutritious and give your digestive enzymes a run for their money. Something about their structure delays and blunts the rise in blood sugar, giving them a low glycemic index. Vegetables and many fruits also have a low GI; we'll discuss them in Phase Three.

Intact Whole Grains

What They Are: Most grains have three parts: bran, endosperm, and germ. (Some, such as barley and oats, are built slightly differently.) The bran, the outer layer, makes up most of the grain. The middle layer is the endosperm, which is starch, and in the center sits the germ, which is rich in protein, fat, vitamins, and minerals. Refining grains means getting rid of all (or most) of the bran and germ—in other words, removing the most nutritious parts, leaving just the starch.

Refining does more than remove nutrients; it also makes foods more apt to send blood sugar levels soaring. That's because the fiber, fat, and other substances in intact grains put up barriers to digestion, making your body work harder and longer at converting food to blood sugar. The germ even contains a compound that blocks the action of amylase, the enzyme in your gut that breaks down starch. Without these roadblocks, refined flour has an easy pass into your system.

Health Bonuses: Diets high in whole grains may cut your heart disease risk by 20 to 40 percent compared to diets that contain very little whole grain. Whole grains provide a wealth of phytonutrients and are a rich source of B vitamins and magnesium, which are critical for a healthy heart and muscles as well as diabetes control.

Buying Tips: Choose the more intact form or coarser cut of the grain. For wheat, that means bulgur wheat (found in health food stores and Middle

Eastern markets) and wheat berries. Always buy 100% whole wheat, whole rye, or other whole grain breads, cold and hot cereals, crackers, crisp-breads, English muffins, bagels, and wraps, and whenever possible choose stone ground, a process that keeps the amylase-blocking substance intact. When choosing oatmeal, get steel-cut, which is the thickest cut, or thick-cut oats. (Steel-cut takes 30 minutes to cook, but some companies sell parboiled versions that are just as good and take only about 5 minutes.) Buy brown rice instead of white and whole corn grits instead of regular, and try some of the other whole grains listed in "Sleuthing Out Whole Grains" on page 129.

Fiber

What It Is: Fiber is one of the components of whole grains that delays the breakdown of starch. Unlike starch and sugar, dietary fiber cannot be broken down by our bodies; we simply don't possess the enzymes. Fiber is either soluble (dissolves in water) or insoluble (does not). Foods high in either type tend to have have a low glycemic index.

Soluble fiber, the type found in oats, barley, psyllium, beans, and cer-tain fruits and vegetables, lowers the GI of a food in a few different ways. When it mixes with liquid and with your own digestive juices, it forms a gel which slows the rate at which your stomach empties. Once in the small intestine, that gel forms a protective layer around starch particles, mak-ing it difficult for enzymes to penetrate. In studies in which people with diabetes took in 10 to 20 milligrams of soluble fiber daily for weeks, their average blood sugar was lowered slightly. After the soluble fiber makes its way to the large intestine, it becomes a meal for friendly bacteria, which convert dietary fiber into short-chain fatty acids that appear to help your blood sugar in two ways. Their presence sends a signal to the liver to stop making glucose and they also appear to increase insulin sensitivity.

Insoluble fiber, the type found in wheat and corn, doesn't form a gel in the upper intestines, but there's some evidence that it might physically stand in the path of starch-pulverizing enzymes. In a study at the German Institute of Human Nutrition in Potsdam-Rehbrücke, Germany, research-ers noted that people who had loaded up on insoluble fiber the previous day had 30 percent lower blood sugar than those who had less insoluble fiber, and other research found that people who consume the most fiber

SLEUTHING OUT WHOLE GRAINS

To hit the "at least half your grains whole" goal, you must determine whether a product actually contains whole grain. Beware: you can't always tell from its packaging. "Made with whole grain" may turn out to mean that the pizza dough, bread, or other food has 30% or less whole grain and the rest is refined flour. Though that's better than no whole grain at all, it may not be what you bargained for. Another term that misleads people: multigrain. The product may have several grains, but often, they're refined.

So unless the front of the package reads "100% whole grain," you'll have to turn to the ingredients list to find out what's really in it. Ingredients are listed by weight from most to least. If the only grains you see are any of the ones listed below, it is a whole grain product. If they're first on the ingredient list and followed by just one other refined grain, the product probably is at least 50% whole grain. If the whole grain comes after the refined grain, it's anyone's guess as to how much whole grain it contains.

If any of these are on the ingredients list, the product contains whole grain:

Amaranth
Barley
Buckwheat
Brown rice
Corn (should say "whole," as in whole cornmeal; popcorn is always whole)
Millet
Oats, including oatmeal
Quinoa
Rye (should say "whole rye")
Sorghum (also called milo)
Teff
Triticale
Wheat (should say "whole wheat"; this includes varieties such as spelt, emmer, farro, einkorn, kamut, and durum; bulgur, cracked wheat, and wheat berries are always whole)
Wild rice

The following terms are used for refined grain:

Flour
Unbleached flour
Enriched flour
Degermed corn flour

> The word "corn flour," "rye," or "wheat" without the word "whole"
> in front of it usually means refined flour. And just because something's
> organic, that doesn't mean it's whole grain!
>
> Some products sport the Whole Grain Stamp, which specifies grams of
> whole grain. In order to receive the stamp, a product must have at least
> 8 grams of whole grain per serving. Clearer is the 100% Whole Grain Stamp,
> which, as it implies, means that all the grain in the product is whole.

from whole grain foods slash their risk of developing type 2 diabetes by
about a third. What helps prevent type 2 can also help manage your blood
sugar once you have either type 1, type 2, or pre-diabetes.

Health Bonuses: Diets high in fiber help keep you slimmer because they
not only make you feel fuller longer but also prevent a small portion of
the calories you eat from being absorbed. Also, soluble fiber reduces LDL
("bad" cholesterol), and both types of fiber help ward off heart disease.
According to a review of the research by scientists at the University of
Minnesota and Harvard University, for every 10 grams of dietary fiber
(both types) eaten per day, the risk of heart disease goes down by 10 to 30
percent. Also, there's compelling evidence that fiber helps prevent colon
cancer and possibly cancer of the esophagus, according to a review by the
American Institute for Cancer Research. Fiber gives the immune system
a boost by feeding the friendly bacteria in your gut (the type in probiotic
supplements), which enhance immunity.

Buying Tips: Add oat and coarsely milled wheat bran (available in natural
food stores and most supermarkets) to cold cereal, muffins, cookies, pizza
dough, and other baked goods. You'll have to add more liquid to the
recipe; otherwise it'll be dry. Check cereal box labels for those containing
at least 4 grams of fiber per 100 calories.

Pasta

What It Is: Most pasta is made from semolina, a coarse cut of wheat.
When semolina is turned into pasta, the granules are embedded in glu-
ten (wheat's protein) forming a web that's tough for your starch-cleaving
enzymes to penetrate. Cook pasta al dente (a little chewy) to keep the GI

low. That may require that you cook it for less time than what's stated on the package, so keep testing to make sure you don't overcook it. However, as with any carbohydrate, even one with a low GI, if you eat too much of it, you will eventually see a big increase in your blood sugar level, so stick with the recommended ½- to 1-cup portions.

Health Bonus: Pair your pasta with tomato sauce or fresh tomatoes and reap the benefits of lycopene, a powerful antioxidant that gives tomatoes their red color. Keep your portion of sauce between ¼ cup (7.5 grams of carbohydrate) and ⅓ cup (about 10 grams of carbohydrate). Add some chicken or shrimp and a little olive oil to help lower the GI of the meal.

Buying Tips: Make sure that "semolina" is in the ingredient list. Although both whole grain and regular pasta have a low glycemic index, whole grain is more nutritious. If you don't like the texture of whole grain, try pasta that's made with extra fiber or is partially whole grain, such as these two Best Life–approved foods: Barilla Whole Grain (51 percent whole grain) and Barilla PLUS (enriched with legume flour, egg whites, fiber, flaxseed, and whole grains).

Legumes
What They Are: These are beans, such as black beans and lentils, which come dried or canned. We've also included edamame (green soybeans) in this group because they share some of the nutrition features of dried beans. Legumes have a very low GI, probably because of their fiber and because they contain resistant starch (see page 132). As with grains, the more intact the bean, the lower the GI. So a side dish of whole, cooked black beans would have a lower GI than a puréed black bean dip, which would have a much lower GI than bean flour.

Health Bonus: Legumes are rich in B vitamins and in minerals associated with improved diabetes management: calcium, magnesium, and zinc. They've been shown to lower LDL cholesterol; this might be their soluble fiber at work (beans have a mix of soluble and insoluble fiber).

Buying Tips: All legumes—black, kidney, pinto, white, cannelloni, garbanzo, adzuki, lentils, soy, pink—are supernutritious, so pick your favorites! Save some money by cooking them from scratch (lentils have the shortest cooking time). If you buy them canned, look for those with no salt added (EdenFoods has a wide variety) or with no more than 120 mg sodium per half cup, such as Goya low-sodium. You'll find edamame in the frozen food section, both with the shell (which you don't eat) or shelled. Toss them into salads and stir-fries or serve marinated as a side dish.

Resistant Starch

What It Is: These are starch granules that escape the clutches of enzymes. Some go untouched because they're part of an intact or very coarsely cut whole grain kernel, protected by the armor of fiber. Cooking and cooling grains and potatoes also creates resistant starch by forming a gel barrier to enzymes. Just-ripe (as opposed to riper, sweeter) bananas contain resistant starch, so if you like your bananas not too ripe, you'll get a little resistant-starch bonus. And legumes are a good source, as mentioned earlier.

Health Bonus: Foods high in resistant starch have a weight-loss edge because they keep you feeling fuller longer for the calories. In a University of Minnesota study comparing the effects of eating morning muffins made from various types of fiber, or those low in fiber or high in resistant starch; the latter type suppressed appetite for an hour longer. Resistant starch is also a fuel for the beneficial bacteria in your gut.

Buying Tips: Whole grains and legumes are good sources of resistant starch. Buy bananas that still have a little green tinge, and eat them before they get mottled and soft (the firmer and less ripe, the more resistant starch). Also, try cooking with Hi-maize, a commercially available corn fiber that is rich in resistant starch. You can substitute about 10 to 25 percent of the flour in recipes with Hi-maize. You can purchase it from King Arthur Flour (www.kingarthurflour.com).

Sourdough Bread

What It Is: This type of bread is made from sourdough starter, a batter of flour, yeast, and good-for-you bacteria. These organisms produce acid, giving sourdough bread its unique taste and a higher acid level than regular bread; the acid lowers the GI.

Health Bonus: Sourdough bread tends to have higher levels of resistant starch than regular bread, driving down the GI even further.

Buying Tip: Look for whole grain sourdough bread to get the full nutrition benefits of whole grain in addition to the GI-lowering effects of sourdough.

OPT FOR LOW-FAT STARCHES

By now you've realized that this plan isn't low-fat, it's just low in saturated fat. That doesn't mean we're not fans of some low-fat foods, especially when it comes to starches. It's best to keep your starches plain, and then add your own healthy fats rather than take your chances with what's served in restaurants and on supermarket shelves.

Make it simple:

- Avoid all French fries, onion rings, and other fried vegetables.

- Eat your vegetables steamed, baked, grilled, or sautéed in a little olive oil.

- Top baked potatoes with a mix of one part reduced-fat sour cream to two parts plain low-fat yogurt. Or use 0% fat Greek yogurt (such as Fage or Stoneyfield Farm's Oikos), which is thicker than regular yogurt and surprisingly creamy-tasting.

- Use the treat calories established in Phase One for cookies, cake, Danishes, and other sweet baked goods. Check the serving size on labels carefully; you're not going to get much of these foods for the number of calories and carbohydrate grams allotted.

- Skip croissants, brioches, and other buttery pastries entirely; it's too hard to have just a little piece.

- Add canola oil instead of melted butter to your pancake batter. Top with a little spread with no partially hydrogenated oil, such as Bestlife Buttery Spread.

- Skip creamy sauces, such as Alfredo and cheese sauces, on pasta unless you find a low-fat version or make it yourself with 1% milk and very-low-fat cheese.

A SAMPLING OF THE GLYCEMIC INDEX

By eating the whole grains, legumes, and the other foods recommended in this section, you will wind up eating mainly low-glycemic-index carbs but it's worth taking a look at a GI chart to find your favorite low-GI foods.

Here's a sampling of GI numbers for grains and starchy vegetables. You'll find a more complete listing, including nonstarchy vegetables, fruit, and dairy products, in the Carbohydrate Counts table on page 343. For a complete searchable database, go to www.glycemicindex.com.

FOOD	GLYCEMIC INDEX
LOW-GI FOODS (55 OR LESS):	
All-Bran cereal	49
Barley	25
Black beans, boiled	30 (most beans range from 30 to 40)
Bulgur wheat	48
Oatmeal (steel-cut)	52
Pasta, regular	44
Pasta, whole wheat	42
Sourdough bread	54
MEDIUM-GI FOODS (56–69)	
Bread, whole wheat	About 52 to 70; a wide range, depending on the brand
Couscous, regular	65
Cream of Wheat	67
Polenta	68
Raisin Bran cereal	61
Rye crispbread	63
HIGH-GI FOODS (70 AND UP)	
Bread, white	Generally over 70, but a wide range
Corn flakes	86
English muffin, white	77
Oatmeal, instant	82
Puffed rice cereal	82

START A "SAFE CARB" COLLECTION

If you follow the Phase Two carbohydrate goals and most of your starches are whole grains with a rougher cut, legumes, and high-fiber cereals, you should start noticing some good after-meal numbers on your blood sugar monitor. Pretty soon you're also going to see patterns. "When I eat a baked potato, my sugar is always high, but when I eat potato salad that has been marinating in vinaigrette for two days, my blood sugar is fine." To make sure it's really a pattern and not a fluke, use your Best Life Diabetes Management Log to record meals (instructions on the log on page 335). If a certain type of carbohydrate-rich food consistently gives you nice blood sugar numbers, it's a keeper. Write it down along with other blood-sugar-friendly foods, and go back to this list when you're working out your menus for the week.

Avoid Fried Foods

It's no mystery why we're asking you to avoid fried foods—they have crazy amounts of calories and are loaded with unhealthy fats that only further add to your already high risk for heart disease. But eliminating *any* food is tricky, especially if it's one that you really like or you use to cope with emotional ups and downs. You don't want to start craving it and then end up feeling deprived—that's a death knell to any weight-loss plan! But how about trying to give them up for just a week? Then, if all goes well, another week. Often, the longer you're away from these foods, the less you'll find you "need" them. And remember, in Phase Three, you can bring them back in measured amounts.

Need a little inspiration? Just look at the scale; the numbers should be heading in a downward direction if you've been a frequent fried food eater and you stop the habit. Here's a comparison of some foods that have been fried and prepared in a leaner manner.

FOOD	CALORIES	FAT (G)	SATURATED FAT (G)	TRANS FAT (G)
POTATOES				
French fries, 4 ounces ("medium"* serving)	380	19	2.5	0–3
Red potatoes, boiled, 4 ounces, tossed with 1½ teaspoons olive oil and lemon juice or vinegar (and spices) to taste	160	7	1	0
Baked potato, 4 ounces (a small baked potato)	110	0	0	0
CHICKEN				
Chicken thigh, with skin, fried	300	24	8	1–3
Chicken thigh, with skin, broiled or baked	159	9	3	0
Chicken thigh, skin removed, broiled or baked	108	6	1.6	0
ONIONS				
Onion rings, 5 ounces ("medium*" serving)	514	27	5	0–2
Onions, sweet, raw, 5 ounces	45	0	0	0

* Large by our standards but considered medium at the fast food chains.

Use the Hunger Scale

Some of the recommendations we've made to help you manage your diabetes have the added benefit of helping manage your hunger, too. For instance, eating regular meals and snacks not only keeps your blood sugar levels stable, it also keeps your hunger in check. Avoiding hunger highs and lows is an important way to prevent overeating. Making the switch to healthier, low-GI carbs has benefits for managing your diabetes, but it also has some weight-loss perks, too: the slow rise in blood sugar that's associated with these foods also helps suppress hunger.

We've already given you a head start on hunger management, but there's still one more essential tool you'll need: the Hunger Scale. Using this subjective 10-point scale, you'll be assigning a point value to your hunger level. Each number represents a different level of hunger or fullness; 1 would be ravenously hungry, and 10 would be nauseatingly stuffed. We've left a column in the Best Life Diabetes Management Log to record hunger, so in addition to finding your meal and blood sugar level patterns, you can also look for patterns of hunger and eating or overeating.

The scale serves two purposes: to signal when it's time to eat and then when it's time to stop. Before you pick up your fork, take a moment to tap into your body's natural cues: how hungry you are, how your stomach feels, if you're having trouble concentrating because you're ready for a bite. This will help you decide if it's really time to eat or not. If you're at 3 or 4, you're just starting to get hungry, or maybe you're feeling a bit uncomfortable. Go ahead and have a snack or meal. Be sure to avoid dropping below 3 or 4; doing so can make it more likely that you'll overeat when you finally do sit down to a meal or snack.

As you're eating, pause during your meal to determine whether you should continue to eat. Stop when you hit 5 on the Hunger Scale; at this point you could eat a little more, but you're not really still hungry. If you put your fork down once you hit this level, you're most likely taking in fewer calories than your body is burning. If you're looking to lose weight, you can bump up the cutoff to a 6, the point at which you feel perfectly satisfied. At this level, you're taking in as much energy as you're expending. Remember: you don't ever want to feel even a tiny bit uncomfortable when eating. You're aiming for satisfied, not uncomfortable.

THE HUNGER SCALE

10 Stuffed: You are so full, you feel nauseated.

9 Very uncomfortably full: You need to loosen your clothes.

8 Uncomfortably full: You feel bloated.

7 Full: You feel a little bit uncomfortable.

6 Perfectly comfortable: You feel satisfied.

5 Comfortable: You're more or less satisfied but could eat a little more.

4 Slightly uncomfortable: You're just beginning to feel signs of hunger.

3 Uncomfortable: Your stomach is rumbling.

2 Very uncomfortable: You feel irritable and are unable to concentrate.

1 Weak and light-headed: Your stomach acid is churning.

The Hunger Scale is easy to use, but it may require a little bit of practice, especially at first. You'll get to the point where it becomes automatic; eating only when you're hungry and stopping when you're comfortable will be almost second nature. Of course, there may be times when the desire to eat will be strong even though your hunger level doesn't indicate it's time to eat. Whenever this happens, try to distract yourself with something else: take a walk, call a friend, write in your journal. You'll probably find that once you get started, you'll forget all about eating.

The Decision to Bring Back Alcohol

One of the factors that can interfere with your assessment of hunger is alcohol. After a drink or two, you might not accurately feel—or might not care about—your level of hunger or fullness. Not to mention, alcohol can also have a major effect on your blood sugar level. So if you decide to bring back alcohol in this phase, do it carefully. Use your treat calories for alcohol, and limit yourself to just a few drinks a week: a drink is 12 ounces of beer, 5 ounces of wine, or 1½ ounces of whiskey, gin, Scotch, or other hard liquor. When you do drink, have no more than one drink per day if you're a woman and no more than two if you're a man.

A few things to keep in mind when you drink:

- Alcohol can send your blood sugar level up or down. Higher-carbohydrate drinks (sweet wine, beer, and mixed drinks made with cola, tonic water, or other sugary mixes) will most likely raise your blood sugar level. But drinks with fewer carbohydrates—light beer, dry wine, and straight gin, whiskey, or other hard liquor—tend to lower your blood sugar level, especially if you drink them on an empty stomach. Remember to eat a balanced meal or snack before you fill your glass, especially with these lower-carb beverages.

- If you're going to be active, like playing golf or dancing at a wedding, while drinking, you'll need to keep an eye on your blood sugar level. Remember that both alcohol and exercise can lower your blood sugar level, so the two together can send the level plunging dangerously.

- Alcohol in combination with certain medicines may trigger a serious low-blood-sugar reaction. We'll talk about this more in the chapter on medications, starting on page 189.

There are times you should probably skip alcohol altogether. Drinking often worsens high blood pressure, so if your blood pressure is not well controlled, you should probably not drink until it has been brought into line. People with diabetes often have abnormal blood lipid levels—high triglycerides and a low HDL or "good" cholesterol level. Even light drinking (about two glasses of wine per week) can elevate the triglycerides even further. Alcohol may also worsen the symptoms of peripheral neuropathy. There are so many specific concerns about alcohol use when you have diabetes or any other medical condition that it's always a good idea to check with your doctor to make sure that you can enjoy alcohol safely.

Nutritional Supplements

Even with the ultranutritious eating plan in this book, you might benefit from taking one or more nutritional supplements. But you certainly don't need a cupboard full of vitamin and mineral pills; we'll help you figure out which supplements are right for you. For research and advice updates on supplements check www.thebestlife.com.

MULTIVITAMINS

Taking a multivitamin/mineral tablet might help you and it probably won't hurt you. While that may not sound like a ringing endorsement, we're still recommending a daily multi. It's true that there's not much evidence that taking a multivitamin does much for anyone, including people with diabetes. Likewise, the evidence isn't all that strong for taking single vitamin tablets, such as vitamin C, or single minerals, such as selenium.

And, in some cases, too much supplementation may actually harm your health (see "When More Is Not Better," page 142). But if there's a chance that a multivitamin can help you, why not take advantage of it?

We're going to be fairly specific about the doses of vitamins and minerals that we think you should take. The goal is to be covered for 100 percent of the recommended levels of vitamins and minerals, especially those linked to better blood sugar control. This is a "multivitamin-as-insurance-policy"; the real nutrition comes from the nutrients you'll get if you eat according to our guidelines. However, if you're on the 1,500- or 1,700-calorie-per-day plan to lose weight, you may not hit 100 percent for every nutrient. Even on the most healthful diet, it's tough to consume all the necessary vitamins and minerals when your calorie consumption is low.

HOW TO PICK A MULTIVITAMIN

Despite what you may see on store shelves, there is no official "diabetes multivitamin." At this point, the assumption is that what's good for the general population is also good for you. In the chart on page 142, we base our numbers on the Institute of Medicine's* recommendations. A perfectly good multivitamin may have a little more or a little less than the institute's recommendations of certain nutrients—that's okay. For instance, the institute recommends 1,000 milligrams of calcium for men and women, but most multivitamins include just 100 to 500 milligrams because any more than that would make the tablet too large to swallow comfortably. Some brands provide higher-than-recommended levels of other nutrients, which is usually fine as long as the nutrient is safe at higher levels.

Before buying a multivitamin, check the supplement facts panel for the serving size. You should have to take only one pill to get the nutrients listed (page 142); put back those requiring two or more tablets. They're often loaded with unnecessary and unproven ingredients. Unlike drugs, supplements are not well regulated, so there's no guarantee that you're

---

* The nonprofit Institute of Medicine, a major U.S. research and advisory organization, sets guidelines for vitamins and minerals. They set these levels based on age and gender; for instance, levels of vitamin C are lower for children than adults, and men need more C than women. The institute also sets the "upper tolerable limit," the most a person can safely consume.

getting a safe and effective product. Generally, the big companies are a good bet. One measure of comfort is if the multivitamin is marked "USP Verified" or has the "USP" symbol. This means an independent organization called the U.S. Pharmacopeia has inspected the plant where the supplements are made and tested the products for purity, potency, and the ability to break down in the digestive tract (otherwise they won't be absorbed into your body). However, some companies with good products opt out of the USP testing.

How can you be sure you're choosing a good multi? Check the supplement facts panel on the label against the guidelines on the following page. At the time of printing, these multis met our guidelines, but check labels, as product formulations change.

Men of all ages and post-menopausal women. Centrum Ultra Men's; Equate (Wal-Mart) Men's Health Formula Daily with lycopene*; the following Nature Made products: Multi for Her 50+,* Multi for Him 50+,* Multi for Him,* Multi Max; One A Day Men's Health Formula; Walgreens One Daily for Men with Lycopene.*

Pre-menopausal women. CVS Daily Multiple Plus Minerals; Nature Made Multi Complete; One A Day Maximum; Puritan's Pride ABC Plus with Lutein and Lycopene; Puritan's Pride Multi-Day Plus Minerals; Sundown Naturals Advanced Formula SunVite; Sundown Naturals Daily Multi; Walgreens Advanced Formula A Thru Z.

Some notes on the terms used on the following chart: "No more than" means that any more might not be safe. If we say "At least" and don't give an upper limit, that means that no upper limit has been set by the Institute of Medicine. If there's no age or gender specification, then the amount given is appropriate for all adults.

---

* Contains no iron. As mentioned on pages 113 and 144, too much iron is bad for your health, but everyone needs some iron. Men and post-menopausal women need 8 mg daily, which most people can get through food. If you have a tendency to be low in iron, or if your doctor suggests that you include iron in your supplement, then choose a supplement with 8 to10 milligrams.

YOUR MULTIVITAMIN SHOULD HAVE . . .

Vitamin A	No more than 3,500 IU
Beta-carotene	No more than 5,000 IU
Vitamin C	60–500 mg
Vitamin D	400–1,000 IU
Vitamin E	30–100 IU
Vitamin K	At least 20 mcg
Thiamin (B1)	At least 1.2 mg
Riboflavin (B2)	At least 1.3 mg
Niacin (B3)	16–35 mg
Vitamin B6	1.7–100 mg
Folic acid	No more than 400 mcg; a premenopausal woman should consume no less than 400 mcg.
Vitamin B12	At least 2.4 mcg. If you're age 51 or older, you might have trouble absorbing B12 so talk to your doctor about whether you need extra. And if you have neuropathy, see information on page 143.
Biotin	At least 30 mcg
Pantothenic acid	At least 5 mg
Calcium (elemental)	At least 100 mg
Iron	No more than 10 mg. If you're a premenopausal woman, have 18 mg.
Magnesium	100–350 mg. If you're a man, you can have up to 420 mg, but most multivitamins don't go that high.
Zinc	8–15 mg
Selenium	20–110 mcg
Copper	0.9–2 mg
Manganese	2–4 mg
Chromium	35 mcg or more; women need less. No upper limit has been established, but up to 120 mcg is considered safe.

WHEN MORE IS NOT BETTER

Vitamins and minerals are essential to health, but in excess, some of them can do a lot of damage. If you stick with the levels we recommend above, you'll be fine, but add other supplements and it might be pos-

VITAMIN B12 AND NEUROPATHY

Tingling, numbness, and pain in the feet often signal peripheral neuropathy, one of the common complications of diabetes and, to a lesser extent, pre-diabetes. But these conditions aren't the only causes of peripheral neuropathy. The same symptoms can be caused by a vitamin B12 deficiency. Severe vitamin B12 deficiency is called pernicious anemia because it can cause a serious fall in the red blood cell count as well as nerve damage. Pernicious anemia results from an autoimmune process that prevents the body from absorbing the vitamin. Having type 1 diabetes, usually an autoimmune problem itself, increases your risk of developing pernicious anemia.

Another reason for B12 deficiency is an age-related decline in absorption. It strikes about 10 to 30 percent of people over age 50 whether they have diabetes or not. This can also cause neuropathy or make the neuropathy of diabetes worse.

Whatever the cause, vitamin B12 deficiency can be treated with vitamin B12 injections or tablets that dissolve under the tongue, where the vitamin bypasses the intestine and is absorbed directly into the bloodstream. If you have neuropathy, your doctor may wish to check your blood levels of vitamin B12 and methylmalonic acid, a marker of vitamin B12 deficiency. Neuropathy is often difficult to treat, so you don't want to miss a problem that could be making it worse.

sible to overdo a few nutrients. Vitamin C, thiamin, riboflavin, pantothenic acid, and biotin are safe at levels many times over the amounts we've listed, but other vitamins, and all the minerals, can be harmful at high levels. So check the labels on the following:

- **Other supplements.** Take a look to see what's in that energy supplement as well as what else might be in the calcium tablet or any other supplements you're taking. Unless prescribed by your doctor, you shouldn't need more than a multivitamin and possibly a vitamin D, calcium, and omega-3 supplement. (Omega-3s are usually not fortified with any other nutrients, but you might as well check.) Do the math, and make sure you don't exceed our recommendations.

- **Fortified foods.** Meal replacements can be fabulous weight-loss tools, but they typically are fortified with a quarter or a third or more of the daily level of many vitamins and minerals. Many cereals are also heavily fortified. Again, do the math and make sure you're not overdoing it. A good rule to follow: if you have one or more fortified foods, skip your multivitamin that day.

■ **Folic acid.** Folic acid is the synthetic form of folate, a B vitamin that's found naturally in foods such as oranges and spinach and is essential for making DNA. This B vitamin is so crucial in preventing a type of birth defect called neural tube defects that in 1998 the U.S. and Canadian governments began adding it to flour, rice, and other grains. It worked—neural tube defects dropped by 20 to 50 percent. The food form has also been linked to protection against cancer, but now it appears that folic acid in supplements may actually promote colon cancer and possibly prostate cancer if taken in excess.

This research is still preliminary, so no major health organization has issued any guidelines on excess folic acid supplementation. As of press time most multis contain 400 mcg, so to be safe, you may want to take a multivitamin every other day if you're a postmenopausal woman or a man of any age. Also, be sure to examine any fortified food carefully to make sure you're not getting too much folic acid from those sources on the day you take your vitamin. As for food sources of folate, keep eating them; they're not linked to any risk.

If you are a premenopausal woman who's even considering becoming pregnant, it's crucial that you get 400 mcg of folic acid every single day via your multi. It may be even more important to get enough of this vitamin before and during conception than afterward.

■ **Iron.** You need iron for proper red blood cell function and to avoid developing anemia, but too much can be risky for the heart, and possibly the brain, as you age. The only adults who need high levels are premenopausal women because they lose iron during menses. After menopause the iron requirement goes from 18 mg to 8 mg; this lower level is also recommended for men age 19 and older. Find a multi that meets your iron requirement, or you can choose an iron-free multi if your doc okays it. Examine any fortified foods; on the days you have foods fortified with 50 percent or more of the daily value for iron (the daily value is 18 mg), skip your multivitamin.

CALCIUM

You need a lot of calcium: 1,000 mg per day for women and men up to age 50 and 1,200 mg after that. Calcium helps preserve and build bone and regulates heart rate, muscle function, and blood pressure. It's also linked to prevention of several types of cancer and type 2 diabetes. You can get it all through your diet, but you have to work at it. Take a look at the guidelines below to determine whether you're getting enough calcium through diet and a multivitamin, or whether you need to supplement. There are a variety of calcium supplements; both calcium carbonate (such as Tums) and calcium citrate (such as Citracal) are well absorbed when taken with a meal. These and other brands have versions that include vitamin D, good choices if you want more than the 400 IU in most multis. But make sure to tally up *all* your daily sources of vitamin D and don't exceed the recommendations on page 142 to avoid vitamin D toxicity.

If you're following the 1,500- or 1,700-calorie meal plans . . .
and are age 50 or younger, you're getting enough calcium if you do all of the following:

- Take in the recommended 2 milk/yogurt servings (which supply 600–700 mg of calcium)

- Eat a varied and nutritious diet like the one we recommend (providing about 300 mg of calcium, not counting dairy servings)

- Take a multivitamin that provides at least 100 mg of calcium

If you are age 51 or older and doing all the above, you'll need to add a 300- to 500-mg calcium supplement.*

If you're following the 2,000- or 2,250-calorie meal plans . . .
and are age 50 or younger, you'll get enough calcium if you:

---

* 300 or 500 mg of calcium are the lowest levels found in most supplements. Even if you need just 200 mg to complete your daily needs, it's okay to get a little more with a 300 mg or 500 mg tablet.

- Take in the recommended 3 milk/yogurt servings daily (which provide 900 mg of calcium or more)

- Get at least 100 mg of calcium from your diet and/or multi

If you are age 51 or older, your diet is varied and nutritious (contributing at least 300 mg of calcium), and your multi provides at least 100 mg of calcium, you probably don't need to supplement, but a 300 mg tablet would guarantee coverage. If your diet isn't reliably nutritious, then take the 300 mg supplement.

No matter what calorie level you're on, if you're not getting the recommended number of milk/yogurt servings, supplement with 300 mg for every serving you skip.

VITAMIN D

Vitamin D was always thought of as the vitamin needed for healthy bones, as it's critical to calcium absorption. But now studies are showing that vitamin D also lowers the risk of cancer and diabetes, and this protection starts early in life. A review of the research by scientists at Booth Hall Children's Hospital, in Manchester, UK, found that infants who were supplemented with vitamin D had a 29 percent lower risk for developing type 1 diabetes than those who weren't. And a large-scale U.S. government study found that adolescents with the lowest levels of vitamin D in their bodies were twice as likely to have high blood pressure; more than twice as likely to have high blood sugar; and four times as likely to have metabolic syndrome, a cluster of problems that includes insulin resistance. Another study, this one from Tufts University, concluded that people consuming higher levels of vitamin D and calcium had a reduced risk of developing type 2 diabetes compared to people consuming low amounts.

You get vitamin D from three main sources: the sun (when its rays hit your skin, your body makes vitamin D), supplements, and foods such as milk that are enriched with vitamin D. If you eat fatty fish such as salmon, mackerel, tuna, and sardines, you're also getting about 100 to 300 IU per 3½-ounce serving. (Fresh wild salmon contains more: 300–1,000 IU.) In winter months, when people get little sunlight and the sun is too weak to have much vitamin D–creating power, about half of Americans are deficient.

How much do you need? Currently, the Institute of Medicine recommends 200 IU for people age 50 and younger, 400 IU for those 51 to 70, and 600 IU from age 71 on up. But those numbers are very likely going to change soon, as most vitamin D experts think we should be taking about 1,000 IU daily—maybe more. Don't take more than 2,000 IU daily from food and supplements combined though, unless your doctor tells you to do so. Too much vitamin D can be toxic.

OMEGA-3 SUPPLEMENTS

The long list of benefits linked to omega-3 fatty acids includes a reduced risk of many of the disorders associated with diabetes: heart disease, depression, and dementia. These fats also are linked to greater intelligence in children, less pain and stiffness in people with rheumatoid arthritis, and a lower risk of breast and colon cancer.

Most of the research into the benefits of omega-3s have not been done on people with diabetes, so we're modeling our recommendations on those of the American Heart Association.

- If you *don't* have coronary heart disease (narrowing or clogging of arteries leading to the heart), eat fatty fish, such as salmon, at least twice a week. Also include foods rich in ALA, the omega-3 found in flaxseeds, canola oil, and walnuts. If you don't get these dietary sources, you can take half a gram (500 mg) of omega-3 daily.

- If you *do* have coronary heart disease, make sure you get about 1 gram (1,000 mg) of EPA and DHA per day, preferably from fatty fish. (See page 109 for fish choices.) Supplementing with EPA and DHA, which are mixed together in capsule form, is also okay, with your doctor's approval.

- If you need to lower your triglyceride level, under a physician's care, you might take 2 to 4 g total of EPA and DHA supplements.

- A warning: check with your doctor before taking omega-3 supplements, especially if you're taking the drug warfarin (brand name Coumadin), because they can cause excessive bleeding.

Choose a supplement that offers the most EPA and DHA per pill; in most cases this will save you money and you won't have to swallow as many supplements. Consumerlab.com, an independent testing company that reports on the quality of nutrition products, examined more than fifty brands for purity and potency, and a large percentage made the grade. Here are some of the high scorers that supply a concentrated amount of omega-3s per pill (manufacturers reformulate, so check labels to make sure the product still contains the right amount). For 500–600 mg of omega-3s per pill: Swanson EFAs Super EPA (mail order only, www.swansonvitamins .com); Carlson Super Omega-3; and Natural Factors Rx Omega-3. The following pills contain 1,000 mg of omega-3s: GNC Triple Strength fish oil and VitalOils 1,000 (mail order only, www.vitalremedymd.com).

THE HYPE ON CHROMIUM AND MAGNESIUM

Deficiencies in the minerals chromium and magnesium as well as potassium and possibly zinc may worsen your blood sugar control. You may have heard that supplementing with chromium or magnesium will improve your condition, but at this point the American Diabetes Association does not recommend supplementing with any of the minerals mentioned above. However, you may need to supplement if tests prove you are deficient. Blood tests can detect if you're low in potassium or magnesium, but it's harder to test for chromium and zinc.

Here's a quick rundown on two minerals that get the most hype when it comes to diabetes.

Chromium

Chromium is essential to enhancing the way insulin works in your body, so you'd think that supplementing with it might be a good idea. But in most studies, supplements did nothing for blood sugar. Indeed, the Food and Drug Administration has concluded that the relationship between chromium supplements and insulin resistance or type 2 diabetes is "highly uncertain." Your best strategy is to eat a varied diet, as small amounts of chromium are contained in many different types of foods. Recommended levels of the mineral are 25 mcg for women and 35 mcg for men up until age 50; 20 mcg for women and 30 mcg for men age 50 and above. Most foods haven't been analyzed for their chromium content, because it's difficult to do so. Following is a list of the chromium content of some of the foods that have been analyzed, adapted from the National Institutes of Health, Office of Dietary Supplements.

FOOD	CHROMIUM (MCG)
Broccoli, ½ cup	11
Grape juice, ½ cup	4
Garlic, dried, 1 teaspoon	3
Basil, dried, 1 tablespoon	2
Beef, 3 ounces	2
Turkey breast, 3 ounces	2
Whole wheat bread, 2 slices	2
Red wine, 5 ounces	1–13
Potatoes, mashed, ½ cup	1.5
English muffin, whole wheat	1.4
Orange juice, ½ cup	1
Apple, unpeeled, 1 medium	1
Banana, 1 medium	1
Green beans, ½ cup	1

Magnesium

Magnesium is involved in more than three hundred biochemical reactions in the body essential for healthy bones, muscle function, normal blood pressure, proper heart rhythm, and many other critical functions. It's also necessary for proper insulin function. The recommended level for men is 420 mg per day; for women, 320 mg. People with diabetes tend to be low in magnesium because they excrete more in the urine, and not having enough of the mineral is linked to lower insulin production and more insulin insensitivity. So should you take a magnesium supplement? If your blood tests show that you are low or deficient, supplementation is warranted. But don't supplement until you find out. Taking too much magnesium causes diarrhea and can harm the bowels. In fact, the Institute of Medicine recommends that people take no more than 350 mg from supplements. (That's just from supplements; it's okay if your daily magnesium intake is higher than 350 mg if you're getting it from foods.) However, if blood tests reveal you're low in magnesium, a dose higher than 350 mg may be necessary and safe. That's for your doctor to decide.

What you *should* be doing is eating magnesium-rich foods—and so should your family members who may be at increased risk of developing diabetes and pre-diabetes. A number of studies show that people who eat a magnesium-rich diet have a lower risk of developing type 2 diabetes. A University of Virginia study showed that obese children who weren't getting enough magnesium in their diets had low blood levels of the mineral and tended to be more insulin-resistant. The following are stellar sources of magnesium:

FOOD	MAGNESIUM (MG)
Nuts and Seeds	
Pumpkin seeds, shells removed, 1 ounce	151
Sunflower seeds, shells removed, 1 ounce	100
Almonds, 1 ounce	78
Cashews, 1 ounce	74
Sesame seeds, 2 tablespoons (⅔ ounce)	65
Peanut butter, 2 tablespoons	50
Peanuts, 1 ounce	48
Walnuts, 1 ounce	45
Fish	
Halibut, cooked, 3 ounces	91
Tuna, yellowfin, cooked, 3 ounces	54
Oysters, cooked, 3 ounces	53
Fruits and Vegetables	
Spinach, cooked, ½ cup	78
Swiss chard, cooked, ½ cup	75
Spinach, raw, 3 cups	71
Grains and Bran	
Wheat bran, crude, ¼ cup	88
Oat bran, cooked, ⅔ cup	58

Legumes and Soy Products

Edamame (green soybeans, available frozen), 3 ounces shelled	81
Roasted soybeans, 1 ounce	64
Tofu, 3 ounces	45
Black beans, ⅓ cup cooked	40

Other

Cocoa, unsweetened, 2 tablespoons	54

UNPROVEN DIABETES SUPPLEMENTS

When you have diabetes, unscrupulous or uninformed people are more than happy to sell you a dizzying array of unproven treatments. A quick Internet search can turn up hundreds of supplements claiming to lower blood sugar and miraculously improve your symptoms. While you know that controlling your diabetes isn't as simple as taking a pill or swigging a tonic, you might be tempted by the more genuine-sounding claims. Sorting out the effective supplements and diet advice from the pure hype isn't easy.

For instance, botanical supplements often found in so-called diabetes supplements, such as fenugreek, bitter melon, gymnema, aloe vera, and ginseng, have been used in world cultures for many years to control blood sugar, but there are still many unanswered questions about their effectiveness, not to mention side effects and dosage safety. Even mainstream vitamins that you can find at any pharmacy, such as vitamins E and C and beta-carotene, are not recommended by the American Diabetes Association because of the lack of strong evidence related to efficacy and concerns about long-term-use safety.

Cinnamon has received a great deal of attention. Although one 2003 study did find that 1 gram (about half a teaspoon) of cinnamon did improve fasting blood glucose, subsequent results from other studies have been mixed. So, until more consistent results can be found, using cinnamon to control your blood sugar isn't recommended.

Something that might help, and costs mere pennies per dose, is vinegar. Vinegar and other acids lower the glycemic index of foods, and research from the University of Arizona suggests that 2 tablespoons of vinegar taken with meals can reduce the post-meal blood sugar spike in people with diabetes. As an added bonus, the same amount of vinegar can also increase satiety, resulting in fewer calories eaten. While it's safe and even encouraged (a vinaigrette dressing tastes great on fresh greens) to use a couple of tablespoons of vinegar to add flavor to meals as part of a healthy diet, more research is needed before experts recommend using it as a treatment for diabetes or pre-diabetes. If you're prone to acid reflux, then it's best to limit the amount of vinegar you eat; its acidity can worsen your symptoms.

At worst, supplements can cause real damage if they are taken improperly; some can have adverse effects with long-term or high-dosage use; and many can react with your diabetes medications. At best, they can be a royal waste of money. If you do decide to use supplements, we cannot emphasize strongly enough how important it is to always run your plan by your health care practitioner. We're going to continue to monitor the science on supplements, and you can watch for updates on www.thebestlife .com as the news comes in.

JUDGING YOUR SUCCESS

Stay in Phase Two for as long as it takes to instill the diet goals, regularly use the Hunger Scale, and figure out which supplements you need. Use the questions below to determine if you've achieved these goals. When you've nailed down all these goals, and are reaping the benefits with better blood sugar, and weight loss (if you need it), then you've successfully completed Phase Two and are ready for Phase Three. If you're not yet ready for Phase Three, go ahead and read through the chapter anyway. The motivation tips can help you stay the course, and the advice on partnering with your doctor will come in handy at your next appointment.

If you answer yes or usually to all of the following questions, you're ready for Phase Three; if you answer no or not usually, then it's best to remain in Phase Two for as long as it takes to adopt the new habits.

1. Is your blood sugar in good control, meaning you're meeting the A1c targets and the home blood sugar monitoring levels that you and your doctor have set?

2. Are you still keeping up the goals of Phase One: monitoring blood sugar if you have diabetes, eating appropriate amounts of carbohydrates, eating three meals and the appropriate amount of snacks, maintaining or increasing activity, and drinking 48 ounces of water daily?

3. Have you become familiar with protein portions and are you eating the recommended level of lean protein for your daily calorie allowance at most meals?

4. Have you familiarized yourself with fat portions and are you having the recommended amounts of healthy fats for your daily calorie allowance at most meals and snacks?

5. Are your starchy carbohydrate foods mainly whole grain and high-fiber, and are you eating beans at least twice a week?

6. Did you avoid fried foods for at least four weeks?

7. Are you using the Hunger Scale?

8. Are you taking a multivitamin/mineral?

9. Are you supplementing with calcium and/or omega-3s if your diet isn't providing the recommended levels of these substances?

10. Are you comfortable enough with the lifestyle changes you've made so far, and are you prepared to take on new challenges?

4

PHASE THREE: LIVING YOUR BEST LIFE

IF YOU'VE FOLLOWED THE diet, exercise, and blood sugar logging guidelines in Phases One and Two, you should be seeing better numbers on your blood glucose monitor and possibly on your A1c and cholesterol lab reports. If you needed to lose weight, you should be seeing results on the scale as well. So what's next? More skills to keep you at your healthiest in the years ahead. In Phase Three, you'll be adjusting your diet just a little bit more to make it as health-promoting as possible. If you haven't started strength training, we'll offer you guidance on that front. And you'll be working on several critical areas that can make or break your long-term success: staying motivated, developing a good relationship with your health care provider, and caring for yourself when you're ill.

PHASE THREE

TIME FRAME: The rest of your life.

WEIGH IN: Weigh yourself once a week.

FOCUS: Developing the skills to stay motivated; further improving your diet and exercise habits; learning to partner with your health care providers and build a good team; and understanding how to care for yourself when you become ill.

OBJECTIVES:

- Maintain all your Phase One and Phase Two goals.

- Work on staying motivated so that you can keep up your healthy habits for life.

- Get enough sleep.

- Continue improving your diet by eating a wider variety of produce and staying within the sodium guidelines.

- Regularly evaluate your exercise routine and make any changes that will help you maintain—or improve—your fitness level.

CHIPAPALOOZA!

When Chip Hiden learned five years ago that he had type 1 diabetes, he was understandably upset. But his familiarity with the disease—both his parents and his two grandmothers have type 1 diabetes—softened the blow. "Being surrounded by positive people who manage the disease well made it much less scary," says the recent college grad and musician. "I realized that people share a limited natural resource—time. That's a heavy thought for a sixteen-year-old! But it didn't sadden me. Instead it energized and repurposed me; I wanted to do something meaningful with my life."

With that impulse, he turned his high school graduation party into a $5-a-ticket fund-raiser for juvenile diabetes research. He convinced a few local bands to play, and "Chipapalooza" was born. Now in it's fifth year, the festival is raising money for both diabetes and environmental causes. Chip parlayed that experience into bigger things at college—booking big musical and comedy acts. And he even founded a radio station, WAC Radio.

"I know this is going to sound weird, but in a way I'm glad I got diabetes. I don't think I would have been as motivated and passionate; it's really made me a go-getter. My advice to anyone with the disease is to take something they're passionate about and use it to fight the disease. Design a Web site for your local diabetes community, or teach others how to make healthy meals. This disease has been life-changing for me, but in a good way."

- Build a health care team tailored to your needs.

- Take proper care when you're sick.

JUDGING YOUR SUCCESS: In the coming months and years, you should remain motivated to live a healthy lifestyle, continue improving your diet, see the right health care providers, and take care of yourself when you get sick. These efforts will result in the best possible outcome of your diabetes or pre-diabetes.

MAINTAIN YOUR MOTIVATION

At age 16, Chip Hiden found out he had type 1 diabetes. His reaction? He started a music festival to raise money for diabetes research. After a lifelong struggle with weight, it was a diabetes diagnosis that finally triggered Nicola Farman to lose 50 pounds—and she's still losing. And Lisa Provenzo tackled her pre-diabetes by becoming a serious runner, which helped bring her blood sugar down to normal levels for seven years. How did these three turn their frightening diagnoses into a positive force in their lives? They'll share their motivation tips with you, and we'll also reveal some of the strategies that have helped our clients and patients stay the course.

Managing diabetes hinges on motivation because the disease asks so much of you. You're sticking yourself with lancets or needles, watching your carbohydrate intake, balancing out the rest of your diet, exercising regularly, and scheduling regular checkups and tests to guard against complications. On top of all this, many of you are also trying to lose weight! Then, there's the fear and uncertainty: Will my diabetes get worse? Will my pre-diabetes become diabetes? Will I develop complications? Can I afford the extra medical expenses? It's a lot to cope with, and it can take its toll emotionally. And when you're overwhelmed or depressed, it's hard to stay motivated to do all the things you need to do to stay healthy.

In this phase, we're offering tools to help keep you on track emotionally. Your head and heart have to be into it for you to manage your diabetes properly in the months and years to come.

I BEAT PRE-DIABETES
(AND DIABETES) FOR SEVEN YEARS

Lisa Provenzo had always been a fairly active person, but her diagnosis of pre-diabetes turned her into a marathoner. "When I found out my sugar and A1c were high, I was determined to beat the disease through lifestyle. I took a diabetes management course at the local suburban Maryland hospital just outside of Washington, D.C., began making more home-cooked meals, and started running. It worked—my sugar went down to just below 100. As long as I kept running and kept my weight below 145, my sugar was under control," recalls the five-foot, four-inch manager at a financial regulatory company. Since then, the 50-year-old has completed two marathons and five half marathons. What keeps her motivated? "My three workout buddies are my main inspiration; we meet at the gym, and we walk and hike together. We have a telephone call tree set up; if I'm not at the gym, one of them calls me. A few times, they've even come and gotten me out of bed!"

But recently, despite her efforts, her fasting blood sugar level climbed to 119—still pre-diabetes but getting closer to the 126 mark—and her A1c climbed to 6.7 after hovering around 6 for years. "When the doctor told me, I cried. I thought I could stave this off forever," says Lisa. Her doctor, she said, surprised her by commenting that she was acting as though she'd failed, when he saw her as a huge success. "He reminded me that I'd staved off both pre-diabetes and diabetes for seven years and that the disease is progressive, and I realized that was actually a big accomplishment." Lisa is taking metformin and is hoping that will bring her blood sugar down, and she's starting to check her blood sugar level regularly, something she hadn't been doing. "I guess the finger pricking symbolized 'disease' and I wasn't quite ready for that reality check," she admits. With two sisters who had gestational diabetes and a grandmother on insulin, she realizes that she's beaten her genetic odds so far. And she plans to continue doing so.

Built-in Mood Boosters

One source of emotional stability is good blood sugar control; levels that are in the healthy range actually enhance your sense of well-being. In addition, the diet and exercise habits that help control blood sugar are themselves mood-boosting. And of course, there's the sweet payoff of fitting back into that pair of jeans or hearing your doctor tell you that your A1c numbers have improved.

You probably know of—or have experienced firsthand—the irritability, lethargy, and confusion that result from hypoglycemia (low blood sugar), but you may not realize that high blood sugar—hyperglycemia—can also throw you for a loop. While hypoglycemia's side effects are well-established, research is starting to document hyperglycemia symptoms. For instance, in a German study, people with type 1 diabetes wore a continuous glucose monitor (a device that senses and records blood sugar levels) for two days while documenting their mood seven times a day. When their blood sugar level rose over 180, people reported being more angry, tense, and unhappy than when it was between 70 and 180. During the study, participants couldn't see the blood sugar readings, so their moods were a true reflection of how they were feeling and not influenced by the numbers.

Exercise is another way to enhance your mood, as numerous studies have shown. It appears to raise levels of feel-good chemicals in the brain and reduces cortisol, the stress hormone. A nutritious diet can also help. Low levels of magnesium, calcium, zinc, chromium, and potassium can worsen insulin resistance and interfere with good blood sugar control. If a poor diet contributes to higher blood sugar levels and higher blood sugar levels dampen mood, you can see how a nutrient-rich diet could give you a psychological lift. The meal plans starting on page 250 are a great example of this type of diet; even if you're not following them to the letter, do look them over for good ideas.

Overcoming Barriers to Motivation

You know you feel better when you exercise, eat right, and are in a good blood sugar zone. But that knowledge doesn't always translate into action—otherwise, there wouldn't be an epidemic of obesity, pre-diabetes, or type 2 diabetes! We hope by the time you've reached this last part of the program, you've stayed motivated enough to meet the goals of Phases One and Two. We want to help you keep that motivation percolating for many, many years to come. Motivation is very individual; people have all sorts of issues and reasons for keeping it or losing it. In our experience with clients and patients, though, many of the same issues come up over and over again.

There are two critical keys to motivation; without them, it's hard to keep at it. They are:

1. Knowing *why* you're doing something—in other words, understanding the benefits. By this point in the book, you should be well aware of the vast benefits of good diabetes management.

2. Believing you can do what it takes. Though a few doubts and uncertainties are perfectly normal before you take on any challenge, you should have the basic confidence that yes, you *can* increase your exercise level; you *can* learn about carbohydrate servings; and you *can* learn to test your blood sugar level and log the results. Psychologists call this "self-efficacy," and people who have it are more successful at changing their behaviors.

Issues and Strategies

You'll notice that for many of the common barriers to healthy eating, exercising, and blood sugar testing outlined on the following pages, we've suggested another underlying issue. See if any of these resonate with you:

"I DON'T HAVE TIME TO . . ." OR "I HATE TO . . ."

You fill in the blank: shop for healthy foods, cook, exercise, or check your blood sugar. People often tell us they simply don't have the time to deal with things or just can't stand doing them. We hear you on the time problem! But people with busy lives who find the time to work out do it because they've made health a priority. They've put healthy habits high up on the list and made room in their crowded schedule.

Everyone gets broadsided once in a while by events that truly make it difficult to stick with a healthy routine. Your mother landed in the hospital on the same week that your report is due at work and your children are off from school. But you could still find time to walk up the hospital steps instead of taking the elevator, park the car a few blocks from the office, or take a quick walk with the kids. And when things calm down a little, truly motivated people go right back to their healthy ways.

But when "I don't have time" is the norm, there's probably another issue at work. Perhaps you are resistant to change or defending the way you're currently living your life. Or, *it could be that you're intimidated by the process.* Maybe you haven't exercised in years; maybe you're not confident in the kitchen. Maybe you've never been good about details, so keeping a blood sugar log seems unmanageable. Remember, one of the keys to motivation is that you have to believe that you can do it.

But what if you simply hate to exercise or cook? What if you dislike the taste of vegetables and other healthful foods or can't stand to prick your finger? When we ask people to think about it carefully, they can usually find something they actually enjoy doing. For instance, unless they have arthritis or another condition that makes walking painful, most people like to walk. (Or at least they do when they're doing something they like, such as playing golf or shopping!) And walking certainly counts as exercise. Or they like to swim or garden or dance. And most people like some sort of healthful food—bananas, carrots, a bowl of shredded wheat cereal.

So take a step back and identify what you can do that's not overwhelming or intimidating. It might mean that you opt for walking instead of the kickboxing class at the gym, or that you sustain your current Activity Level for a while until you're ready to tackle the next level. Maybe you eat just three types of fruits and vegetables instead of a wide variety, at least at the beginning. We're not suggesting you shortchange yourself or that you don't aim high; just don't aim so high that it feels hopeless and overwhelming.

Also, be very specific about your goals and how you're going to achieve them. Women who used the following goal-setting exercise doubled their weekly workout time compared to a similar group of women who did not use the technique. (The study was a joint effort by Columbia University in New York City and the University of Konstanz in Germany.)

Write down the following questions and then answer them as specifically as you can. We've offered an exercise example to show you how it's done, but you can apply this technique to carb counting, food shopping, blood sugar testing, and any other healthful habit.

1. What is my exercise goal in the next 24 hours?

Find a goal you know you can achieve.

Example: "Getting 30 minutes of exercise in the morning."

2. What's the most positive outcome of achieving this goal?

This is crucial—you *must* be able to name and imagine a benefit; otherwise, this technique won't work.

Example: "Doing this regularly will get me into better shape and help me manage my diabetes better."

3. What's the main obstacle standing in the way?

Example: "I don't have enough time to work out in the morning."

4. How can I overcome the obstacle?

Be very specific, noting when and where the obstacle occurs.

Example: "In the morning (when), I can skip reading the newspaper at the kitchen table (where), which will give me 20 more minutes. At night, I can turn off the TV and get to bed an hour earlier so I can wake up earlier and give myself another 15 minutes in the morning."

5. How can I prevent the obstacle from occurring?

Again, be specific about the when and where.

Example: "I could make 10 P.M. my new bedtime and from now on read the newspaper later in the day."

6. How, specifically, can I achieve my exercise goal?

Focus specifically on when and where it will happen.

Example: "Between 6:30 and 7 A.M., I'll exercise with a 30-minute aerobics video in my living room and then take a shower."

Twenty-four hours later, repeat this exercise, but this time, when you answer question 1, give yourself a two-week goal. It could be the same goal—exercising for 30 minutes—or another goal, such as taking the stairs instead of the elevator.

SEEING HERSELF THROUGH HER DAUGHTER'S EYES

"I thought my pregnancy, my sanity, and my entire life was at risk when I got diagnosed with gestational diabetes," says Nicola Farman, a 47-year-old wife, mother, and online project manager living in Long Island, New York. With the help of insulin, she got her gestational diabetes under control, but after she gave birth, the diabetes remained. She tried managing it with oral medications for a few years, but when her A1c hit a whopping 12 with typical morning blood sugar levels of 240, she added insulin to her drug regimen. "The insulin helped enormously. My A1c is still a bit high at 6.5 to 7, but it's been going down as my weight has dropped. I've lost 50 pounds—it's taken years to get below 250 pounds. I struggle every day, but I'm determined to reach 175 and maintain it. I've got a great support system in my family and my certified diabetes educator."

Nicola's routine includes a breakfast of oatmeal and a salad with turkey breast for lunch. "Since I started packing that same lunch for my husband, he's lost 70 pounds," she notes. She cooks a light dinner and has given up alcohol. "While I've never been a big drinker, I did like the occasional glass of wine, but even that puts my sugars in orbit."

What's also helped peel off pounds: the 3/4-mile walk from the Long Island Railroad station to her job, in addition to swimming, taking the dog on long walks, and doing yoga. To fit it all in, she traded in supermarket shopping for online grocery delivery, which not only bought her an extra two hours but also cut down on junk food impulse buys. She also gave up something she loved—choral singing; there wasn't enough time to practice and perform. "But it's all been worth it. What keeps me most motivated is looking at my daughter and seeing myself through her eyes. I'm doing this because I want to be a good role model for her and have a long, healthy life."

"THERE'S TOO MUCH STRUCTURE" OR "THERE'S NOT ENOUGH STRUCTURE"

If you're really serious about fighting diabetes, you have no choice but to improve your diet and exercise habits, and monitor your blood sugar. (And for pre-diabetes, the first two are musts.) But you do have many options as to how to go about it, especially on a program as flexible as this one. You'll be most successful if you hit upon the right amount of structure for your personality type. "I tell my clients to ask themselves, 'What's easier to manage—a set plan that's prescribed for me or making my own choices? Or somewhere in between?' " says Jody Brand Levine, LCSW-C, a psychotherapist specializing in the treatment of people with diabetes based in Potomac, Maryland. "Some people do better when they have lots of choice; a set program makes them feel deprived and controlled. But for others, too much choice simply creates more stress. This is especially true for perfectionists. With too much choice, they veer from what they view as perfection to imperfection, which can take a toll on their self-esteem."

Within the eating, exercising, and blood-sugar-testing guidelines of the Best Life program, there is a wide range of structure. We urge you to tailor it to your style. You can design your own diet or follow our meal plans. Use our 12-week exercise plan, or find your own path to moving up the Activity Scale. Go ahead and adjust your blood sugar testing schedule to your own needs, or use our model on page 45. Find your structure comfort zone and run with it!

"I FEEL GUILTY TAKING SO MUCH TIME FOR MYSELF"

"But how can I take time away from my family, friends, or job to exercise or log my blood sugar and meals?" is a question we hear all the time. We ask you to take Nicola Farman's approach (see box on page 162) and remind yourself that you will be a better parent, spouse, sibling, friend, and employee if you're happy and healthy yourself. When you closely examine your schedule, there may be places other than family or work to trim from—perhaps cutting out a television show or happy hour. It's hard to sacrifice something you enjoy, but chances are, you'll enjoy exercising, or, at the very least, you'll have a tremendous feeling of satisfaction at the end of your workout. And sometimes you can schedule exercise with family and friends or cook with them (a great skill to pass on)—a win-win for all.

If you still can't justify the time for yourself, the underlying issue might be that your self-worth is too tied into taking care of others. Part of that is not valuing yourself enough. This can be a difficult issue to resolve, but a good first step is to reframe the way you think about yourself. "With practice, you literally can become the person that you think you should be. For instance, if you tell yourself that you're valuable and that you deserve that hour at the gym, you will start to value yourself. And by actually going to the gym, you are now a person who takes time out and goes to the gym. Our actions become who we are," advises Jody Brand Levine.

"MY POOR HEALTH PREVENTS ME FROM EXERCISING"

Neuropathy, retinopathy, arthritis, an amputated limb, heart disease, or other diabetes-related conditions make exercise particularly challenging. In fact, there are some types of physical activity you *shouldn't* do when you have these conditions. But in every case, there are some safe ways to get moving. Check out our suggestions in "Exercising with Complications of Diabetes" on page 241.

"I DON'T NEED TO MAKE ALL THESE CHANGES"

When Lisa Provenzo (see page 157) was first diagnosed with diabetes, she wasn't diligent about checking blood sugar. "I didn't check all that often. In fact, I lost the blood glucose monitor and had to get a new one," she admits. "I thought I could stave off diabetes forever, and so I guess I couldn't admit to myself that I really had it and had to check blood sugar." It could be that, like Lisa, you haven't accepted your disease and you're in some denial. That's a normal reaction, but keep in mind that the longer you wait to make healthy lifestyle changes, the riskier your disease becomes.

Educate yourself about diabetes, and focus on the positives. Write down what you're doing to help yourself in regard to diet, exercise, blood sugar testing, and logging results. Where are you coming up blank? For instance, are you not testing your blood sugar? Make a commitment to work on that one area for a week. You can use the goal-setting technique on page 160 to help you come up with a workable plan. Then deal with the other areas.

Focusing on one issue at a time is less overwhelming than trying to piece together the entire picture. For instance, if you haven't gotten your blood sugar monitor out in a while, commit to starting that again. If you also need to move to the next Activity Level, tell yourself it's a move you'll *eventually* make, even if it's not for a few weeks or even months. By not putting pressure on yourself to change everything immediately, you can move from denial to thinking about making changes at a comfortable pace. As you make progress on your first goal, you will feel more motivated and confident to tackle the more challenging health behaviors down the road.

You don't have to jump to the top of the mountain in one leap; just keep putting one foot in front of the other, and you'll make progress.

"I CAN'T STOP EATING"

Why do you reach for that cookie when you're not hungry, or automatically open the fridge door even after coming home from a restaurant stuffed? And why did you get stuffed in the first place? Overeating is driven by a powerful combination of physiological and emotional forces. But just because it's complicated doesn't mean you can't outfox it.

On the emotional side, food is soothing and comforting; it helps reduce stress and eases painful feelings, such as loneliness and hurt. When you head to the vending machine to quell the deadline jitters or open a box of cookies in the evenings when you feel lonely, you're trying to help yourself—a good thing—but you're using the wrong coping tool.

There is also a slew of hormones, brain chemicals, and other physiological forces behind overeating that scientists are just beginning to sort out. But whether it's physiological or emotional, ultimately your body is asking to be soothed and comforted and to be given some pleasure. You can achieve this without food. Start making a list of all the other things that make you feel good. Going out with friends, calling a friend, reading, and watching movies are all great ways to boost your mood without boosting your calorie and carbohydrate intake. And we know that excercise *burns* calories and carbohydrates, and boosts mood.

Meanwhile, get the worst food offenders away from you. Purge the house of cookies, chips, and other foods that get you into calorie trouble. To avoid feeling deprived, you might keep one small treat around, and make sure to have it only when you'll enjoy it most—not in front of the TV, when you're barely paying attention to what you're eating, or when you're running out the door and don't have time to savor it. Don't get into a routine with unhealthy foods. For instance, after a few days of eating chips in the midafternoon, your body will come to expect the treat. So although it might be okay to have those chips, on occasion, don't always have them at the same time. That way, you'll have one less trigger to fight.

"I CAN'T GO IT ALONE"

The more support you have, the better you'll do, so go ahead and ask for help—family members can pitch in by helping you shop and cook and joining you on walks, hikes, bike rides, and other outings. Take a cue from Lisa Provenzo (page 157)—her three workout buddies have literally gotten her out of bed to work out. Online support groups can also be very comforting and motivating; we have lots of them at www.thebestlife.com.

"I'M DEPRESSED"

An estimated 20 to 40 percent of people with diabetes also have some level of depression, about double the rate of the general population. Along with the emotional pain, depression can worsen blood sugar control and raise the risk of complications. People experience depression differently, but there are common symptoms, including a loss of pleasure in things you once enjoyed, changes in eating or sleeping patterns, feelings of hopelessness or guilt, or trouble concentrating.

The conventional wisdom is that having diabetes triggers depression and vice versa—but a recent review of the research challenges that assumption, at least when it comes to type 2 diabetes. The joint University of Michigan–Ann Arbor and Johns Hopkins University in Baltimore review found that being depressed raises the risk of type 2 diabetes by 60 percent, but having type 2 diabetes doesn't increase your odds of developing depression. It's possible depression is also a trigger of pre-diabetes. Research is showing that depression often leads to weight gain, particularly of visceral fat, the type of belly fat that leads to insulin resistance, pre-diabetes, and type 2 diabetes. Being depressed also causes the release of higher levels of cortisol, the so-called stress hormone. This, in turn, promotes the accumulation of visceral fat—the more cortisol you have in your body, the more visceral fat gets laid down. Plus, inflammation is on the upswing and other systems go awry during depression, which may worsen insulin resistance and spur on type 2 diabetes and pre-diabetes. But why is depression more prevalent in type 1 diabetes? Unlike type 2, in people with type 1 diabetes, it's the disease that may be driving the blues.

If you're a woman with diabetes, you're more likely to have depression than a man with the same diagnosis. However, regardless of gender, having a low educational status and living without a partner are both significantly associated with depression in people with diabetes.

The impact of feeling blue is significant to diabetes management. The depression-diabetes duo creates a vicious cycle, making it more difficult to gain control over the disease and your weight. In a study of nearly 4,500 people with type 2 diabetes conducted by the University of Washington in Seattle in conjunction with a health maintenance organization, those with depression exercised less, ate more fat and fewer fruits and vegetables, and were less likely to adhere to their prescriptions of blood-sugar-lowering, cholesterol-lowering, and antihypertensive medications.

Not surprisingly, dropping the ball on key aspects of diabetes management bodes poorly for your disease. "Being depressed raises your risk for diabetic complications, such as retinopathy, neuropathy, kidney disease, heart disease, and sexual dysfunction, in part because depressed people have a harder time motivating themselves to exercise, eat right, and perform the other tasks that good diabetes management requires," explains Kristin S. Vickers Douglas, PhD, LP, associate professor of psychology at the Mayo Clinic College of Medicine in Rochester, Minnesota. Because exercise is a way to lift mood and treat depression, being physically active is especially critical when you have depression and diabetes. But Dr. Vickers Douglas's research on people with type 2 diabetes shows that depression gets in the way of your ability to get moving. "Compared to people with type 2 who are not depressed, those with depression exercise less, count fewer pros and more cons to exercise (such as seeing exercise as difficult or too time-consuming), are less confident that they can perform the exercise or stick with a program, and don't view exercise as being as beneficial."

The biggest difference her research detected between those with depression and those without is that depressed people had a harder time getting back on track after breaking their exercise routine; there was a lot of self-blame and feelings of failure. "Whether it's exercise, healthy eating, blood sugar testing, or other elements of healthy living, you need to be more forgiving of lapses. They are a natural part of the process of change. Responding with guilt, frustration, and self-hatred is only going to erode your confidence and make it harder to stay on track. Instead, treat yourself as you would a good friend: be supportive, encouraging, and motivating," advises Dr. Vickers Douglas. She says the goal-setting exercise described on page 160 could be very helpful after a lapse.

If you are depressed, do your part to help yourself, and don't hesitate to get help from a psychologist or other mental health professional. Ask your primary care physician, friends, and local diabetes support groups for referrals. Psychotherapy, such as cognitive behavioral therapy, and antidepressant medications are effective in treating depression. The National Institute of Mental Health (www.mentalhealth.gov) has free reading materials to help you understand depression and lists local mental health services in your area. The National Mental Health Information Center of the Substance Abuse and Mental Health Services Administration has an online services locator that can help you find local resources for emotional well-being (www.mentalhealth.samhsa.gov). Treatment cost, availability, the severity of depressive symptoms, and treatment preferences are all considerations when determining the best treatment; your doctor can help you sort through your options.

Additionally, ask your doctor about supplementing with omega-3 fatty acids; recent research suggests that they may reduce the incidence of, as well as treat, depression in people with type 2 diabetes.

Don't let depression consume you and derail your diabetes management efforts. Be assured that with help, you'll feel better and diabetes management will become easier.

GET SOME SLEEP!

Exercise, diet, blood sugar testing . . . and sleep? You might not have expected to see sleep as part of our program, but it has a strong impact on your health. We're treating sleep very seriously in this book because it touches on so many aspects of diabetes management. Lack of sleep can not only sap your energy and motivation to stick with the program, but can affect your hormones, actually promoting insulin resistance, obesity, and diabetes.

Americans are becoming more sleep-deprived, and it's taking a toll on our health—and our waistlines. A poll by the National Sleep Foundation showed that the number of Americans who sleep less than six hours a night jumped from 13 percent in 2001 to 20 percent in 2009, and those who reported sleeping eight hours or more dropped from 38 percent to 28 percent in the same time period. New research at the University of Buffalo in New York found that study participants who averaged less than six hours of sleep per night, compared to those who got six to eight hours, were nearly five times as likely to develop pre-diabetes. In addition, an analysis of recent studies suggests that sleep deprivation makes it harder to control appetite because leptin (one of the hormones that signals that you've had enough to eat) levels drop, while ghrelin (a hormone that stimulates hunger) levels rise, creating a double-whammy diet buster.

But it's not just the *lack* of sleep that increases diabetes risk, it's the *quality* of the sleep you get, too. A study from the University of Chicago found that after just three nights of disturbed sleep (think: pets scurrying in your bedroom, a snoring partner, children waking you in the night), insulin sensitivity decreased in study participants; this change had the same metabolic effect as gaining 20 to 30 pounds. And that's in people *without* diabetes or pre-diabetes.

If you already have diabetes, logging enough quality shut-eye is even more important because sleep also appears to moderate the hormones that regulate blood glucose, and losing out can contribute to elevated hemoglobin A1c levels in people with the disease. In fact, a 2006 University of Chicago study found a clear association between poor quality and quantity of sleep and reduced blood sugar control. As many people with diabetes can attest, sleep is often interrupted in the night because of frequent trips to the bathroom or nerve pain. Obstructive sleep apnea, when breathing stops during sleeping, is a condition that is frequently associated with diabetes and obesity; however, studies show that when obstructive sleep apnea is treated with continuous positive airway pressure (CPAP; a device that helps keep airways open so you can breathe more easily), overnight blood glucose levels are stabilized.

So try switching off the late-night news and settling in to snooze. If you aren't getting enough hours of sleep or suffer from low-quality sleep due to related symptoms, work with your doctor to find some shut-eye solutions. And try these tips from the National Sleep Foundation to hit your nightly goal of seven hours:

- Create a regular, relaxing bedtime routine and lights-out time. A comfortable bed and a cool, dark, quiet sleeping space are most conducive to quality rest.

- Aim to wrap up your exercise routine at least three hours before bedtime. Too much activity right before bed can make it hard to wind down and feel sleepy.

- Skip caffeinated beverages, or switch to decaf eight hours before your anticipated bedtime, and avoid alcohol a few hours before you hit the hay. Both can disrupt sleep.

- Avoid using your bedroom for non–sleep related activities. Piles of undone laundry, a computer desk brimming with work to be done, and a big, blaring TV don't foster an ideal sleeping environment.

CONTINUE IMPROVING YOUR DIET

If you've been following the guidelines in the last two phases, you should have a great diet by now. But you're not finished; most of you can make your eating plan even more nutritious, tastier, more varied, and even better for your blood sugar levels and your long-term health.

Vary Your Produce Picks

If the same fruits and vegetables dominate your fruit basket and refrigerator, it's time to expand your repertoire. Bringing in more variety is not only more interesting for the taste buds but helps you cast a wider nutrient net. Scientists estimate that there may be 100,000 phytonutrients (beneficial plant compounds other than vitamins and minerals), and they're not all in apples or bananas! One way to help ensure you get this diversity is to eat fruits and vegetables of every color. As you can see from the table on page 171, similarly colored produce generally shares some of the same phytonutrients. That's because the pigments that give them their hue are themselves phytonutrients. For instance,

Nutrition in Every Hue

A fruit's or vegetable's color is a good indicator of the different vitamins, minerals, and phytonutrients it contains. Put a rainbow on your plate, and you're going to cover a lot of your nutrient bases. Here's a color-by-color breakdown.

FRUIT/VEGETABLE COLOR OR TYPE	SUCH AS . . .	WHAT THEY BRING TO THE TABLE
Green	Asparagus, beet greens, broccoli, Brussels sprouts, collard greens, dandelion greens, green beans, honeydew melon, kale, kiwi, mustard greens, okra, parsley, peas, peppers, spinach, Swiss chard, romaine lettuce, and zucchini	Lutein and zeaxanthin, powerful antioxidants (especially lutein) linked to reducing the risk for two eye diseases: cataracts and macular degeneration, the leading cause of blindness. Many are also good sources of beta-carotene.
White/green	Artichokes, asparagus, celery, chives, endive, garlic, green pears, mushrooms, onions, and scallions	Onions, potatoes, and garlic are especially rich in allyl sulfides, which help prevent stomach and colon cancer and may lower cholesterol. Onions are also a good source of quercetin, which protects against cancer and possibly heart disease. The rest contain flavonoids, a large class of phytonutrients linked to preventing heart disease.
Cruciferous (a family of mostly green-white vegetables)	Arugula, bok choy, broccoflower (a broccoli-and-cauliflower hybrid), broccoli, Brussels sprouts, cabbage (all types), cauliflower, collard greens, kale, mustard greens, rutabaga, Swiss chard, turnips, turnip greens, and watercress	Cancer-fighting compounds called indoles and isothiocyanates.

FRUIT/VEGETABLE COLOR OR TYPE	SUCH AS . . .	WHAT THEY BRING TO THE TABLE
Yellow/orange	Apricots, butternut squash, cantaloupe, carrots, citrus fruit, mangoes, papayas, peaches, pumpkin, and sweet potatoes	Bioflavonoids, which may help protect against cancer and heart disease, and vitamin C. Citrus peel contains limonene, which also helps fight cancer. Some have beta- and alpha-carotene, antioxidants that are linked to reducing the risk of cancer and heart disease.
Red	Pink grapefruit, red tomatoes, salsa, tomato-based juices, tomato-based pasta sauce, tomato soup, and watermelon	Vitamin C and lycopene, a powerful antioxidant linked to protection from cancer and heart disease.
Purple/blue/deep red	Blackberries, blueberries, cherries, cranberries, eggplant, grape juice, plums, prunes, raisins, red apples, red beans, red beets, red cabbage, red or purple grapes, red onions, red pears, red wines, and strawberries	Anthocyanins, a potent group of antioxidants that helps prevent blood clots and may improve brain function.

lycopene, a powerful antioxidant linked to a lower risk of heart disease, gives tomatoes and watermelon their red color. Beta-carotene, which the body converts to vitamin A as needed, gives carrots, butternut squash, and cantaloupe their intense orange color. There are some exceptions; broccoli, for instance, is rich in beta-carotene, but its green pigment masks the orange color, and vegetables containing the same type of phytonutrient, such as cauliflower and radishes, aren't necessarily the same color.

So far, you've been eating two fruit servings daily and six or seven vegetables, depending on your daily calorie level. For a refresher go back to "Daily Servings" on page 53. At 15 grams of carbohydrate per serving, fruit has triple the carbohydrates of a serving of vegetables, which is why we've limited your daily fruit servings. However, you may be able to eat more fruit if you find that it doesn't spike your blood sugar level, and you can certainly have an extra fruit as your daily dessert, as long as you meet the carbohydrate limit, which is 10 grams for the 1,700-calorie plan and 15 grams for the 2,000- and 2,250-calorie plans.

As for vegetables, take your cue from the U.S. Department of Agriculture's Dietary Guidelines:

Dark green vegetables: 3 cups per week

Orange vegetables: 2 cups per week

Legumes (dry beans): 3 cups per week

Starchy vegetables: 3 cups per week

Other vegetables: 6½ cups per week

Remember that legumes and starchy vegetables belong under the grain/starchy vegetable group. If you need a reminder as to the number of servings you get from this group, check the tables on pages 53 and 55.

PROTECTIVE PRODUCE

If you have pre-diabetes, listen up! Research is showing that eating more fruits and vegetables can substantially reduce the risk of developing type 2 diabetes.

One reason for the protective effect: fruits and vegetables are low in calories for their size, helping you keep your weight down, which, in turn, improves insulin resistance. They're also loaded with antioxidants, which are particularly important for people with diabetes and pre-diabetes.

Stay Within the Sodium Guidelines

One of the triggers of heart disease and stroke is high blood pressure, or hypertension. Eating too much sodium raises blood pressure—to some degree in most people and to a larger degree in sodium-sensitive people. The American Heart Association and other health authorities recommend maxing out at 2,300 milligrams to 2,400 milligrams of sodium daily. If you already have high blood pressure, going down to 1,500 milligrams may be even more helpful.

COFFEE, TEA, AND DIABETES

Fruits and vegetables aren't the only source of phytonutrients; coffee and tea are also major contributors. In fact, for people who don't eat many fruits and vegetables, these beverages are their primary source of phytonutrients.

A number of studies show that coffee drinkers are less likely to develop pre-diabetes and type 2 diabetes than those who don't sip. Drinking as little as one cup of coffee daily reduced the risk of type 2 diabetes by 60 percent compared to people who never drank coffee. This applied both to people with normal blood sugar as well as those with pre-diabetes, according to a study from the University of California at San Diego. The protective effect was seen in both current coffee drinkers as well as those who used to regularly drink but quit. Decaf coffee also appeared to be protective, but there wasn't enough data to prove a definitive benefit. Tea drinkers may also reap some perks, thanks to the brew's antioxidants. (Both regular and decaffeinated versions should reduce the risk.)

But there's a caffeine caution: Caffeinated beverages can spike blood sugar for about thirty minutes after consuming them, so some experts suggest switching to decaf coffee if you have diabetes, or drinking tea, which has considerably less caffeine than coffee (or drink decaffeinated tea). Try making the switch yourself and see whether your blood sugar improves. (Wean yourself off caffeine gradually to avoid the unpleasant side effects, such as headaches and fatigue.) If you don't notice an improvement in a few months, and you're really wedded to regular coffee, cap it at two cups per day. More than that may not only affect blood sugar, but it can also interfere with your Phase Three sleep goal.

On the Best Life meal plans, 2,300 mg of sodium is the limit on the 1,500-, 1,700-, and 2,000-calorie-per-day plans. We went up to 2,400 mg daily on the 2,250-calorie plan because it's nearly impossible to consume that many calories and keep your sodium intake below 2,300 mg. If it was hard for *us* to work within that limit, it's no wonder that an average person struggles to keep a lid on sodium consumption. In fact, the average American consumes about 4,000 mg of sodium for every 2,000 calories (and you know that most people are consuming more than 2,000 calories per day!).

When you think "sodium," you think "salt"; it's true, about 90 percent of the sodium in our diet comes from salt. (By weight, salt is 40 percent

WHERE'S ALL THE SODIUM COMING FROM?

Here's a small sampling of popular high-sodium foods, courtesy of the USDA's Agricultural Research Service. Notice the wide range of sodium content for the same food; that's why it's so important to compare labels.

FOOD	SERVING SIZE	RANGE (MG)
Bread, all types	1 ounce (a medium slice)	95–210
Frozen cheese pizza, plain, cheese	4 ounces	450–1,200
Frozen vegetables, all types	½ cup	2–360
Pretzels	1 ounce (28.4 g)	290–560
Salad dressing, regular-fat, all types	2 tablespoons	110–505
Salsa	2 tablespoons	150–240
Soup (tomato), reconstituted	8 ounces	700–1,260
Tomato juice	8 ounces (1 cup)	340–1,040
Tortilla chips	1 ounce (28.4 g)	105–160

According to the Centers for Disease Control National Health and Nutrition Examination Survey, the top sources of sodium in the American diet are (ranked in order of which foods provide the most sodium):

1. Pizza topped with meat
2. White bread
3. Processed cheese
4. Hot dogs
5. Spaghetti with sauce
6. Ham
7. Catsup
8. Salty snacks/corn chips
9. Whole milk*
10. Pizza topped with just cheese
11. Noodle soups
12. Eggs (whole/fried/scrambled)
13. Macaroni with cheese
14. Milk, 2%*

* Fat-free milk has just as much sodium as other types of milk but is not listed here because (unfortunately) it's not as widely consumed as the fattier milks.

sodium and 60 percent chloride.) The rest comes from other sodium-containing chemicals added to food. But most of the salt we consume doesn't come from the salt shaker. Instead, it's estimated that 77 percent of the salt in our diet comes from processed foods. Naturally occurring sodium may constitute another 12 percent of intake. For instance, did you know that a cup of milk has 103 milligrams of sodium and there are 125 milligrams of sodium in 3 ounces of shrimp? Another 12 percent or so is added during cooking, and only 6 percent comes from the salt shaker at the table. (Unless you're one of those people who starts shaking heavily before even tasting the food!)

Too much sodium used to get all the blame for raising blood pressure, but now it's clear that too little potassium is also a culprit. Because potassium is found mainly in fruits and vegetables, which most Americans don't eat enough of, and sodium is found in processed foods, which Americans eat too much of, you can see why the average American has a 90 percent likelihood of developing hypertension in his or her lifetime. So, in addition to cutting back on sodium, you must also eat more potassium. If you eat the amount of fruits and vegetables recommended on this plan, you'll do just fine.

If you like salty foods, you might be groaning about now, but if you're worried that you'll never enjoy food again, you're wrong. Your taste buds will adjust, and pretty soon, foods you used to like will seem unpleasantly salty. And then there's the salt shaker trick: the strongest salt sensation comes from salt crystals hitting your tongue. The salt taste sort of disappears when cooked. But take a fresh, ripe tomato, which is virtually salt-free, and add just a few sprinkles of salt, and you get that satisfying salty sensation with just a smidgen of sodium.

Use these tips to help reduce your sodium intake:

AT THE GROCERY STORE

- Read labels; sodium shows up in surprising places.

- Compare labels and buy products with less sodium. Pay particular attention to staple items, such as bread and cereal; there's a wide range of sodium content in these products. Beware of canned soups—most are loaded with sodium. Buy those with no more than 500 milligrams per cup.

- Whenever possible, buy "low-sodium" or, even better, "no-salt-added" foods, such as beans and frozen and canned vegetables.

- Buy raw fish, poultry, and meat instead of cooked, processed versions.

- Make 700 mg of sodium your cutoff for frozen meals; the lower the sodium content, the better.

- Remember: Sea salt and kosher salts are still salt. Buy them if you like them, but use them as sparingly as regular salt.

IN THE KITCHEN

- Gradually reduce the amount of salt you use to season your recipes so your taste buds can adjust.

- When cooking foods that need some salt, use this rule of thumb: ⅛ teaspoon (250 mg sodium) for every four servings. Let people salt to taste at the table.

- Rely on lemon juice and vinegar to add flavor to salads, marinades, and sauces.

- Use fresh and dried herbs, pepper, and citrus peel to season cooked and fresh dishes.

- Make plain rice or other grains and add your own spices instead of using sodium-filled spice mixes.

- Rinse salt from canned food, even tuna.

AT THE TABLE

- Serve food unsalted or very lightly salted. If you need a little salt, add a few grains to the food just before eating.

- Keep fresh lemon or lime wedges on hand—a squirt on chicken, meat, fish, salads, and soups can add enough flavor that you might not need salt.

▪ Balance high-sodium items with foods lower in sodium. When you do have a high-sodium food (for instance, soup), balance it out with low-sodium items such as grilled vegetables and plain rice.

EVALUATE YOUR EXERCISE ROUTINE

Every few months, take some time to evaluate your exercise routine. Do you need to mix it up and try new forms of physical activity to keep you motivated? Is it too easy—do you need to push yourself a little harder? If you're following our twelve-week fitness plan (page 355), you still have a few weeks to go. You may be just beginning the strength-training section. If you are using your own routine, now might be a good time to add in some strength training if you haven't done so already. If you've never used weights or machines, it might seem a little intimidating. But people tell us all the time that once they begin, they're hooked! For anyone trying to lose weight or maintain weight loss, strength training is indispensable— nothing does a better job of reshaping your body and helping to keep your metabolism in high gear.

There are literally hundreds of different strength-training exercises, but don't let the abundance of options confuse you. If you're feeling overwhelmed, there are eight moves that will accomplish everything you need. The Basic Eight strength-training moves hit all the major muscle groups and ensure that you develop strength, power, and endurance equally. Together these exercises give your muscles the ability to perform quickly and efficiently while also preventing the loss of muscle tissue that occurs naturally through aging and disuse.

The Basic Eight are simple to perform and, best of all, don't take much time; you can go through them in about 20 minutes. That's little time to invest for what will be a huge payoff!

Whether you've never lifted weights before or are an experienced exerciser who has never found the right strength-training regimen, you'll find the Basic Eight a simple and efficient exercise routine. The basic moves are:

1. Squats, which work the upper legs (quadriceps and hamstrings)

2. Lunges, which work the upper and lower legs (quadriceps, hamstrings, and calves)

3. Chest Press, which works the chest (pectorals) and back of upper arms (triceps)

4. Shoulder Press, which works the shoulder muscles (deltoids)

5. Butterfly, which works the upper back muscles (trapezius and latissimus dorsi)

6. Dumbbell Fly, which works the chest muscles (pectorals)

7. Biceps Curl, which works the upper arms (biceps)

8. Triceps Extension, which works the backs of the upper arms (triceps)

You can perform all Basic Eight moves with dumbbells, although if you belong to a well-equipped gym, all of the moves have a machine alternative. (Visit the exercise video library at www.thebestlife.com to see demonstrations for each exercise.) Whether you're using dumbbells or a weight machine, keep in mind that the weight needs to be heavy enough to fatigue your muscles after 8 to 10 repetitions.

Here's a good progression for both beginners and experienced exercisers to follow:

- Begin with 1 or 2 sets per exercise, 8 to 10 repetitions per set, at least two times a week. Take no more than 20 to 30 seconds in between sets. You may find you can't make 8 to 10 reps in the second set, but that's okay; it's evidence you're working hard enough in the first set to produce changes in your muscles. As your strength improves, you'll eventually make the reps.

- After about four weeks, reassess. If you're making all your sets easily, add another. Also check your weights. Are they heavy enough?

■ Keep reassessing every four to six weeks, and when you're ready for a new challenge, add another day. Your ultimate goal: 3 sets of each exercise, 8 to 10 reps, every other day.

As you advance and increase your activity level to Level 4 or 5, you may want to add additional exercises to your routine. Find some good examples on the Best Life Web site.

PARTNER WITH YOUR DOCTOR

Your doctor should be your number one partner in the effort to manage your diabetes or to stop your pre-diabetes from making the transition to full-fledged diabetes. We're going to offer some pointers on making that partnership as smooth and productive as possible. (We'll usually say "doctor" in this chapter, just for convenience's sake, but this could mean a nurse practitioner, physician's assistant, or other health care provider.)

It sounds kind of obvious, but the first thing is that you should have a good, mutually respectful relationship with your physician. You should have confidence in your doctor's knowledge and experience. Her judgment is critical: is this an urgent matter, or something that can be addressed gradually? Her manner should be reassuring and respectful; just as you have high regard for your doctor's professional training, she should listen to your concerns and value those things of special importance to you. You have vital information and important insight into your health, especially if you've been working hard to live a healthy lifestyle by making the kinds of changes we've suggested. A good doctor will want to know what you've been doing and how you think you can best help yourself.

At the same time, it's important to be realistic. Even the most highly professional, motivated, and compassionate doctor has limited time to spend with you. People often feel rushed through appointments with their doctor and assume that the doctor doesn't care or isn't aware of how they feel. Believe us on this one: doctors and other health care providers are just as frustrated as their patients at the need to see a large volume of people everyday. But given this reality, it's very important to come to the visit prepared so you can get the most out of the time allotted. The following steps are key:

- **Bring an up-to-date list of all your medications to every doctor's appointment.** Include the name of each medication, the tablet or capsule strength, how many tablets or capsules you take, and when you take them. Update the list every time there is a change. If you take insulin, indicate what type, how many units, and when you take it. Be sure to also include any over-the-counter medicines, vitamins, or supplements you take.

    There are several reasons to keep a medication list. For one thing, studies show surprisingly poor communication between physicians and their patients regarding medications. Maybe the doctor thought she said to take the pill twice a day, but you understood it to be once a day. And if, like most people, you see more than one doctor, you're probably the only one who knows what they've all prescribed. Last, medical records are often incomplete or inaccurate. Your list can set things right.

- **Get your blood tests done before your visit.** It's important for you and your doctor to have laboratory results available to you when you're actually in the office; you and your doctor will see the effects of any shifts in diet, exercise, or drugs that have occurred over the past several months. You should go for blood tests a week or two before your appointment and ask the lab to send a copy to you and to the doctor. Bring your copy to the visit, just in case the doctor's copy didn't make its way into your folder. At the end of the appointment, ask for the lab order form that will allow you to have blood work done prior to your next visit.

- **Bring your finger-stick blood glucose test results with you to each office visit.** The results should be recorded neatly in the Best Life Doctor's Log or in a similar manner.

    You should review your blood sugar level before you see the doctor, looking for patterns—what makes it go too high, what sends it too low? What effect does exercise have? Are there particular meals that cause a problem? Your doctor should look at the results, but you're the one with time to really study them. You may very well identify patterns or see problems that should lead to adjustment in your medications. Don't be afraid to point these out.

- **Write down your questions and concerns before your appointment.** Bring a list, but keep it short—two or three issues are probably all that can be addressed at most visits—and make sure to discuss the most important things first. For instance, if you've been having frequent low-blood-sugar reactions, chest pain, or shortness of breath, or if you've had episodes where you felt faint, these need to be discussed before the pain in your wrist. Don't be embarrassed about asking questions or bringing up subjects such as sexual function that might seem a little awkward. If your interest in sex has diminished or you're having difficulty with erections or orgasms, let your doctor know. And don't expect her to ask—doctors tend to fail to ask about sexual issues. You shouldn't feel uncomfortable about discussing the cost of your medical care, either. Your health is your first priority, but your doctor may not realize that your medications are costing more than you can afford or that you've lost your job and are paying out of pocket. She may be able to find a lower-cost generic drug for you or eliminate some laboratory tests that aren't as critical.

Build a Great Team

More than almost any other medical problem, diabetes often requires a team approach. Unfortunately, multiple caregivers also means more expense and, sometimes, conflicting recommendations. Your particular health issues will dictate how many team members you need. If you have mild diabetes with no complications, a primary care provider might be the only person you see regularly, along with a yearly eye checkup by the ophthalmologist. But if you have a heart condition, you may be seeing a cardiologist as regularly as you do your primary care physician. Significant neuropathy may mean you'll need to see a podiatrist several times a year.

HEALTH PRACTITIONERS EVERYONE NEEDS TO SEE:

- **Primary Care Provider (PCP).** Your PCP can be an MD; usually people see a general or family practitioner or an internist; occasionally, an endocrinologist (see page 183) fills this role. Or, you may be under the care of a nurse practitioner or a physician's assistant. More important than the credentials following his name is whether your

PCP is looking at the whole range of your health issues, including your blood sugar levels, blood pressure, and cholesterol levels, as well as whether he's thorough and interested in your success.

- **Ophthalmologist or Optometrist.** Retinal disease and vision loss are common—and, understandably, feared—problems in diabetes. If you have diabetes or pre-diabetes you'll need to see an ophthalmologist or optometrist at least once a year; be sure to tell the eye doctor you have diabetes. Getting the tests to check vision or determine the lens prescription for your glasses is not enough; you'll need a retina exam and screening for glaucoma. If you see an optometrist, make sure that he includes these tests. Some PCP offices or clinics may have the equipment to take photos of your retina; these images can be sent to an eye specialist for evaluation.

SPECIALISTS YOU MAY NEED TO SEE:

- **Endocrinologist.** An endocrinologist is a physician who specializes in treating diseases of the hormone-producing glands. As insulin is a hormone, diabetes is considered a hormonal disorder. Endocrinologists also treat thyroid disease, pituitary disorders, high or low blood calcium, adrenal problems, and low testosterone or other sex hormone disorders. Some endocrinologists specialize in fertility issues, including the treatment of polycystic ovary syndrome, a common condition in women of childbearing age that often coexists with pre-diabetes. In many areas of the country there is a shortage of endocrinologists, particularly given the rapid increase in the prevalence of diabetes. Most people with type 2 diabetes will not need to see an endocrinologist, but many people with type 1 diabetes and those with type 2 who have had difficulty managing their blood sugar levels will benefit from seeing someone in this specialty.

- **Podiatrist.** A podiatrist or doctor of podiatric medicine (DPM) is a physician and surgeon specializing in foot and ankle care, including the treatment of diabetes-related conditions. People with peripheral neuropathy and sensory loss may get foot ulcers, or calluses that can become ulcerated if they are not treated. Surgery is sometimes necessary to correct a bad bunion or hammertoe to prevent ulcer formation. A podiatrist may trim the toenails of someone who has neuropathy and is at risk of injuring him- or herself. He may prescribe orthotics—specialized shoe inserts—or prescription shoes with increased depth in the toe cap to prevent irritation or skin breakdown.

- **Registered Dietitian or Nutritionist.** As complete as the diet advice in the Best Life program is, you may still benefit from added counseling from a nutrition expert. Because anyone can call herself a nutritionist, you need to seek out a person with the proper credentials. You know you're in good hands if your nutritionist is a registered dietitian (RD) because, at minimum, she has a bachelor's degree in nutrition or a related field, has completed an internship in the nutrition field, and passed a comprehensive nutrition exam. Like MDs, RDs must stay up to date in their field to keep their license. A nutritionist who is not an RD is also usually a perfectly good choice as long as she has a nutrition degree from an accredited college. Your nutritionist can give you the extra help necessary to lose weight or bring your prediabetes, diabetes, blood pressure, or cholesterol under control. She can also help you with any special dietary needs if you have kidney or liver disease.

- **Certified Diabetes Educator (CDE).** A CDE is someone who has special training and experience in counseling people on all aspects of their diabetes care. Most certified diabetes educators are nurses or registered dietitians who undergo additional training. They know their stuff: they've had to log many hours of teaching and counseling people with diabetes before taking a certification exam. Like nutritionists, many work in hospital settings, but some are in private practice. They are often key people in the diabetes self-education programs run by many hospitals and other health care organizations. They counsel pregnant women with diabetes and many times are the frontline health care providers who, under a physician's supervision, help people with type 1 diabetes adjust their insulin regimens.

- **Mental Health Professional.** If stress, depression, or anxiety become too much for you to handle, you may need some professional help. Psychiatrists, psychologists, social workers, therapists, and even life coaches can help you. Counseling may be all that is necessary, but some people may need antidepressant or antianxiety medication. Remember, though, that many studies have shown that regular exercise is a powerful tool in the battle against depression and anxiety. If you're feeling blue, try ramping up your exercise as the first step.

- **Other Medical and Surgical Specialists.** Sometimes specialists are needed for the evaluation or treatment of problems resulting from diabetes. If you're having chest pain or shortness of breath, you may need to see a cardiologist to diagnose the problem. Blocked arteries to the heart can be treated by the cardiologist with angioplasty, in which the blockage is opened by a balloon, often with a stent or flexible tube put in place to prevent it from coming back. Blockages in arteries to the heart that can't be treated with angioplasty may require a cardiothoracic surgeon to do coronary artery bypass graft surgery. Blocked arteries to the brain or lower extremities may require evaluation by a vascular surgeon, and angioplasty or bypass can be done in these arteries too. In most cases your PCP or endocrinologist can treat painful neuropathy, but if your symptoms are unusual in some way or are not responding to treatment, you may need to see a neurologist.

- **Personal Trainer.** Although not technically a health care practitioner, an exercise expert can make a big impact on your well-being. He can ensure that a routine is safe, effective, and tailored to fit you and your needs. He will also help you fine-tune your workouts so you'll get results without wasting a lot of time or energy. For instance, he can help you build on the twelve-week program on page 355 and show you proper technique for the Basic Eight on page 179. Finally, he can help you set realistic goals and keep you motivated. Prices vary widely from about $30 to $250 per hour, so shop around. To cut costs, you can invest in just one session to help familiarize yourself with the machines at your gym or you can round up a few friends for group sessions and split the fee. Your trainer should hold a current certification in CPR and be certified by an organization such as the ACSM (American College of Sports Medicine) or ACE (American Council on Exercise); visit their Web sites to search online for certified trainers near you.

WHEN YOU'RE SICK . . .

In most people with stable diabetes, minor illnesses are not a big deal. You'll be able to weather a cold or flulike problem without too much difficulty. The real issue is recognizing when things are getting to be more than you can safely handle at home and when you need to contact your doctor.

Common sense will tell you the main thing you need to know about being sick with diabetes: you have to monitor yourself much more frequently and be prepared to get help if you're getting worse. When you're sick, your body becomes less responsive to insulin, which means that your blood sugar level is probably going to go higher. If you have pre-diabetes, your blood sugar level may well rise into the clearly diabetic range, and many people first learn that they have diabetes during an illness. If you have diabetes and are on oral medication, you shouldn't take more without talking to your doctor. If you're on insulin, and especially if you have type 1 diabetes, you are probably accustomed to adjusting your insulin doses regularly. When you are sick, you may need a big increase in your insulin dosage, but it's really impossible to predict ahead of time how much more you'll need.

The single biggest risk for anyone with diabetes who is sick is dehydration. Dehydration is a problem for anyone who is ill; everyone has received the advice to "get enough rest and drink plenty of fluids." But the issue with diabetes is much more serious: If your blood sugar levels go very high, you will start to lose glucose in your urine, and this will cause your body to produce more urine. If you have a fever, you will be losing even more water in your sweat and in the air you exhale when breathing. People who are admitted to the hospital with out-of-control diabetes have often lost 10 pounds or more of fluid from their bodies.

Severely out-of-control blood sugar levels in diabetes accompanied by dehydration can cause conditions referred to as either diabetic ketoacidosis (DKA), mostly in people with type 1 diabetes, or the hyperglycemic hyperosmolar state (HHS) in those with type 2. Both of these conditions are characterized by very high blood sugar levels and severe dehydration. The main difference is that in DKA there is no effective insulin action and the glucose can't get into cells at all. This causes your body to make ketones, substances used as alternative sources of fuel when your body can't use insulin. Ketones are acidic and in large amounts cause major chemical changes in your blood, making you even sicker. You can check for ketones in your body, usually using a dipstick urine test. The presence of ketones, especially in large quantities, means you should contact your doctor or seek medical attention.

If you have diabetes and you're sick, here are the basic things you need to do:

- Make sure you get lots of fluids so you don't get dehydrated. You should weigh yourself to make sure you're not losing a lot of water weight. You'll need to take in enough salt to keep the water in your system, so you may need to eat some chicken broth or other clear soup.

- Get enough calories and carbohydrates to meet your energy needs. You may need to eat foods that are simple to digest, such as crackers or gelatin. Try to get 50 grams of carbohydrate into your system every three or four hours. If you can't eat because of nausea or stomach upset, you may have to drink sugar-containing liquids such as regular ginger ale—something we don't normally want you to do—just to get enough carbohydrates.

- Test your blood sugar level more frequently, at least every three to four hours. If you have type 1 diabetes, be prepared to take extra insulin.

- If you have type 1 diabetes, test the ketone level in your urine or blood. If it's high, make sure it comes down as you take in more fluid and insulin.

You should call your doctor:

- If your sugars are above about 250 for more than twenty-four hours.

- If your ketones are high and won't come down after several hours of treatment.

- If you're losing weight.

- If you can't keep down fluids or are losing more fluids with vomiting or diarrhea than you can keep down.

- If you develop abdominal pain.

- If you notice a change in your breathing.

- If you have a high fever that won't come down.

- If you or a family member find that you are confused or sleepy and difficult to awaken.

These all may be signs of DKA or HHS. If you can't reach your doctor and your situation is not getting better, you may have to call 911 or have someone take you to a hospital emergency room. Diabetes that's badly out of control is a medical emergency. It's a problem that's easy to treat in its early stages, but more difficult to manage and sometimes even fatal if allowed to go on.

JUDGING YOUR SUCCESS

To know if you're successful at Phase Three, you'll need to examine more than a checklist of goals; you have to look at the totality of your life. Do you think you're "Living Your Best Life"? Part of it is having blood sugar in the good range, staying healthy, and avoiding the complications of diabetes and pre-diabetes with a great diet, a challenging exercise plan, regularly scheduled doctor's appointments, and all the other components of this program. But, as you well know, there's more to feeling happy and success-ful: good relationships, a stimulating environment, a sense of satisfaction, and all the other facets that round out a good life. We've given you many of the tools needed to live your best life; keep using them to carve out this work in progress.

5

DRUGS USED TO TREAT DIABETES AND PREVENT COMPLICATIONS

NO SUBJECT GENERATES MORE questions among people with diabetes than the medicines they take. It's no wonder: diabetes drugs are powerful—even lifesaving—but they can have major side effects and are often expensive. The number of medications available for treating diabetes has increased tremendously, so even physicians sometimes find it hard to keep up with all the options now available. With the number of people affected increasing so rapidly, the list of medication options will continue to grow as drug companies dedicate more of their research effort to diabetes treatment. In addition, most people with diabetes take more than one medication. In this chapter, we're going to review all the medications available to treat diabetes and focus on practical aspects that you need to know.

The medical management of your disease may not end with diabetes drugs. You could be taking drugs to treat or prevent conditions that accompany diabetes and pre-diabetes, such as high blood pressure or heart disease. Or you may be seeing specialists to help ward off—or treat—neuropathy, retinopathy, erectile dysfunction, kidney disease, or other complications. The second part of this chapter guides you through the medical aspects of preventing complications and offers some advice on treatment. If you don't have any complications (and hopefully this program will help prevent them), you'll still get a lot out of reading about them. You'll know what symptoms to look for, and which tests you need to detect any issues early, when you can nip them in the bud. And finally, you'll learn about the exciting directions for treating—maybe even curing—diabetes in the future.

Throughout this book, we've emphasized good dietary and exercise habits as the keys to reversing pre-diabetes and preventing diabetes and the complications it can cause. But it's important to remember that needing medication does not mean that your efforts have failed. We said right from the opening pages that taking care of diabetes requires the strength of three pillars: diet, exercise, and medication. It's great if a person can keep his blood sugar, blood pressure, and cholesterol under control without medicine. But sometimes even someone who's done everything right will need medication. At the same time, being on medication doesn't lessen the importance of a healthy lifestyle.

Let's give an example: Cheryl is overweight and has a family history of diabetes. She sees her doctor for a regular checkup and learns that she has pre-diabetes, with a fasting blood glucose of 116. She's told to change her lifestyle, eat more healthful food, and exercise. She does so, and as a result she loses a lot of her belly fat. When she sees her doctor again in six months, her blood sugar level is normal. Cheryl is thrilled and dedicates herself to continued good behavior. Her blood glucose level, blood pressure, and cholesterol levels all stay where they should at her regular doctor visits.

Four years later, Cheryl is told that her blood sugar level has risen again, even though she has maintained all of the healthy habits that initially helped lower her blood sugar. After another year, her fasting glucose level has risen to 152. On repeat testing, the value is 136. Her doctor tells Cheryl she has diabetes and recommends that she start taking metformin.

What did Cheryl do wrong? Nothing. Unfortunately, as time passed, her body made less insulin, and even though she has kept her weight at a healthy level and exercised regularly, the amount of insulin her pancreas can manufacture is no longer enough to keep her blood sugar levels normal. Does this mean her efforts over the past several years have been wasted? Absolutely not! First, she delayed the start of medication for several years, and she will need much less medicine because she has a healthy diet and is physically active. Second, her weight loss has reduced her insulin resistance, helping to keep her blood pressure and cholesterol at healthy levels—two feats that blood sugar control through medication alone would not have accomplished. Her efforts have been well worth it. She knows it and plans to keep it up.

Often people ask whether they can ever go off of medication for diabetes once it has been started. The answer for people with type 1 diabetes is no because they completely or almost completely lack insulin production. For those with type 2, the answer varies depending on the particular situation. In someone who has insulin resistance as the primary problem, significant weight loss can mean putting away the medicine, perhaps even permanently. In a person whose insulin production has declined, it may be more difficult to come off the medication altogether, but often the number of medications can be reduced or the doses cut back. And some people who require insulin may be able to shift to oral medication.

What about drug treatment of pre-diabetes? Only recently have doctors recognized that pre-diabetes is associated with serious medical problems, especially an increased risk of heart disease, and there are no medications that are specifically designed for those with pre-diabetes. The emphasis with medication therapy has been to keep blood sugar levels near normal in those with diabetes, but blood sugar control alone doesn't address the insulin resistance that is the basis for the increased risk of vascular disease in pre-diabetes. Reducing your intra-abdominal fat through diet and exercise is the best way to improve insulin resistance, but certain medications may be of value for those with pre-diabetes. Metformin (see page 196), in particular, may be appropriate for the treatment of pre-diabetes. As we go through the various medications in the following pages, we'll highlight how drugs affect insulin resistance and their potential value in those whose blood sugar levels have yet to rise into the diabetic range.

HOW YOUR DOCTOR THINKS
ABOUT DIABETES MEDICATIONS

People tend to lump diabetes medicines into two categories, pills or insulin, but in order to understand why a specific medication makes sense in a given situation, you need to ask *why* the sugar is high (insulin resistance, insulin deficiency, or both) and *when* the sugar is high (whether you have a greater elevation of fasting glucose, or the sugars are highest after eating, or whether both are a problem). These are the questions your doctor tries to answer when he or she is making decisions about diabetes medications.

For someone with type 1 diabetes, the *why* question has a clear answer: the person is not making insulin and will need insulin treatment. For someone with type 2 diabetes, the answer is not always so simple. Someone with significant abdominal obesity is likely to benefit from a medication targeting insulin resistance. Someone who is relatively slender may have diabetes that results from impaired insulin production, and a medication that increases the amount of insulin made by the body may be more effective. Many people with type 2 diabetes have both problems, and medications attacking both are often used in combination.

When can be answered only by you, and requires that you do finger-stick blood glucose tests and keep a careful record of the results. Remember that the glucose in your blood comes from two sources: the food you eat, and during periods of fasting, glucose released by the liver. In some people with diabetes, their blood sugar spikes following meals; in others, the spike is caused by excess glucose released by the liver. Some medications target one problem more effectively than the other, so knowing when blood sugar levels are highest is essential to using medications for diabetes intelligently. Conversely, knowing when blood sugar levels may be going low can help prevent serious hypoglycemic reactions. By providing your doctor with finger-stick test results that reveal patterns in glucose fluctuations, you can become a partner in making good medication decisions.

One specific pattern needs special consideration: high fasting blood glucose values. It seems perfectly logical for blood sugar levels to rise after eating, but many people are surprised to find that they have higher glucose levels when they get up than they do before other meals of the day, such as dinner. Higher blood sugar levels in the morning mean that you have less insulin action in your body overnight. We often see this in people treated with medications such as the sulfonylureas (page 194), which are more effective at promoting insulin release following eating than during prolonged fasting.

In addition, there are two special conditions that may raise fasting glucose levels. The first is called the dawn phenomenon, which results from an increase in certain hormones in the body, especially the stress hormone cortisol, beginning at three or four o'clock in the morning. Cortisol increases insulin resistance, often causing a rise in blood sugar values. The other problem is called the Somogyi effect. This refers to a blood sugar level that rises in the early morning after the person experiences an unrecognized hypoglycemic event during the night. High morning glucose values should prompt some testing at bedtime and then a few tests at 2 or 3 A.M., just to rule out nocturnal hypoglycemia. Clues to nighttime hypoglycemia include fitful sleep, nightmares, or awakening drenched in sweat.

MEDICATIONS USED IN THE TREATMENT OF TYPE 2 DIABETES

Let's talk about the specific medications used to treat diabetes; we'll discuss these by class. A class of drugs is a group whose members are similar in terms of how they work and what side effects they tend to have. A few notes on some of the information we've included on the following pages: The cost information comes from *Consumer Reports* and from a survey of national pharmacy chains. We include the generic (or chemical) names of medications throughout, whether or not it is available to purchase instead of the brand name. We want you to know the generic names because something that isn't available as a generic today will probably be available as a less expensive generic in the future.

As we describe each class of drugs, we suggest you focus on the "why"—the underlying cause or causes—of a person's diabetes and the "when" of high or low blood sugars. Our goal is for you to be well informed about your medications and thoughtful about the patterns in your blood sugars. This will allow you to work with your doctor or other health care provider in figuring out the best regimen of medications for you.

Medications That Increase Insulin Production

Sulfonylureas—Glyburide, Glipizide, and Glimepiride

	GENERIC NAME	BRAND NAME	TOTAL DAILY DOSE
Drug names	Glyburide	Micronase, DiaBeta, Glynase	1.25–20 mg
	Glipizide	Glucotrol, Glucotrol XL	2.5–20 mg
	Glimepiride	Amaryl	1–8 mg
Cost per month	$4–$12	$35–$94	
When to take	30 minutes prior to meals, either once daily or divided into two doses		
Side effects	Hypoglycemia		
Effect on weight	Moderate tendency for weight gain		
Special concerns	Alcohol increases the risk of hypoglycemia		

Sulfonylureas are the oldest class of medications other than insulin used for diabetes treatment. These medicines work by helping the body make more of its own insulin, and, provided the pancreas is still functioning, the medications are often very effective. All of the drugs are available generically, and they are inexpensive. They are most effective in treating the rise in glucose that occurs after you've eaten (postprandial glucose, to use medical terminology). Knowing whether the medications are effective involves doing after-meal finger-stick testing, and if, two hours after eating, the glucose level is higher than desired (under 140 is ideal; up to about 180 may be acceptable), the dose may need to be increased or there may need to be a change in medication.

Sulfonylurea medicines should be taken before eating. If you take the medicines once daily, about 30 minutes before breakfast is best. If you are on a twice-daily schedule, you should take the medicine 30 minutes before breakfast and 30 minutes before dinner. Sometimes confusion arises because the bottle may have a sticker that says, "Take with food." That's actually a bit misleading. The medicine is labeled this way to prevent a low-blood-sugar reaction if you take the medicine and then don't eat anything for several hours.

In fact, hypoglycemic reactions are by far the most serious side effect of the sulfonylureas. They can occur anytime, including at night in some people. Some doctors have their patients use these medicines before bed in order to lower their fasting glucose values. This works for some people, but in others can lead to episodes of hypoglycemia while sleeping, which may be dangerous. These drugs have a moderate risk of weight gain, and that risk is partly related to the potential to cause a low-blood-sugar reaction, which can lead to overeating.

It is important to note that alcohol intensifies the risk of hypoglycemia with the sulfonylureas. People with diabetes often ask whether they can drink. If you're taking one of these drugs, you'll need to be careful about alcohol consumption, especially if you haven't eaten. When there's alcohol in your bloodstream, the sulfonylureas trigger an even greater insulin release than they do under normal circumstances, so your blood sugar can go much too low.

Meglitinides—Prandin and Starlix

	GENERIC NAME	BRAND NAME	TOTAL DAILY DOSE
Drug names	Repaglinide	Prandin	0.5–4 mg before each meal
	Nateglinide	Starlix	60–120 mg before each meal
Cost per month	N.A.	$174–$195	
When to take	From 30 minutes up to immediately before each meal		
Side effects	Hypoglycemia (though the risk is lower than with the sulfonylureas)		
Effect on weight	Modest tendency for weight gain		

Meglitinides are similar to the sulfonylureas in many ways. They also prompt the body to make more insulin, though they do so in a chemically different way from the sulfonylureas, so they are considered a different class of medication. They are faster-acting than the sulfonylureas, and their effect doesn't last as long. This means that they have to be taken more often, and in most cases, they should be taken with each meal. This makes them less convenient, but it also means they are less likely to cause severe hypoglycemia. Meglitinides are also less potent. This would be a disadvantage in most people, but in those prone to hypoglycemia, Prandin and Starlix may be safer than the sulfonylureas. Overall, Prandin and Starlix are prescribed much less often than the sulfonylurea medicines because they're more expensive, less potent, and have to be taken more frequently.

Medicines That Reduce Insulin Resistance

Metformin

	GENERIC NAME	BRAND NAME	TOTAL DAILY DOSE
Drug names	Metformin	Glucophage, Glucophage XR, Glumetza, Fortamet, Riomet	500–2,500 mg daily, usually in divided doses
Cost per month	$9–$18	$77–$154	
When to take	Effective anytime but best tolerated if taken with food		
Side effects	Bloating, gas, diarrhea		
Effect on weight	Moderate tendency for weight loss		
Specific concerns	Cannot be used by people with kidney disease		

Metformin is literally in a class by itself, at least in the United States, where no other member of this family of drugs is available. It is the medication that is used most as a first-line drug treatment for diabetes, and for good reasons. The medication is very effective in many people, an inexpensive generic is available, and, unlike many diabetes medications, it tends to promote weight loss rather than weight gain. Metformin works by reducing the amount of glucose that is produced by the liver. Unlike the sulfonylureas and meglitinides, metformin does not have to be taken before meals to be effective. The major problem with metformin is that it causes significant gastrointestinal side effects in many people, especially bloating, gas, and diarrhea. These side effects can be reduced by (1) starting at a low dose and gradually working up to a larger one; (2) taking the medication with food or even after eating; and (3) using the extended-release form of the medication. Sometimes people who have tolerated the drug for a long time get a stomach flu or something similar and find that they can no longer take metformin without experiencing lots of gastrointestinal symptoms. In these cases, the medication can be stopped temporarily and then restarted, sometimes at a low dose, and increased as tolerated. Even though the extended-release form is tolerated better, many physicians prefer to start with the regular form because it is often associated with more weight loss. Some of the weight loss may relate to gastrointestinal symptoms, and it may be that the people who lose weight most effectively are those with mild queasiness—not enough to be a problem but just enough to reduce the appetite.

As we discussed in the opening chapter, insulin resistance is one of the key factors leading to diabetes, but it is increasingly recognized as an important issue in other settings as well. Insulin resistance itself increases the risk of cardiovascular disease, and most physicians now consider pre-diabetes to be a serious condition, not only because of the likely progression to diabetes but also because heart disease risk is higher in people with blood sugars in the pre-diabetic range than in those with normal blood sugar levels. Many physicians and diabetes researchers think it's appropriate to the treat people with pre-diabetes with metformin, and some even advocate the use of metformin in a person with abdominal obesity, even if he or she has normal blood sugar levels. In addition, polycystic ovary syndrome (PCOS) is often treated with metformin. PCOS is a metabolic disorder that affects women of childbearing age. The symptoms include irregular periods and infertility, as well as excessive facial and body hair, acne, and hair loss from the scalp. PCOS is a complex disorder and not fully understood, but a major part of its cause appears to be insulin resistance. A high percentage of women with PCOS are also overweight. Metformin treatment sometimes helps with weight loss, often corrects irregular menstrual periods, and definitely improves fertility. In fact, because PCOS is one of the most common causes of infertility, metformin, a medication thought of as a diabetes drug, is also one of the most widely used infertility treatments. It's important to emphasize that all uses of metformin other than the treatment of diabetes are "off label." That is, the Food and Drug Administration (FDA) has not approved metformin for use in these areas, but it is often of benefit and physicians frequently prescribe it for these purposes.

Metformin carries a low risk of lactic acidosis, a very serious side effect. Lactic acid is a chemical made by muscle cells; the kidneys must get rid of lactic acid, otherwise it builds up in the blood. When too much lactic acid accumulates in the blood, a person develops lactic acidosis. The symptoms are not very specific: abnormal breathing, nausea and vomiting, abdominal pain, and confusion are all common. The condition is very treatable if it is detected early but may lead to organ damage or even death if not corrected. Metformin increases lactic acid production. If the kidneys are working properly, this isn't a problem. However, in people who have kidney disease, usually with an elevated creatinine level (see page 238), metformin increases the risk of lactic acidosis, so the drug should not be used. In other situations where the kidney function may be reduced, such as in people who have heart failure or are on diuretics, a doctor may recommend against using metformin. The intravenous dye given for CT scans and certain other X-ray tests may damage the kidneys, so the usual recommendation is to stop metformin for about twenty-four to forty-eight hours around the time of the test, until it's clear that the kidneys weren't harmed. Some doctors are hesitant to use metformin in older people— usually those over 80—because they often have some underlying kidney dysfunction and are prone to dehydration; both are conditions that can make kidney function even worse if they become ill.

Here's an important point: people who are told about the risk of lactic acidosis often come away with the message that "metformin is bad for your kidneys." This is not correct. Metformin doesn't *cause* kidney damage; it just can't be used in those who already have kidney damage for some other reason, such as diabetes or high blood pressure.

There's one last intriguing fact about metformin: it may increase longevity. Some of you may know that severe calorie restriction, sometimes referred to as a "starvation diet," extends the life expectancy of almost all animals. Severe calorie restriction increases the function of a cell protein called AMP kinase, which in turn improves cell survival. Metformin has the same effect on AMP kinase. Studies have shown that mice treated with metformin live longer than those that are not given the medicine. This is research to watch for in the future.

Thiazolidinediones (TZDs)—Actos and Avandia

	GENERIC NAME	BRAND NAME	TOTAL DAILY DOSE
Drug names	Pioglitazone	Actos	15–45 mg
	Rosiglitazone	Avandia	2–8 mg
Cost per month	N.A.	$80–$274	
When to take	Once daily at any time, with or without food		
Side effects	Fluid retention, swelling		
Effect on weight	Often cause weight gain		
Special concerns	May worsen edema or heart failure		

Actos and Avandia are drugs that help your body respond better to insulin; they work by increasing the amount of glucose taken up into muscle cells in response to insulin. They are unique among diabetes drugs in that you need to wait a minimum of two or three weeks in most cases to see any effect, and it may take six weeks or even longer in some cases to see the full benefit. The same is true when they're stopped: you will have to wait several weeks for the effects, and often the side effects, to go away. They are easy to take, and, given how long they last, it is never necessary to take them more than once a day.

The thiazolidinediones, also called TZD drugs or glitazones, are highly effective for diabetes, but endocrinologists have differing views on these medications: some are strong advocates, while others are cautious about their use because of side effects. On the positive side, the drugs seem to maintain their blood sugar–lowering benefits longer than many of the others. For example, the study known as A Diabetes Outcome Progression Trial, or ADOPT, published in late 2006, showed that people treated with Avandia as their only diabetes medication maintained better blood sugar levels and had more sustained improvement in insulin resistance over five years than those treated with either glyburide or metformin. There have been some data suggesting that these drugs help maintain the function of beta cells (the insulin-producing cells in the pancreas) over time, and many doctors believe that this is key to the management of diabetes in the long term. On the negative side, there is often weight gain with these medications, sometimes quite significant. The drugs tend to cause salt and water retention, and they frequently worsen edema, or swelling of the legs, and congestive heart failure.

There is also controversy over whether one of the drugs, Avandia, is associated with an increased risk of heart disease. The concern was first raised by a highly publicized review of data from many studies published in 2007. Follow-up research has yielded mixed results, but the FDA now requires a "black box" warning about possible heart disease risk on the package insert for Avandia. In July 2010, an advisory panel to the FDA recommended that Avandia remain on the market, though panel members were highly divided on the question. As of press time, the FDA has not reached a decision about whether to keep Avandia on the market. Similar studies have not identified an increased risk of heart disease for those using Actos, though the reason for this difference is not clear.

Obviously, the decision to start any medication is a highly individual one, and this is especially true when there is any controversy surrounding a particular drug. In many people, Actos and Avandia provide superb control of blood sugar with no side effects whatsoever and possibly with benefits that other medications cannot provide. In other people, side effects such as worsening of heart failure are clear reasons not to use the medicines. As with all medications, if your doctor prescribes either of the TZDs, familiarize yourself with the advantages and disadvantages and watch to make sure that things are going as you and your doctor had hoped. It's worth asking your doctor periodically whether any new information concerning these medications has become available, as there are ongoing studies involving both that will help us know over the longer term whether the safety concerns are justified or were exaggerated.

Drugs Related to Hormones Other than Insulin

Insulin may be the main hormone that helps to regulate blood sugar, but there are others that have an important role in keeping glucose levels within the healthy range. There are three that are important where diabetes medications are concerned: glucagon, glucagon-like peptide-1 (usually called GLP-1) and amylin.

Glucagon is the second most important hormone related to blood sugar control. Unlike insulin, which lowers blood sugar, glucagon raises it, and it can be used for the treatment of low blood sugar in an emergency. Under normal circumstances, glucagon is one of the hormones that helps balance insulin, preventing the blood sugar level from going too low. While glucagon plays an important role in balancing insulin under normal circumstances, there is evidence that too much glucagon production contributes to high blood sugar levels in many people with diabetes.

GLP-1 gets its name from the fact that it is chemically similar to glucagon, but, like insulin, it lowers blood sugar. GLP-1 is made by cells in the intestine after eating, and it travels via the bloodstream to the pancreas, where it increases the amount of insulin that's made and also reduces the amount of glucagon. Several medications available to treat diabetes increase the effects of GLP-1: Januvia and Onglyza, oral medications, and Byetta and Victoza, given by injection.

The same beta cells in the pancreas that make insulin also make amylin. Amylin lowers blood sugar primarily by reducing the amount of glucagon that is made. Symlin, a medication that must be given by injection, mimics the action of amylin in helping to keep blood sugar levels low.

DPP4-Inhibitors—Januvia and Onglyza

	GENERIC NAME	BRAND NAME	TOTAL DAILY DOSE
Drug names	Sitagliptin	Januvia	25–100 mg
	Saxagliptin	Onglyza	2.5–5 mg
Cost per month	N.A.	$225	
When to take	Once daily at any time, with or without food		
Side effects	Few side effects in most people		
Effect on weight	Usually no change in weight		

Januvia and Onglyza increase the amount of GLP-1 in the body. Under normal circumstances, GLP-1 lasts only a few minutes in the blood before an enzyme called dipeptidyl peptidase 4, or DPP-4, breaks it down. Januvia and Onglyza prevent DPP-4 from breaking down GLP-1, so the GLP-1 stays in the blood longer; in response, the body makes more insulin and less glucagon than it would without these drugs. Together, these actions lower the blood sugar level.

Januvia and Onglyza are easy to take and generally have few side effects. They're expensive but have less of a tendency to cause weight gain than some of the other medications and carry a fairly low risk of hypoglycemia. Januvia has been approved for use in the United States only since late 2006, and so far, its safety track record is good, though a recent study reported that Januvia may cause pancreatitis (see page 203) in experiments with rats. Interestingly, giving metformin along with Januvia seemed to protect against this problem. Onglyza became available in 2009.

Hormone Analogs—Byetta, Victoza, and Symlin

	GENERIC NAME	BRAND NAME	TOTAL DAILY DOSE
Drug names	Exenatide	Byetta	5–10 mcg twice daily
	Liraglutide	Victoza	0.6–1.8 mcg once daily
	Pramlintide	Symlin	15–120 mcg three times daily
Cost per month	N.A.	$220–$276	
When to take	Approximately 1 hour before meals twice daily for Byetta; once daily at any time for Victoza; immediately before each meal for Symlin		
Side effects	Nausea and worsening of acid reflux; hypoglycemia		
Effect on weight	Often promote weight loss		
Special concerns	Rare cases of pancreatitis have been reported with Byetta		

Byetta and Victoza are similar to the hormone GLP-1, and Symlin is similar to the hormone amylin. Like insulin, they are proteins and would be broken down by acid in the stomach if taken orally, so they must be injected under the skin. Byetta and Victoza come in pen form; Symlin comes both in pens and in vials for use with syringes.

Since it was introduced in 2006, Byetta has been prescribed widely. Two words tell the story of its popularity: weight loss. In addition to increasing insulin and reducing glucagon, GLP-1 slows stomach emptying, leading to a feeling of fullness, and may suppress the appetite center in the brain. Even with Januvia, the levels of naturally occurring GLP-1 are not high enough to have a significant impact on appetite, but the GLP-1 effect with Byetta is great enough to reduce appetite. Not everyone loses weight on the drug, and among those who do lose weight, the amounts vary enormously—from as little as a couple of pounds to as much as 20 or 30 pounds or even more. Victoza, which has very similar effects, became available in 2010. A once-weekly form of Byetta and long-acting forms of similar products are in late-stage development at the present time and may be approved for use over the next several years.

Byetta and Victoza have significant side effects. Because they slow stomach emptying, they cause nausea in many people, though this problem tends to improve with time. Byetta and Victoza may make acid reflux (heartburn) worse. This can be a serious problem in someone with diabetic gastroparesis, a form of neuropathy in which the stomach already empties too slowly. A relatively rare but serious side effect reported with these drugs is pancreatitis, an inflammatory condition of the pancreas characterized by severe pain. Pancreatitis can result in chronic pain, digestive problems, and further worsening of diabetes. Severe cases are sometimes fatal. Pancreatitis appears to happen in fewer than 1 in 1,000 people on these medications, and for now there is no absolute proof that the drugs increase the risk of this condition. However, since it's such a serious problem, it's essential to tell your doctor if you have abdominal pain while taking either Byetta or Victoza.

Symlin works like Byetta except that it doesn't increase insulin production. It suppresses glucagon release following meals, slows stomach emptying, and lessens appetite. It is given before each meal, rather than just twice daily. Like all the drugs we're discussing, it's approved for use in people with type 2 diabetes, but it's the only medication other than insulin that's also approved for use in patients with type 1, where it is given in conjunction with insulin (see page 230). Symlin is available in both pens and vials and has a wider range of doses available than Byetta or Victoza. Sometimes people who can't tolerate Byetta or Victoza can take Symlin at very low doses. It's important to emphasize that though Byetta, Victoza, and Symlin facilitate weight loss in some people, they're approved only to treat diabetes. The drugs are presently being studied for the treatment of pre-diabetes and obesity.

Drugs That Slow the Digestion of Starch
Alpha-Glucosidase Inhibitors—Precose and Glyset

	GENERIC NAME	BRAND NAME	TOTAL DAILY DOSE
Drug names	Acarbose	Precose	25–100 mg
	Miglitol	Glyset	25–100 mg
Cost per month	$84–$108	$111–$132	
When to take	At the start of each meal containing starch		
Side effects	Bloating, gas, diarrhea		
Effect on weight	Modest tendency to promote weight loss		

Precose and Glyset are unusual in that they do not actually have to be absorbed into the body to have an effect. Instead, they interfere with enzymes in the intestine, such as alpha-glucosidase, that break down starches and sucrose (cane sugar) into the glucose and other simple sugar molecules that your body absorbs. The enzymes still work, but less rapidly, so your blood sugar doesn't rise as much or as quickly as it would following a meal containing starch. They are the only oral medications whose effects on blood sugar are not related to an increase in insulin or improvement in the body's response to insulin.

Precose and Glyset are not used as much as other diabetes medications because they frequently cause gastrointestinal side effects. These drugs work by interfering with the digestive process. This tends to promote weight loss, but also commonly results in intestinal side effects that resemble the symptoms of lactose intolerance, a condition in which people have difficulty digesting the milk sugar lactose. Most people have to start with a low dose, sometimes even just once daily, and work their way up.

When used alone, Precose or Glyset don't cause hypoglycemia, but they can worsen hypoglycemia caused by other drugs, such as the sulfonylureas, when used in combination. People who take Precose or Glyset should always carry glucose tablets or a glucose-containing gel for the treatment of hypoglycemia. That's because glucose is absorbed directly by the intestine into the bloodstream, but sucrose, the sugar in most foods and in our sugar bowls, must be broken down into simple sugars by alpha-glucosidase before being absorbed. Precose and Glyset slow this process down, delaying recovery from a hypoglycemic reaction if a sugar or starch other than glucose is used.

Other Medications

Welchol

	GENERIC NAME	BRAND NAME	TOTAL DAILY DOSE
Drug names	Colesevelam	Welchol	3.8 mg
Cost per month	N.A.	$238–$259	
When to take	Once or twice daily with food		
Side effects	Constipation, elevated triglycerides		
Effect on weight	Not much change		
Special concerns	May reduce the absorption of other medications		

Welchol is a bile-acid sequestrant, a class of medications used to treat high cholesterol, also discussed on page 236. The drug has also been approved by the FDA for the treatment of diabetes, but only in combination with metformin, the sulfonylureas, or insulin. The blood-sugar-lowering effect is relatively small, and standard treatment requires six pills per day. It would seem ideal to have a single drug that lowers both blood sugar and blood cholesterol, but given the cost, gastrointestinal side effects, and large number of tablets required for treatment, the medication is not considered first-line for either problem.

Bromocriptine

	GENERIC NAME	BRAND NAME	TOTAL DAILY DOSE
Drug names	Bromocriptine	Cycloset	0.8–4.8 mg
Cost per month	N.A.	N.A.	
When to take	Once daily in the morning		
Side effects	Nausea and vomiting, fatigue, dizziness, headache		
Effect on weight	Tends to cause weight loss		

In May 2009, the FDA approved the drug bromocriptine, brand name Cycloset, for the treatment of type 2 diabetes. Bromocriptine is not a new drug; it has been used for many years to treat certain kinds of pituitary tumors and, more recently, for the treatment of Parkinson's disease. Studies have shown that people with diabetes have reduced levels of dopamine, and low levels of dopamine are thought by some to contribute to insulin resistance. Bromocriptine mimics the action of dopamine in the brain, though it's not entirely clear whether this is the reason the drug lowers blood sugar levels. The role of this medication in diabetes management will become clear only over time.

As of the writing of this book, the form of the drug approved for use in diabetes has not yet come to market, so there is no widespread experience in using the medication for diabetes treatment and no information concerning cost. The side effects noted above are recognized with current use of the medication for other problems.

COMBINATION DIABETES DRUGS

Many of the drugs we've discussed are available in combinations of two drugs in one tablet. Listed below are the combination diabetes medications presently available in the United States. (The brand name is given in parentheses if the generic is not available.)

GlucoVance	Glyburide and metformin
Metaglip	Glipizide and metformin
Avandamet	Rosiglitazone (Avandia) and metformin
Avandaryl	Rosiglitazone (Avandia) and glimepiride
Actosplus Met	Pioglitazone (Actos) and metformin
Duetact	Pioglitazone (Actos) and glimepiride
Janumet	Sitagliptin (Januvia) and metformin

Understanding combination medicines involves nothing more than understanding the two separate components; combining them in one pill doesn't change how they work or what they do. The advantage of a combination medicine is that it's easier to take one pill than two, especially if you are on several medicines. The main disadvantage is that it isn't as easy to adjust medication doses. For example, if a patient is taking GlucoVance but is experiencing frequent episodes of hypoglycemia, the doctor may wish to reduce the glyburide dose but not the metformin dose. There are various dosage combinations of GlucoVance available, so the dosage adjustment could probably be made without changing medications, but a new prescription would be required. If the person were taking the two drugs separately, simply reducing the number of pills of glyburide or cutting a pill in half would achieve the same result.

Insulin

Virtually nothing about diabetes is as misunderstood as insulin treatment. Almost everyone who's unfamiliar with diabetes views insulin in negative terms; we often hear people say things like "I'll do anything but take insulin." We've talked about all the evidence showing that lowering blood sugar helps prevent blindness, kidney disease, and other serious problems. When someone says, "anything but insulin," does she really mean she would rather risk kidney failure and the need for dialysis than to take insulin? We don't think so, but that's the kind of anxiety that is raised by the idea of insulin treatment.

Here are some of the common myths about insulin treatment and the realities behind them:

Myth: Being on insulin means that you have a more severe disease than if you are on pills.	**Reality:** Disease severity is measured by the number and level of complications and by blood sugar swings, not by which medication you're on.
Myth: Insulin injections are painful.	**Reality:** Insulin shots hurt very little. Most people find that the finger-stick tests are actually more uncomfortable than insulin shots.

Myth: Insulin is a last resort. Your doctor should try every other diabetes drug before using insulin.

Reality: Even in type 2 diabetes, early treatment with insulin is often the best choice. Insulin should be used when it will work better at a lower cost and with fewer side effects than other drugs.

Myth: Insulin treatment can never be stopped.

Reality: People with type 1 diabetes will always need insulin treatment, but if a person with type 2 diabetes eats a proper diet, loses weight, and exercises regularly, he or she may be able to stop insulin treatment.

Here's something to consider: before insulin treatment, diabetes in children was uniformly fatal within months, and dramatically reduced the life span of adults who were diagnosed. Insulin therapy transformed this completely. In 1996 the Joslin Diabetes Center, a leading institution in diabetes research and treatment, handed out its first medal honoring someone who had survived seventy-five years with type 1 diabetes. The recipient developed diabetes in 1921, the year insulin was discovered.

Now think how you'd react if you woke up tomorrow and read the following newspaper headline: DOCTORS ANNOUNCE SUCCESSFUL TREATMENT FOR BREAST CANCER, and the article described how people diagnosed with breast cancer who injected themselves under the skin one or more times a day could have a nearly normal life expectancy. Would you think, "I wouldn't do that" or "I wouldn't want my mother or sister to do that." Of course not. You'd be ecstatic for anyone in your life who might have breast cancer. In the 1920s, insulin transformed diabetes in just this way, yet almost ninety years later, many people fear the very thing that has saved countless lives. Instead of fearing insulin, we need to return to fearing the consequences of uncontrolled diabetes, and recognizing the role insulin can play in helping prevent them.

We're not saying that insulin is the perfect treatment; it has to be prescribed correctly and used carefully, but it's no different from any other medication in this respect.

There are whole books on the subject of how to use insulin correctly; obviously we can't hope to cover all the aspects of insulin treatment in just a few paragraphs. Instead, we'll give a brief overview of the kinds of insulin that are available and cover some basic aspects of how it's used, especially for people with type 2 diabetes. (We'll talk about insulin treatment for people with type 1 diabetes on page 219.)

BASICS OF INSULIN TREATMENT FOR TYPE 2 DIABETES

All forms of insulin lower blood sugar levels, both by helping cells take up more glucose and, in the muscles and liver, by promoting the storage of that glucose as glycogen. In the liver, insulin also reduces the release of glucose into the blood plasma. In the past, insulin was extracted from animal pancreas tissue, but now virtually all insulin is made synthetically. The available forms of insulin either are identical to human insulin or are insulin analogs, meaning that they have slight chemical changes designed to give them special properties. Insulins differ primarily in terms of how long after injection they reach their maximum, or peak, activity and their total duration of action. At present, all insulin available in the United States must be given by injection. Insulin is available in an individual form or premixed. Premixed insulins combine the intermediate-acting NPH insulin with a faster-acting insulin in the hope of providing the benefits of both types with a single injection. The major insulins available in the United States are:

TYPE OF INSULIN	GENERIC	BRAND	PEAK ACTION	DURATION OF ACTION
Very-fast-acting	Lispro	Humalog	30–90 minutes	3–5 hours
	Aspart	NovoLog	40–50 minutes	3–5 hours
	Glulisine	Apidra	60–120 minutes	3–5 hours
Fast-acting	Regular or "R"	Humulin R	2–3 hours	5–8 hours
		Novolin R	2–3 hours	5–8 hours
Intermediate-acting	NPH or "N"	Humulin N	8 hours	20 hours
		Novolin N	8 hours	20 hours
	Lente	Humulin L	7–15 hours	18–24 hours
		Novolin L	7–15 hours	18–24 hours

(*continued on next page*)

TYPE OF INSULIN	GENERIC	BRAND	PEAK ACTION	DURATION OF ACTION
Long-acting	Glargine	Lantus	N.A.	24 hours
	Detemir	Levemir	N.A.	Up to 24 hours
Cost per month	Varies with the type of insulin and the dose. The least expensive are regular, NPH, and Lente. Humalog, NovoLog, Apidra, Lantus, and Levemir are available as brand name only.			
When to take	Varies; see below			
Side effects	Hypoglycemia			
Effect on weight	Tends to promote weight gain			

Premixed Insulins

BRAND NAME	IS A MIXTURE OF
Humulin 70/30, Novolin 70/30	70% NPH, 30% regular
Humulin 50/50	50% NPH, 50% regular
Humalog Mix 75/25	75% NPH-like, 25% Humalog
Humalog Mix 50/50	50% NPH-like, 50% Humalog
NovoLog Mix 70/30	70% NPH-like, 30% NovoLog

Normally insulin is made in your pancreas, and the best way to think about how to use insulin is to ask yourself what your pancreas would do if everything were working properly. When most people without diabetes fast, the glucose level remains fairly stable and the body makes a rather steady amount of insulin. Doctors refer to this as the basal insulin production, meaning the insulin that is around as a base or background all the time. When you eat a meal, your blood sugar rises; how quickly and how high depends on what you've eaten. In this situation, the body makes extra insulin to match the rising sugar. Doctors call this bolus insulin; the word "bolus" means an amount of food or medicine given all at once. Injected insulin can be used to meet your basal or background needs, your bolus or meal-related needs, or both. In people who make little or no insulin, such as many people with late-stage type 2 diabetes or anyone with type 1 diabetes, both insulin needs must be met, and doctors refer to this as basal-bolus insulin treatment (see page 220).

In people with type 2 diabetes, insulin is often used in combination with other medications. (The FDA may not specifically have approved some of these combinations, but doctors can still use the medications together and it's a sure bet that every conceivable combination has been used in someone.) One of the most common uses for insulin in type 2 diabetes is in someone who wakes up with a high blood sugar level but doesn't have as much of a problem later in the day. Most of the medications that work to help your body make more insulin, especially the sulfonylurea drugs such as glipizide, have a greater effect on meal-related insulin production than on fasting insulin production. The result is that many people, especially those on drugs such as glipizide, have higher glucose values in the morning than they do later in the day. A long-acting form of insulin, such as Lantus, will work very effectively to lower morning glucose values in this situation.

Let's take Bill's case, which is very typical. Bill was on 1,000 milligrams of metformin twice a day and 5 milligrams of glipizide in the morning before breakfast. His hemoglobin A1c level was 7.1, so his control overall was not bad, but his fasting glucose values were routinely over 140. His glucose values before dinner were lower—often in the 90s. His doctor wanted to lower his hemoglobin A1c and initially recommended increasing his glipizide, since his dose was less than the maximum. After three months on this, Bill did indeed have a lower A1c—it had fallen to 6.6—but his morning blood sugar levels hadn't changed very much and he was having frequent hypoglycemic episodes in the afternoon. He had also gained weight, partly because he was eating more to prevent the low blood sugar levels.

Bill was referred to an endocrinologist, who suggested he start on a long-acting insulin. At first Bill was shocked: "I didn't think my diabetes was that bad!" The endocrinologist reassured him that it had nothing to do with having "bad" diabetes but that the insulin would better prevent the rise in his overnight fasting blood sugar level. Bill reluctantly agreed. The doctor stopped Bill's glipizide and prescribed long-acting Lantus insulin at a low dose of 12 units per day. Bill was told that the initial amount of insulin would probably not do much but that he should go up on the dose by 1 unit every day until his blood sugar levels fell to under about 100.

Over the next several weeks, Bill did exactly as instructed. The first thing that surprised him was how easy the insulin shots were and how little they hurt. As he had been told, initially his blood sugar levels in the morning were still high, and the values before dinner were initially higher than they had been because he no longer had glipizide on board to help lower them later in the day. After about a month, when he was up to just over 40 units of insulin, his fasting glucose values started to fall and the predinner numbers fell along with them. He had his first fasting glucose test under 100 when he got to 56 units and stopped there for a few days before going up even more slowly until he settled at 60 units. Several months later, after he had been on a stable dose of insulin and metformin, his hemoglobin A1c was 6.7 and he had fasting glucose levels averaging about 90 and predinner numbers averaging about 105. His overall control was improved, he had a better balance in his premeal glucose levels throughout the day, he was no longer having episodes of hypoglycemia, and he had even lost some of the weight he had gained on the increased glipizide. Overall, his situation was clearly better.

A long-acting insulin, such as Lantus, can be used very effectively to bring down high morning glucose values and can be administered at any time of the day because the effect usually lasts twenty-four hours or more. The same result can often be achieved by using NPH insulin at bedtime; it is started at a low dose and increased gradually, just as with the long-acting insulin. The advantage of NPH insulin is that it's less expensive, but it's much more likely to cause a low-blood-sugar reaction overnight because its action rises to a peak level before starting to fall, whereas the Lantus has a much more consistent effect.

While many people with type 2 diabetes have high morning blood sugar levels, others have high glucose values after meals. Most oral medications, especially the sulfonylureas, work best to help with meal-related rises in blood glucose, but sometimes even a combination of oral medications doesn't prevent big spikes in glucose after meals. Other times, a person may have to take so much oral medication to control the rise in glucose that she experiences frequent episodes of hypoglycemia later. In either case, a rapid-acting insulin, such as Humalog, NovoLog, or Apidra, might be a good choice. People with type 1 diabetes usually take very-fast-acting insulin before each of their meals, as we discuss beginning on page 219.

People with type 2 diabetes often need this only with certain meals. For example, if your blood sugar level typically rises only to the high 100s after breakfast and lunch but is nearly 300 regularly after dinner, you might benefit from taking a rapid-acting form of insulin before the evening meal. This can be a very effective approach to keeping blood sugar levels down, but you have to be careful not to use it as a way to overeat while maintaining good blood sugar levels.

All of the insulins listed in the box on page 209 other than Lantus and Levemir can be mixed in the same injection and still retain their individual properties. There are several insulin combinations that come premixed in vials or syringes. These combine an intermediate-acting insulin, NPH, with a faster-acting insulin. The faster-acting insulin may be regular or "R" insulin or one of the very-fast-acting analogs, Humalog or NovoLog. Premixed insulins are designed to provide the benefit of both long-acting and short-acting insulin in the same shot. Most of the time, they are used twice daily, before breakfast and before dinner, with the idea that the short-acting insulin will help with the meal-related glucose rise and the longer-acting insulin will provide background coverage between meals. Their obvious advantage is convenience, and when they work well, it is certainly easier to use a premixed insulin than to take separate shots or mix the insulins yourself. The disadvantage is that the proportion of the two insulins is fixed and there is no way to take more short-acting insulin for a larger meal without also increasing the longer-acting insulin. Also, because the NPH rises to a peak of action, the mixed insulins are much more likely to cause hypoglycemia between meals than when a very-long-acting insulin, such as Lantus, and a very-short-acting insulin are given as separate shots.

By far the most serious side effect of any form of insulin therapy is hypoglycemia. Before the widespread availability of home glucose monitors, this was much more of a concern. In fact, until the 1980s people were often hospitalized for several days when insulin treatment was initiated because there was no other practical way to get numerous blood sugar readings in the course of a day to help with dosage adjustment. Now that people can monitor their glucose levels at home, insulin dosages can be adjusted with much greater confidence and much less anxiety. Still, low-blood-sugar reactions remain a concern, and as you increase your physical activity or improve your diet, there is a good likelihood that your insulin dose will need to be reduced, unless your blood sugar levels were not well controlled before you made the lifestyle changes.

The other major negative aspect of insulin treatment is weight gain—but it's not a foregone conclusion that you will pack on the pounds. Weight gain while using insulin depends on two factors. The first is how much your blood sugar falls after starting treatment. For instance, a person who starts with an A1c of 10 and falls to 7 on treatment is more likely to gain weight than someone who starts with an A1c of 7.5 and falls to 7, regardless of whether the person is treated with oral medications or insulin. What's the connection between improved blood sugar levels and weight gain? You know that a common symptom of out-of-control diabetes is excessive urination; when this happens you lose glucose, and calories, in your urine. The higher your blood sugar level, the more calories you're losing. Your body compensates for this loss by ramping up your appetite. If you start taking a medication that lowers your blood sugar quickly, you'll no longer lose glucose and calories in the urine, but your appetite won't reset for a while. It's during this time that people are most prone to gain weight. The higher your starting A1c, the more weight you are likely to gain. This is a strong argument for not allowing yourself to get out of control in the first place. The second factor is whether you are experiencing hypoglycemic episodes, which tend to cause overeating; avoiding hypoglycemia will help minimize weight gain. Sometimes people gain less weight with insulin than they do with oral medications because if insulin is used properly it may be less prone to cause low blood sugar levels than some pills.

Even though we've spent several pages discussing insulin, we haven't addressed the practical, day-to-day aspect of using insulin, such as how and where to inject, how to mix insulins, and proper storage and travel considerations. Your doctor, diabetes educator, or pharmacist can give you lots of information on these aspects of insulin treatment, and they are also covered in the diabetes self-management courses offered by many hospitals. The pharmaceutical companies that manufacture insulin can also provide booklets and even DVDs demonstrating the injection techniques. The complicated part of insulin use is emotional: overcoming the anxiety about insulin treatment that is so common. Once most people establish a routine, they find the reality of insulin treatment easy.

INSULIN PENS, PUMPS, PATCHES, PUFFERS, AND PILLS

When many people think of insulin, they envision syringes and vials, alcohol swabs, and big needles. In actuality, insulin is very easy to use, and the needles have become so small that most people report little discomfort. All insulin available in the United States must be given by injection, but there are several injection options and researchers are working on developing noninjection systems. Let's take a look at what is available now or will be on the market shortly.

- **Insulin pens.** All the major insulins are available in disposable preloaded pens or in cartridges that fit into reusable pens. Insulin pens—which look pretty much like ballpoint pens when the caps are on—are small and very easy to use. The pen or cartridge is reused until empty and then discarded. You attach a fresh, sterile needle at each use. These needles are generally even smaller and thinner than those available on syringes, and most people say they hardly feel the needle go in. The correct dose is administered by turning a dial at the end of the pen opposite the needle, and for each unit there is a click as the user turns the dial, so one can confirm that the dose is correct by both look and feel. Pens are especially convenient for people who need meal-related insulin, because they can be stored at room temperature for up to four weeks. The user can keep the pen in his jacket pocket or her purse and use it at the start of a meal.

- **Insulin pumps.** See page 226.

- **Hide-and-seek for syringes.** "Inject-Ease" is a spring-loaded device that pushes the syringe into the skin so that the user doesn't have to, and the device hides the needle while it's going in for those who really have a hard time overcoming their anxiety about injections.

- **Insulin jet injectors.** Jet injectors force insulin through the skin under high pressure without actually using a needle. The insulin comes out under very high pressure in a very narrow stream and is forced directly through the skin. The user has to fill the device with insulin, but once filled it can deliver injections for two to three weeks. Even though there are no needles, there is still sometimes discomfort or bruising because of the high pressure, though for some people this is less than with needles. Jet injectors are larger than insulin pens and more expensive.

(*continued on next page*)

■ **Inhaled insulin.** Insulin cannot be taken in standard pill form because the stomach acid and enzymes in the digestive tract break it down, but insulin can be absorbed directly through the lining of the lungs or the oral membranes where protein digestion does not take place. Exubera, a type of insulin taken by inhalation, was available in the U.S. for about two years until it was withdrawn in late 2007 because of poor sales. Research is ongoing to develop inhaled forms of insulin that are easier to use and meet the needs of a larger number of people.

■ **Other options.** Some companies are working to develop pills that will pass through the stomach and dissolve in the small intestine, where the insulin can be absorbed into the blood without being broken down by stomach acid. Other companies are working on patches that allow insulin to be absorbed directly through the skin. Insulin is a large molecule, so it does not pass through the skin easily. Researchers are looking into using electrical currents or ultrasonic waves applied to the skin to improve the absorption of the insulin molecule.

The Right Medicines for You

As you can see, there are a lot of medication choices, and deciding which ones make sense for a given person with type 2 diabetes isn't always easy, especially if he or she needs more than one medicine. One common mistake people make is to think that in the early stages of a medical problem (and not necessarily just diabetes) doctors use medicines that are somehow not as effective as others and that the strongest medicines should be saved for when things get bad. That's completely incorrect. Your doctor will give you what she thinks is the best medicine for your condition from the outset, but you have to recognize that best doesn't simply mean strongest and certainly doesn't always mean newest. The best medicine is the one that overall has the greatest benefit with the fewest problems. This might vary from one person to another. For example, both glipizide and Byetta tend to lower blood sugar levels after meals. Glipizide is an oral medication and is available as an inexpensive generic, but it also tends to cause a little weight gain and more severe hypoglycemia. Byetta must be given by injection and is very expensive, but it often helps people lose weight. Which is the best drug? For someone who's on a tight budget or is paying out of pocket for medications, glipizide makes the most sense. In a situation where weight loss is the paramount concern, Byetta may be a good choice. These are some key considerations that your doctor or other health care provider must take into account when deciding how best to manage your diabetes medications:

1. If someone diagnosed with diabetes is slender or has little or no abdominal obesity, is relatively young (in the late 20s, 30s, or 40s), has a family history of type 1 diabetes, or just isn't responding as expected to oral medications, the person may actually have late-onset type 1 diabetes. In this case, it's best to start insulin treatment early.

2. Most people with type 2 diabetes, especially those with some abdominal obesity or insulin resistance, should be given metformin as their initial medication. It's inexpensive, improves the body's responsiveness to insulin, and often results in weight loss. However, it cannot be given to someone with kidney problems.

3. In most cases, it's better to maximize the benefit of one medication before starting a second. This means the dose of one medication should be increased to the maximum, or to the maximum that a person can tolerate, before adding a second drug. For example, the dosage range for metformin is from 500 to 2,500 milligrams per day, and most people achieve the maximum benefit on doses of 2,000 to 2,500 milligrams per day. If your doctor has prescribed metformin, in most cases it makes sense to increase the dose to that level before adding a second medicine. On the other hand, if someone has diarrhea that simply won't go away at doses higher than 1,000 or 1,500 milligrams, it's not appropriate to go higher than that dose. Once a second drug is added, in most cases the same approach should be used with that drug before adding a third drug. There are, of course, exceptions, and some prominent diabetes researchers think that combination therapy right from the beginning offers significant advantages. However, using fewer medications keeps the cost down and reduces the likelihood of drug interactions.

4. If a second or more than two drugs are needed, it's important to chose medicines from different classes to be certain that their benefit is cumulative, not redundant. For example, Byetta has the same actions as GLP-1 in the body, and Januvia raises the body's own level of GLP-1. Because both drugs work in a similar manner, it doesn't make sense to use them together. Similarly, you wouldn't use Actos as the first drug and Avandia as the second or glipizide as the first drug and glimepiride as the second; in each case, the two drugs come from the same class.

5. If metformin alone isn't doing the job, there is no clear "next best" medication to add, and practice differs very much from one doctor to another. Guidelines from the American Diabetes Association and the European Association for the Study of Diabetes recommend insulin, a sulfonylurea (glyburide, glipizide, or glimepiride), Actos or Byetta as appropriate second-line drugs, and the American Association of Clinical Endocrinologists urges doctors to consider using insulin earlier rather than later if controlling a person's blood sugar levels is proving difficult. If someone has primarily elevated fasting glucose levels—higher before breakfast than before dinner—a long-acting insulin is often the most effective therapy. If someone has high glucose values mostly after meals, a sulfonylurea or Byetta will work well provided the person is still making enough insulin. The TZD drugs, such as Actos, have a sustained benefit in controlling blood sugar levels and may help prolong the survival of beta cells in the pancreas. Each, therefore, has some advantages, but each also has potential problems, as we've discussed. The proper choice can be made only by a doctor who really knows you and your diabetes.

6. Finally, even if a combination of medicines is working well, it may have to be adjusted at some point. Obviously, if the medication regimen no longer keeps your blood sugar under control, it needs to be reevaluated. But the opposite is equally true; if you follow our Best Life program, you are almost certainly going to have lower blood sugar levels and you may very well lose weight. These changes may mean that your medication will have to be reduced or possibly some medication even eliminated.

Insulin Treatment for Type 1 Diabetes

Properly using insulin to treat type 1 diabetes is the subject of many books, and we're not going to be able to cover everything in the next few pages. The principles are pretty straightforward, though, and achieving good results is something that comes from working hard to find the right dosing schedule for each person. If you skipped ahead to this section, you should go back and read the section about insulin (beginning on page 207) where we discuss many of the basic elements of insulin therapy.

It wasn't so many years ago that having type 1 diabetes meant you were tied to a rigid schedule of meals, and often to meals that were very similar, so that you could have some idea of how your blood sugar level would respond. The widespread use of home glucose meters and the ability to give insulin in a way that matches the body's usual requirements fairly closely have changed this.

Insulin treatment of type 1 diabetes is sometimes called "intensive insulin therapy," but we think that's kind of misleading because it suggests that when you're treating type 2 diabetes you're somehow less concerned about the outcome than you are in someone with type 1. What makes insulin treatment for type 1 diabetes "intensive" is that the person either needs to take several injections per day or needs to use an insulin pump. We'll talk about these separately because there are important practical differences between the two approaches. Of course, the manner in which the insulin is administered is a secondary concern. What's most important is meeting the physiological need for insulin in a manner that is as close to a normally functioning pancreas as possible, replacing both the background (or basal) insulin that the body normally makes all the time and the meal-related (or bolus) insulin that accompanies carbohydrate intake. The components of this approach to insulin treatment (which we mentioned briefly on page 210) are summarized in the box titled "Basal-Bolus Insulin Therapy" on page 220, and a detailed explanation of how to use insulin in this way follows in the next several pages.

BASAL-BOLUS INSULIN THERAPY

Basal Insulin Meets the body's need for insulin during the overnight fast and between meals. If you're on injections, you'll use a very-long-acting insulin such as Lantus or Levemir. If you're using a pump, a small amount of fast- or very-fast-acting insulin given continuously provides basal insulin. (See below for how to adjust your basal insulin.)

Bolus Insulin Meets the body's need for additional insulin when you eat. Bolus insulin has two components that are added together to give the total dose:

- Meal-related insulin, necessary for the carbohydrates in the food you're eating. Often people use an "insulin-to-carbohydrate ratio" to determine their meal-related insulin needs. (See page 221 for how to establish your insulin-to-carbohydrate ratio.)

- Correction insulin, used to compensate for a high premeal glucose level. (See page 224 for figuring your correction factor.)

INSULIN BY INJECTION

Type 1 diabetes can be treated with multiple daily injections of insulin, often abbreviated MDI. In this case, a combination of two different kinds of insulin are used. One insulin, most often Lantus or Levemir, is long-acting. These insulins are relatively "flat" in their action, which means that after injection, the amount of insulin in the blood rises relatively slowly and stays fairly constant over many hours. Lantus insulin usually lasts twenty-four hours or more; Levemir often lasts up to twenty-four hours, though in some people, two separate shots are necessary. The goal with these insulins is to match the body's basal or background insulin production. This works pretty well as long as the background insulin requirement is more-or-less steady during a twenty-four-hour period, and this is true for many people. In these situations, the long-acting insulin is adjusted to get the fasting sugar level under control exactly as was described for Bill (see page 211).

In some people, the background insulin requirement varies quite a bit and it can be hard to match their individual pattern with one or two shots per day. The most common reason for this is the "dawn phenome-non," in which hormones released by the body in the early morning hours cause the blood sugar to rise. In this case, if the dose of long-acting insulin were high enough to meet the body's requirements in the early morning, it would almost certainly be too high later in the day and would cause hy-poglycemia. If the dose were lowered to prevent hypoglycemic reactions in the afternoon or early evening, then the morning numbers would remain too high. A person in this situation would probably be managed better with an insulin pump, which we discuss on page 226.

In order to match the rise and fall in blood sugar that results from eating carbohydrates, you need to use short-acting insulin. In most cases these days, the very-short-acting insulin analogs—Humalog, NovoLog, or Apidra—are used for this purpose. They have the advantage of working quickly enough that they can be taken from about fifteen minutes before a meal up to immediately before eating or sometimes even at the end of a meal. This rapid action is a big advantage for people with type 1 diabetes because it means that they can be totally spontaneous about when they eat. Before these very-fast-acting insulins were available, regular, or "R," insulin had to be used for this purpose. This type of insulin needs to be given thirty to forty-five minutes prior to eating, which means you have to know well in advance when you're going to eat. Regular insulin also lasts much longer than the very-fast-acting insulins, so it commonly causes hy-poglycemia several hours after the meal.

Figuring out the doses for meal-related insulin can be a challenge, and there are a lot of different approaches you can take. Basically, you're trying to match the amount of insulin you inject with what your body will need to deal with the rise in glucose that will occur with your meal. If you eat a high-carbohydrate meal, you're going to need a lot more insulin than if you eat a meal with very few carbohydrates. That sounds simple enough, but in reality it can be very hard to figure out exactly how much insulin that is.

The gold standard in most people's minds for giving meal-related insulin uses carbohydrate counting. When you count carbohydrates, you tally up all the carbohydrates in the meal you're about to eat or have just eaten if you're taking the insulin at the end of the meal. (We give you a carbohydrate count for many common foods in the "Carbohydrate

Counts" chart on page 343, and you can search thousands of foods for their carbohydrate content at www.thebestlife.com.) Let's take the Trout with Roasted Vegetables served with couscous, and raspberries for dessert, the Day 3 dinner in our meal plan (see page 264). The carbohydrate count for that meal is about 45 grams.

In order to determine how much insulin you need for this meal (or for any meal containing 45 grams of carbohydrate), you need to figure out your insulin-to-carbohydrate ratio, the amount of insulin your body needs to metabolize a certain amount of carbohydrate. This number varies from individual to individual, but the average person needs somewhere around 1 unit of insulin for every 5 to 10 grams of carbohydrate, so a 45-gram carbohydrate meal will require somewhere between 4 and 9 units of insulin. The person who needs 1 unit of insulin for every 10 grams of carbohydrate will require 4.5 units (45 grams divided by 10 grams/unit). With most standard insulin syringes or pens, you can give only whole units, so you'd have to round down to 4 or up to 5. If you need more insulin—say 1 unit for every 5 grams of carbohydrate—you'd divide 45 grams by 5 grams/unit to get 9 units. If you have an insulin-to-carbohydrate ratio of 1 to 5 and you eat a meal containing 40 grams of carbohydrate, you'd need 8 units. If you eat a meal containing 65 grams, you'd need about 13 units.

A common recommendation that doctors, diabetes educators, and dietitians make is to start with 1 unit of meal-related insulin for 10 grams of carbohydrate and see whether your blood sugar levels are reasonably well controlled. Do before-meal and after-meal finger-stick tests. A normal before-meal blood sugar level would be under about 100 for most people, and two hours after meals, the goal would be less than 140. (These are targets to shoot for; they'll be very hard to achieve initially, so don't get discouraged.) If you eat the Trout with Roasted Vegetables, couscous, and raspberries, you'd start by taking 4 units. If your before-meal blood sugar level is 115, which is pretty good, and your after-dinner number is 155, which is also pretty good, you're in the right ballpark. If your before-meal blood glucose level is 115 but two hours later it's 283, you know that 4 units of insulin wasn't nearly enough. The next time you have a meal with 45 grams of carbohydrate, you'll probably need more insulin (unless you were much more physically active that day or some other factor changed), so you could try 1 unit of insulin for every 9 grams of carbohydrate instead of 10, which would give you exactly 5 units. If that proved to not be enough, the next time you could try going to 1 to 8, which would give you 5.6 units (45 divided by 8 equals 5.6), which you'd have to round up to 6 units. Or you could just go up by 1 unit and see how your numbers respond. If you do this a few times with different meals, eventually you'll have a pretty good sense of how much insulin you need for how many grams of carbohydrate.

After reading this, you might feel as though you need a PhD just to have dinner. We know that it can be frustrating, but don't let the idea of having to do some simple math frighten you away from trying to control your sugar. Most people who end up doing a good job with meal-related insulin dosing start out by counting carbohydrates but eventually develop a method that works for them; they know from experience how their blood sugar responds to certain foods or meals and go back to formal carbohydrate counting for foods that they don't normally eat or if it seems as though they're going off track a bit. That's the same kind of advice a football coach or piano teacher would give: if your game is off, go back to basic drills; if you're hitting the wrong notes, go back to practicing scales. There are a lot of tools that can help you with these calculations, and we'll talk about some of them below when we discuss insulin pump therapy (page 226) and continuous glucose monitors (page 228).

Knowing your insulin-to-carbohydrate ratio is a good start, but it's not quite the whole story. First of all, there isn't a person in the world with type 1 diabetes who always has normal premeal glucose numbers. Your goal is to have your numbers as close to normal after the meal as you can get them, but it's obvious that if you are high before a meal, the usual amount of insulin isn't going to be enough. Let's say you figure out that for the trout-couscous-raspberry meal you need 8 units of insulin, meaning that your insulin-to-carbohydrate ratio is about 1 unit for about every 5.5 grams of carbohydrate. If one day you sit down to dinner and your blood sugar level is 105, and then you take 8 units of insulin, two hours later your blood sugar level is likely to be in a pretty fair range—maybe in the mid-100s or lower. On the other hand, if you sit down to eat and your blood sugar level before dinner is 230, 8 units of insulin would be enough to cover the food, but if you factor in the high premeal reading it will be too little. If you want to reduce your blood sugar level to a decent range, you'll need to increase your dose.

Extra insulin taken because of a high blood sugar level before a meal is called correction insulin. Just as you need to establish an insulin-to-carbohydrate ratio, you should try to figure out your individual correction factor, the approximate fall in blood glucose level that you expect from a unit of insulin. Obviously, no one can ever know that number exactly because it will vary somewhat from one situation to another. But with a little trial and error, you can usually figure out that 1 unit of insulin will lower your blood sugar by about 25 points, by 30 points, or by whatever you determine to be your number. You'll have to go through some trial-and-error testing, keeping careful records, just as you did with the insulin-to-carbohydrate ratio for food. For most people, it's reasonable to start with the assumption that 1 unit of insulin will lower the glucose by 50 points and then set a target for the upper-limit premeal number you'll accept. For example, you might decide to correct for any glucose number over 120 before meals and assume at the beginning that 1 unit of insulin will drop you by 50 points. If your premeal blood sugar level is between 121 and 170, or up to 50 points above the 120 mark, you'd take 1 extra unit of insulin; if it is between 171 and 220, or between 51 and 100 points above the 120 mark, you'd take 2 extra units; if it is between 221 and 270, or between 101 and 150 points above the 120 mark, you'd take 3 extra units, and so on. So if your blood sugar level before that trout dinner is 88 or 92 or 114, you'd take 8 units—8 units for the food and nothing extra because you started out in a good range. But if your predinner number is 146, you would take 9 units—8 units for the food and 1 extra unit because you are starting out within the 121-to-170 range, within 50 points of your premeal target. If your predinner number is 228, you'd take 11 units—8 units for the food and 3 extra units for the high blood sugar level, which is between 101 and 150 units above your premeal target. You get the picture.

If your correction insulin isn't lowering your sugar as much as it should or is lowering it too much, you'll have to adjust your correction factor up or down. For example, if before the trout dinner your blood sugar level is 228 and you take 11 units of insulin (8 for the food and 3 extra for the high sugar level) and after eating your number is 154, your correction factor is about right. But if after the meal your sugar is still in the high 200s, your correction insulin wasn't sufficient. You'll have to try 1 unit for every 30 points of glucose above your target or 1 unit for 25 points until you can reliably reach the proper range. You may have to subtract some insulin from the amount you would normally take if your premeal number is low.

Often people with type 1 diabetes are given detailed instruction on how to establish an insulin-to-carbohydrate ratio, but they're led to believe that somehow this number is written in stone and applicable at all times. Well, guess what: a person's insulin sensitivity, and therefore his or her insulin-to-carbohydrate ratio, may change over time. If someone loses weight, for example, the same dose of insulin will go further. In addition, the insulin sensitivity may be different at different times of the day. Usually people are more insulin-resistant in the morning, and they often need more insulin for the same amount of carbohydrate with breakfast than they do for the same amount of carbohydrate, or even the exact same meal, at dinner. This, too, is something that you can learn only from experience.

If we step back and try to look at the forest here, things are not as scary as the individual trees would make them seem. If you have type 1 diabetes and decide you'd like to treat it with multiple daily injections, you'll have to take a dose of long-acting insulin such as Lantus or Levemir, starting at a low dose and working up until your fasting blood sugar level is normal. Plus you'll also have to take a dose of very-short-acting insulin, such as Humalog, NovoLog, or Apidra, before each of your meals, matched to your carbohydrate intake and adjusted for premeal high or low values. It's a big pain at the beginning, and even after you've had type 1 diabetes for a long time you'll still often be frustrated by how unpredictable things seem. But figuring out your insulin doses eventually becomes somewhat second nature. Many people with type 1 diabetes achieve really excellent blood sugar control in this way, and we've known many people who have maintained nearly normal hemoglobin A1c levels and are in terrific shape with no complications over long periods of time. Remember: no one expects you to figure all this out on your own. Your doctor, nurse practitioner, or diabetes educator will guide you with insulin dosing, especially at the beginning. And don't expect to get things perfectly right at the outset. If you make small changes and keep careful track of what happens to your blood sugar levels, eventually you'll figure out what works.

INSULIN PUMPS

The other way to manage type 1 diabetes is with an insulin pump. An insulin pump is a device that administers insulin continuously under the skin. There are no individual injections, and only fast-acting insulin is used. The background insulin requirement is met by an infusion of the insulin on a continuous basis. While someone who is using injections may take 24 units of Lantus or Levemir once daily, a person on an insulin pump may get 1 unit per hour round-the-clock of Humalog, NovoLog, or Apidra (all very-fast-acting insulins), which amounts to pretty much the same thing. Meal-related insulin is given by programming the pump to administer a certain amount of insulin at mealtime, using the same strategy we talked about for the insulin-to-carbohydrate ratio and correction factor.

Insulin pump technology has progressed amazingly over the past couple of decades. Today, several insulin pumps are available, including those manufactured by Medtronic, Animas, and Disetronic, among others. They are about the size of a cell phone, and most of them are very easy to use. Even a person who does not consider him- or herself a "techie" can use an insulin pump very easily. Most pumps require the wearer to insert a small plastic tube or catheter about a half inch long into the fat under the skin using a needle in the center of the tube. After insertion, the needle is removed, leaving just the soft plastic catheter in place. Usually the catheter is inserted into the abdomen or upper thigh, but other areas can be used as well. Flexible plastic tubing connects the catheter to the insulin pump, which is then clipped to a belt or carried in a pocket, and the insulin is pumped through the tubing and into the fat under the skin. The catheter, also called an infusion set, is usually changed about every three days. One pump, the OmniPod, is placed directly against the skin, so there is no connection tubing, and the catheter inserts itself automatically. The pump is worn twenty-four hours a day; pumps can either be waterproof or water resistant or can be detached for short periods of time for bathing.

Deciding how much insulin to give with an insulin pump is the same as when insulin is given by injection, but insulin pump manufacturers have worked hard to give people tools to figure out their insulin requirements. Most of the pumps in use today are so-called smart pumps, meaning that they not only respond to commands that you enter telling them how much insulin to give, but they also help collect information and do calculations to assist with insulin dosing. Most of the pumps communicate directly, usually via infrared light (the same kind that's used in your television remote control) with select glucose meters. Many of the smart pumps and the meters that work with them keep databases of the carbohydrate content of various foods. If you program in your insulin-to-carbohydrate ratio and correction factor, beam glucose test data to the pump, and then tell the pump what you are about to eat, it will calculate how much insulin you need to take. The pumps also keep track of how much insulin you've been given in the preceding several hours, which helps prevent an overdose of insulin that would cause hypoglycemia. Most of the pumps have software that allows the user to download all the finger-stick glucose and insulin data to a computer and analyze the information. Sometimes in doing this, patterns emerge that were not obvious when the person was just responding to individual numbers. Some of the pumps now work with continuous glucose monitors (see page 228).

Most insulin pump users are devoted to the idea that a pump is the only real way to treat type 1 diabetes properly. Certainly, in the days before the very-fast-acting and long-lasting insulin analogs were available it was nearly impossible to have the same control and flexibility with injections as with an insulin pump, but this is much less true with the newer insulins. At this stage, the choice between multiple daily injection therapy and an insulin pump is largely a matter of personal preference, and there are pros and cons to either approach. Pump treatment offers the greatest flexibility in insulin dosing, and the tools for deciding how much insulin to give are getting better and easier to use all the time. A pump does become necessary if someone has lots of variability in his or her background insulin requirement. For example, for someone with a significant dawn phenomenon, it's usually impossible to get the fasting sugars under control with a once-daily long-acting insulin shot without causing hypoglycemia at other times of the day. On the other hand, a pump wearer can simply program the device to give a larger amount of basal insulin during the early-morning hours and correct the problem pretty easily.

The main downside to insulin pump treatment is the need to be attached to a bit of technology all the time. Of course, you can choose to go off the insulin pump and onto shots for short periods of time in select circumstances, such as when you're going to the beach for a few days on vacation and don't want to get the pump wet. The advantage of shots is that you're not attached to anything in between injections, but the major disadvantage is the fact that injections need to be given several times each day and, as we've said, certain patterns in glucose fluctuation just can't be treated as effectively with insulin given by injection. Remember, too, that although we've chosen to discuss this in the type 1 diabetes section, both multiple daily injection therapy and insulin pump treatment are appropriate for some people with type 2 diabetes. The percentage of pump users who have type 2 diabetes is relatively small—fewer than 10 percent—but is likely to grow over time.

CONTINUOUS GLUCOSE MONITORS

Throughout this book, we've urged you to test your blood sugar level regularly using your glucose meter, but we have to say that the present technology for monitoring blood sugar levels—although it has gotten a lot better—isn't perfect. Though the finger-stick tests are not terribly painful, it would be nice to be able to check your sugar without any discomfort at all. And interrupting your daily routine to do a test is not very convenient. Finally, it's expensive to get a lot of data; test strips typically cost 75 cents or more *each*. Many companies are trying to come up with a better solution. There's a lot at stake, given how many people have diabetes.

We are just at the beginning of some significant advances in glucose monitoring, and one of the most exciting is the development of continuous glucose monitors, or CGMs. There are several CGM systems currently available, including those made by Medtronic, DexCom, and Abbott Laboratories. These devices rely on a small, flexible catheter placed into the fat under the skin, similar to the tube through which insulin flows from an insulin pump. Glucose levels in the fluid between the fat cells, called interstitial fluid, are measured, and the results are sent by radio waves to a separate receiver. These measurements are fairly close to blood glucose readings. Measurements are made every one to five minutes, and the receiver displays the current glucose reading as well as a graph of how the glucose levels are changing. At present, CGM systems are not as accurate as finger-stick blood glucose test results, so some finger-stick testing is still required for validation of the results and is recommended whenever there is a high or low number that would require action on the part of the wearer. The devices have audio and vibrating alarms that can be set for glucose levels above or below a certain number, and one of the most valuable roles for these CGMs is to provide a warning alarm for low-blood-sugar reactions in people who do not have symptoms during hypoglycemia (a condition called hypoglycemic unawareness).

One system, the MiniMed Paradigm REAL-Time Revel System, integrates a continuous glucose monitor and an insulin pump. The Paradigm smart pump receives information from the continuous monitor, so that there is no need to separately input finger-stick information when preparing to give meal-related insulin. The manufacturers of the DexCom CGM and the Animas insulin pump are working on integration of their systems as well, and this is clearly a trend that will continue with other manufacturers.

Of course, the real goal in integrating a CGM and an insulin pump is to create an artificial pancreas, or what medical professionals call a closed-loop system. The loop refers to the continuous cycle of feedback information: the blood glucose level changes; the change is detected by the CGM; the CGM sends information to the insulin pump, which adjusts its insulin output; and the blood glucose level changes again in response to the insulin. The loop is closed when this happens automatically. At present CGM–insulin pump systems are not closed-loop because the person has to make the decision of how much insulin to give rather than this happening automatically. It's hard to predict when such a system will actually become available, but prototype systems are already being used in experimental settings. One problem with these systems is that the glucose level in the tissue fluid doesn't change as quickly as the blood glucose level, and it takes some time for insulin injected into subcutaneous fat to take effect. As a result, the insulin effect always lags somewhat compared to insulin that's made by a normally functioning pancreas, where changes in blood glucose are sensed instantaneously and the insulin is released directly into the blood. Given the serious problems—glucose levels that are dangerously high or dangerously low—that can result if the wrong dose of insulin is given, such systems will have to be studied extensively before they are made available for widespread use. But we're optimistic that the technical hurdles will be overcome. Along with islet cell transplantation (see page 247), closed-loop insulin delivery systems offer the promise of revolutionizing the management of type 1 diabetes.

Drugs Other than Insulin for Type 1 Diabetes

The only medication specifically approved by the FDA for treating those with type 1 diabetes other than insulin is Symlin, which we discussed on pages 202 to 203. Symlin has several effects in those with type 1 diabetes, including reducing the meal-related release of glucagon, a hormone that raises blood sugar levels. This helps control the rise in glucose after meals, and many patients who use Symlin along with insulin find that their blood glucose levels fluctuate less than with insulin alone. As we mentioned before, Symlin also slows stomach emptying and helps people feel full more quickly. As a result, it sometimes helps people with type 1 diabetes lose weight.

Some doctors use metformin (see page 196) to help treat type 1 diabetes, even though it is not FDA-approved for this purpose. Metformin does not replace insulin, of course; people with type 1 still need basal-bolus insulin therapy. Metformin is used in this situation to help improve the body's response to the insulin that is used for treatment. Unfortunately, having the insulin deficiency of type 1 diabetes does not necessarily prevent someone from developing abdominal obesity and insulin resistance. In this case, the insulin resistance isn't the cause of the diabetes, but it may make the diabetes more difficult to control and contributes to other problems. It is likely that improving insulin resistance is beneficial for those with type 1 diabetes just as it is with people who have type 2, because the insulin resistance itself is associated with an increased risk of cardiovascular disease and other conditions.

BEYOND BLOOD SUGAR: PREVENTING COMPLICATIONS

In addition to the blood-sugar-lowering drugs discussed in the first part of this chapter, you may be taking medications to help control cholesterol, blood pressure, erectile dysfunction, and other complications of pre-diabetes or diabetes. You'll read about some of these medications in this section, but even more important, you'll read about how to prevent complications so that you may not need these drugs at all.

Keep Your Heart Healthy

Besides insulin resistance, the other major risk factors for heart and vascular disease are high blood pressure, or hypertension, and abnormal levels of blood fats or lipids, which are the cholesterol and triglycerides that circulate in your bloodstream. Controlling these two problems is critical to preventing heart disease. If lifestyle changes like those in the Best Life program don't get these problems under control, you'll need medication. If you're already taking medication, you might be able to lower the dose or go off the drugs completely with the lifestyle changes outlined in this book. That's for you and your doctor to determine.

TREAT HIGH BLOOD PRESSURE

Your blood pressure deserves every bit as much attention as your blood sugar if you have diabetes; if you have pre-diabetes, high blood pressure may even be a bigger issue than your blood sugar level, at least initially. High blood pressure is often called the silent killer because in most cases there are no symptoms. Hypertension increases the risk of blocked arteries to the heart, brain, and lower extremities and is a major contributor to kidney disease and eye disease in people with both diabetes and pre-diabetes. Hypertension is epidemic in the U.S.: an estimated 27 percent of adults have it, and another 31 percent of adults have prehypertension, or borderline elevation in blood pressure, according to the most recent government survey.

Normal blood pressure is generally considered no higher than about

120 for the top or systolic number and no higher than 80 for the bottom or diastolic number. This would be written 120/80, and the doctor or nurse would tell you that your blood pressure is "120 over 80." There's clear evidence that lowering blood pressure with medication reduces the risk of heart disease, stroke, and kidney damage. Most doctors will start someone on blood pressure medication if her pressure remains higher than 130 to 140 for the systolic pressure or 85 to 90 for the diastolic pressure.

There are many drugs to treat high blood pressure; we'll focus on two main classes: the ACE inhibitors and ARB medications, both of which have special benefits for people with diabetes. The "A" in both groups of drugs stands for angiotensin. Angiotensin is a hormone that raises blood pressure, especially in the small vessels in the kidney where blood is filtered during the first stage of urine production. ACE stands for angiotensin-converting enzyme, and ACE inhibitors (often written either as "ACEs" or "ACEIs," though people usually say "aces") prevent the production of angiotensin. ARB stands for angiotensin receptor blocker (people usually say "arbs"), and these medicines block the action of angiotensin. There are many medicines in each category; those available in the United States are:

ACE INHIBITORS			ARB MEDICATIONS	
GENERIC NAME	BRAND NAME		GENERIC NAME	BRAND NAME
Benazepril	Lotensin		Candesartan	Atacand
Captopril	Capoten		Eprosartan	Teveten
Enalapril	Vasotec		Irbesartan	Avapro
Fosinopril	Monopril		Losartan	Cozaar
Lisinopril	Zestril, Prinivil		Olmesartan	Benicar
Moexipril	Univasc		Telmisartan	Micardis
Perindopril	Aceon		Valsartan	Diovan
Quinapril	Accupril			
Ramipril	Altace			
Trandolapril	Mavik			

ACEs and ARBs lower blood pressure and specifically help to reduce pressure within the kidneys, so they have a special benefit in preventing kidney disease in diabetes. The ACEs are an older class of drugs and most are available as generics, so they are relatively inexpensive. By far the most common side effect of these drugs is a dry cough that just doesn't go away. The ARBs are newer, and none is available as a generic at present; consequently, they are more expensive. The patent on Cozaar, the first ARB available in the United States, will expire in 2010, so generic versions of these medications will be available within the next few years. Neither ACEs nor ARBs can be used during pregnancy because they may harm the growth and development of the fetus. Otherwise, a drug from one of these classes should usually be the first line medication for high blood pressure in someone with diabetes because of the special benefit to the kidneys.

An important study published in 2007 called the ADVANCE (Action in Diabetes and Vascular Disease) trial found that treatment with an ACE inhibitor in combination with a diuretic reduced the risk of heart disease in those with diabetes, even if they did not have hypertension. Many doctors and diabetes researchers have begun to ask whether blood-pressure-lowering meds should be considered for every person with diabetes or pre-diabetes, or every person deemed at high risk of heart disease, rather than just those who have high blood pressure. Another major study published in 2008 (the ACCOMPLISH trial, short for "Avoiding Cardiovascular Events through Combination Therapy in Patients Living with Systolic Hypertension") found that using a combination of an ACE inhibitor with amlodipine, a blood pressure medicine from a different class called the calcium channel blockers, was even more effective in reducing cardiovascular disease risk than the combination of an ACE inhibitor with a diuretic.

Getting high blood pressure under control is more difficult than you might think, and many people need two, three, or more medications to get blood pressures that are near normal; when you have pre-diabetes or diabetes, you may be taking these drugs on top of other medications to lower your blood sugar and cholesterol levels and control other conditions. The need for so many medications is one of the most frustrating things to many people with diabetes. That's why lifestyle is such a key element: it may eliminate or at least limit the amount of medication you require. To track your progress, we suggest that you get a simple, automated blood pressure machine that you can use at home. Take the machine with you when you see your doctor so that you can tell whether the results correlate with those at the medical office or clinic. Your blood pressure should be something you follow just as carefully as your blood sugar.

BRING DOWN YOUR BLOOD LIPID LEVELS

Almost everybody knows that high cholesterol increases your risk for heart disease, and by now you've heard us say in a hundred ways that having pre-diabetes or diabetes adds to that risk. Cholesterol and triglycerides are the two major forms of fat that circulate in the blood, and together they are referred to as lipids. You know that oil and water don't mix, and so it is with cholesterol or triglycerides and blood. These fats don't dissolve in the blood, but are packaged into particles along with special proteins. There are different types of particles, and each has a different metabolic part to play. The major particles are termed high-density lipoprotein, or HDL; low-density lipoprotein, or LDL; and very-low-density lipoprotein, or VLDL. All cholesterol is chemically the same, but when it's packaged in one type of particle it does one thing, and when packaged in a different kind of particle it does another. HDL particles help remove cholesterol from the linings of blood vessels, so the higher the HDL cholesterol level, the lower the risk of heart disease. HDL is usually termed "good" cholesterol for this reason. LDL particles put more cholesterol into the plaques lining arteries, so the higher the LDL cholesterol level, the greater the risk of heart disease. LDL cholesterol is therefore called "bad" cholesterol. VLDL particles contain mostly triglycerides, which we'll talk about on page 237. HDL cholesterol levels of 40 mg/dL or more for a man and 50 or more for a woman are generally considered normal, but the higher you go the better off you are. Similarly, LDL cholesterol levels should be less than 100 to be normal, but there is evidence that even lower values help reduce your risk of heart disease.

If you follow our Best Life meal plans, you're already doing a lot to improve your cholesterol level. That's because they are low in saturated fat, which raises LDL or bad cholesterol levels, and high in monounsaturated and polyunsaturated fats, which tend to raise HDL or "good" cholesterol levels. If you can't get to a satisfactory level with lifestyle changes alone, it may be that you have a hereditary cause of your elevated bad cholesterol. In that case, you might need medication.

The major cholesterol-lowering drugs are the statins, (technically called HMG CoA reductase inhibitors), and they are some of the most widely prescribed medicines around. The statin drugs available in the United States (listed in order of descending potency) are:

GENERIC	BRAND		GENERIC	BRAND
Rosuvastatin	Crestor		Lovastatin	Mevacor
Atorvastatin	Lipitor		Pravastatin	Pravachol
Simvastatin	Zocor		Fluvastatin	Lescol, Lescol XL

Statin drugs target primarily LDL cholesterol. Some of these drugs are available generically, others only as brand name. There have been many studies showing the benefit of cholesterol lowering with statin drugs in those with diabetes, and because the data are so strong and the risk of heart disease is so high in people with diabetes, the American Diabetes Association recommends that a statin drug be used in any person with diabetes and known heart disease or any person with diabetes and another risk factor for heart disease, such as high blood pressure, even if the cholesterol levels are normal. Although less than 100 is regarded as normal, many doctors consider an LDL of less than 70 to be the target with statin treatment for those with diabetes because pushing the LDL lower provides even more benefit.

Statin drugs are very powerful in cutting the risk of heart disease, but of course they're not perfect. Many people who take them complain of muscle pain, and people often say they feel the way they do the day after a hard workout, even when they haven't been physically active. Sometimes this just shows up as fatigue. On rare occasions statins can cause muscle damage, so tell your doctor if the muscle pain is severe or persistent. Occasionally the drugs cause liver problems, but it is far more common for people with pre-diabetes or diabetes to have abnormal liver blood tests due to fatty liver, which is an accumulation of insulin resistance–causing fat within the liver. Studies show that statin drugs can be used safely in people who have liver test abnormalities from fatty liver, and there is even some evidence that the drugs may improve the problem by lowering fat levels in the blood. Statin drugs have also been reported to cause cognitive impairment, such as difficulties with memory, and they may cause or worsen peripheral neuropathy in some people. It can be a challenge for people with diabetes to know exactly what to do when there is overwhelming evidence of benefit, as there is with the statin drugs, but some real concerns about safety and side effects. This is the kind of issue that needs to be addressed by each person individually and a clear example of why it's important to work with a doctor you trust and who will listen to your concerns and answer your questions.

There are several other classes of medications that can help lower LDL cholesterol levels, and some of these medications may also have beneficial effects on triglycerides and HDL cholesterol levels, though the effects are usually small. Ezetimibe (brand name Zetia) blocks the absorption of cholesterol from the intestine. Used with statin drugs, this medication lowers LDL cholesterol impressively, and the drug Vytorin contains a combination of simvastatin along with ezetimibe. However, studies have yielded somewhat conflicting results in terms of whether ezetimibe reduces the risk of heart and vascular disease. Since there is strong evidence that the statins reduce the risk of heart disease, most experts in this field suggest that a person be treated first with a statin, and that the statin drug be increased as necessary until the cholesterol is controlled. Zetia should be added if the statin drug alone is not adequate to control the cholesterol, or if the person cannot tolerate high-dose statin therapy because of side effects.

Other drugs also lower LDL cholesterol. Niacin (also called nicotinic acid) is a B vitamin; at high doses it lowers LDL cholesterol and triglycerides, and it's more effective at raising HDL cholesterol than other cholesterol-lowering drugs. There are many brands, and the main side effect is an uncomfortable flushing. Niacin comes in immediate-release and slow-release forms, and the latter may reduce the flushing somewhat. Many niacin preparations are sold as supplements and are not subject to the same degree of oversight by the FDA as prescription drugs. Some over-the-counter forms of slow-release niacin have been associated with liver damage, but the prescription form Niaspan has not. Niacin sometimes raises blood sugar levels, so it has to be used cautiously in people with diabetes.

The bile acid sequestrants, including the drugs cholestyramine (Questran, Questran Light, Prevalite, Locholest, and Locholest Light), colestipol (Colestid), and colesevelam (Welchol), lower LDL cholesterol, but the drugs cause severe constipation in many people and often raise triglyceride levels. As discussed earlier, Welchol is also approved for the treatment of diabetes.

The insulin resistance syndrome causes low HDL cholesterol and high triglyceride levels. High triglyceride levels increase the risk of peripheral vascular disease and can lead to pancreatitis. Triglyceride levels can vary over time in the same person, and they may rise or fall depending on whether the blood sugar is under good control or not. Normal triglyceride levels are under about 150 mg/dL, but levels in the 500s, 600s, or even over 1,000 are seen commonly in people with uncontrolled high blood sugar levels. The statin drugs do not lower triglycerides very effectively, but another class of medication, the fibrates, lowers triglycerides very well; to a lesser degree, these drugs also lower LDL cholesterol and raise HDL cholesterol. Fibrate drugs include gemfibrozil (Lopid), clofibrate (Atromid-S), and fenofibrate (Tricor, Lofibra, Triglide, and Antara). You may be a good candidate for one of these drugs if you have a low LDL cholesterol level but a high triglyceride level. If both the LDL cholesterol and the triglyceride levels are elevated, a fibrate may need to be given along with a statin drug. The main side effect is muscle pain, just as with the statin drugs, and using the two kinds of medication together does increase the possibility of muscle damage, so you must be monitored carefully.

Stay on Top of Other Complications

The microvascular complications of pre-diabetes and diabetes are mostly related to high blood sugar levels, but high blood pressure often plays a role as well, especially in diseases of the eyes and kidneys.

RETINOPATHY: THE MOST SERIOUS FORM OF EYE DISEASE IN DIABETES

Diabetes remains one of the most common causes of vision loss. If you have diabetes, it's crucial that you see an ophthalmologist or optometrist at least annually, and the examination needs to include glaucoma screening and a careful examination of your retina. If your eye doctor thinks that there is evidence of retinal disease, he will refer you to a retina specialist. The specialist may decide you need a fluorescein angiogram. This is a test in which a special dye is injected into a vein; it allows the doctor to see where your blood vessels may be leaking blood or fluid or where there may be aneurysms, small areas of weakness in the vessel walls that cause the vessels to bulge and possibly rupture. If the test confirms any of these problems, you may be a candidate for laser photocoagulation, a treatment that helps seal off leaking vessels. Laser treatment can also reduce neovascularization, also called proliferative retinopathy. This is a condition in which the retina, which is not getting enough oxygen, makes a hormone called vascular endothelial growth factor, or VEGF. VEGF causes new blood vessels to grow, and it usually helps tissues recover after injury. However, in the eye the new vessels are prone to leak blood and fluid into the retina and surrounding tissues. Laser treatment can often eliminate these vessels. If bleeding into the eye is severe, the person may need a vitrectomy, the surgical removal of the gel in front of the retina. The gel is normally clear but may become clouded by blood. After removal, the gel is replaced with a clear saltwater solution.

A new treatment for proliferative retinopathy uses drugs that block VEGF, originally developed for cancer chemotherapy, to prevent new blood vessels from growing. Two such medications are available: Avastin (generic name bevacizumab) and Lucentis (generic name ranibizumab). These medications are normally injected directly into the eye tissues, though there are ongoing studies to determine if they will work if given intravenously.

NEPHROPATHY: KIDNEY DISEASE CAUSED BY DIABETES

Ongoing monitoring of your kidney function is an essential part of regular diabetes care. Both high blood sugar levels and high blood pressure damage the kidneys, and diabetes and hypertension are the two most common causes of kidney failure. There are several simple tests that will determine how well your kidneys are working.

Most doctors measure a blood creatinine level two to four times per year, each time a hemoglobin A1c level is done. Creatinine is a by-product of muscle metabolism and is normally eliminated from the body through the kidneys. If your kidneys are working properly, they filter out most of the creatinine, and the levels in the blood will remain low. Normal levels vary with age and gender, but a normal creatinine level is up to about

1.5 mg/dL or so in an adult man and up to about 1.2 in an adult woman. If your blood creatinine level is high, you cannot take metformin, which is the most common medication used to treat diabetes, because of the possibility of a rare side effect called lactic acidosis.

The most precise measure of kidney function is the glomerular filtration rate, or GFR. Using a person's age, gender, and blood creatinine level, an estimated GFR (written eGFR) can be calculated. The formulas used to do this calculation are slightly different depending on race, because creatinine is made in muscle cells, and African Americans have a greater muscle mass on average than do Caucasians or Asians. When you look at the lab report, you are likely to see an eGFR reported for both African Americans and non–African Americans, because the lab isn't usually given information about your race. A measurement called a creatinine clearance is very close to an actual GFR and can be done if more precise information about kidney function is needed. To measure a creatinine clearance, you'll need to collect all your urine for twenty-four hours in a container from the lab and have your blood drawn when you bring it in.

A simple and useful test for identifying very early kidney problems in diabetes is the measurement of microalbuminuria. This is a simple test that requires only a small urine sample. Albumin is the major protein in the blood; microalbuminuria means small (micro-) amounts of albumin protein (-albumin-) in the urine (-uria). Normally, the kidneys filter blood but don't allow any albumin protein to pass into the urine; a kidney that's been damaged by diabetes allows some of that albumin to pass into the urine. If the amount of albumin in the urine is increased, it signifies kidney damage. You should have a test for microalbuminuria once a year. The ACE and ARB blood pressure medicines we discussed on page 232 will help prevent or reduce urinary albumin excretion. If you have albumin in your urine, you should be treated with one of these medications.

NEUROPATHY: NERVE DAMAGE CAUSED BY DIABETES

Diabetes is a common cause of neuropathy, or nerve damage, and we now know that significant nerve damage often develops in the pre-diabetic phase. There are many forms of neuropathy. The most common, peripheral neuropathy, causes tingling, numbness, and pain in the feet. As the condition progresses, the symptoms may spread up the legs. The hands

240 THE BEST LIFE GUIDE TO MANAGING DIABETES

may be affected as well, usually after the symptoms in the legs and feet have become fairly severe. Numbness in the feet may mean that you don't feel when your feet are rubbing against your shoes, causing calluses or skin ulcers that can become infected. In severe cases, infection may spread to the underlying bone. This is often difficult to treat and may require prolonged antibiotic therapy. Sometimes hospitalization is necessary, and if an infection is extremely resistant, surgery to remove infected bone or even amputation may be required. These very serious problems usually occur when a person has both neuropathy and poor circulation, so it's critical to prevent both problems by keeping blood sugar levels, blood pressure, and cholesterol under control.

The doctor usually knows about retinopathy or nephropathy before a person with diabetes does because the problems show up on a retinal exam or lab tests before there are any symptoms. Neuropathy is different; usually the person has symptoms before the doctor sees any evidence of the problem. In the office, the only test that's usually done is to use a small, slightly stiff nylon fiber, a microfilament, to test sensation. Basically the doctor touches the microfilament to certain areas, usually on the sole of the foot, to see whether the person can feel it. This test is not very sensitive: many people with early neuropathy still have enough nerve function to feel the microfilament. Specialized nerve testing called electromyography and nerve conduction studies can identify very early neuropathy, but in most cases these tests are not necessary and don't really change the treatment. The only additional studies that need to be done in most cases are simple blood tests to exclude other causes of neuropathy, such as thyroid problems or a vitamin B12 deficiency. Just looking at the feet really gives the most important information: you might see areas of redness, calluses, ingrown nails, or skin ulceration. If you have neuropathy, examine your feet daily in bright light, and use a handheld mirror to look at the areas you can't see otherwise. If you have any of the problems we mentioned above, you should see a podiatrist.

The pain of neuropathy can really cause suffering; people describe it as a burning or electrical-type pain in their feet. Neuropathic pain is usually worst at night as one is trying to fall asleep. People often say that even the covers lying on their feet cause pain. Good blood sugar control often reduces the pain of neuropathy, and many medications are effective for pain relief, including antidepressants such as nortriptyline (Pamelor) and duloxetine (Cymbalta), and anti-seizure drugs such as gabapentin (Neurontin) and pregabalin (Lyrica).

Autonomic neuropathy is another form of nerve damage. The autonomic nervous system controls the body functions that are automatic, such as how fast or slow your heart is beating, the constriction of your blood vessels to keep your blood pressure stable as you go from lying to sitting to standing, and the rhythmic contractions of your intestine as it moves food through your digestive tract. Autonomic neuropathy means that there's damage to these nerves, and the result may be abnormal regulation of the heart, blood pressure, or intestinal function. The most common problem is gastroparesis, meaning reduced stomach emptying. People with gastroparesis have severe acid reflux symptoms, a diminished appetite, or frequent nausea and vomiting. Some people with autonomic neuropathy have lower intestinal symptoms, such as frequent constipation or diarrhea. Blood pressure and heart rate may not respond as they should to posture change, and some people develop what's called orthostatic hypotension, meaning a fall in blood pressure when going from lying to sitting or standing, that can lead to dizziness, lightheadedness, or fainting. These problems are sometimes difficult to manage, but medications designed to block stomach acid production, promote stomach emptying, treat constipation or diarrhea, regulate the heart rhythm, and raise the blood pressure can often be used to reduce the severity of the symptoms.

EXERCISING WITH COMPLICATIONS OF DIABETES

The right amount and kind of exercise can benefit everyone with diabetes. But there are specific concerns for people with some of the complications we've outlined on the previous pages.

- **Heart and vascular disease.** If you have known heart disease and you've not been exercising, it is important to get your doctor's approval before starting an exercise program. He may ask you to undergo a stress test if you haven't had one in a while: that will help him know whether the blockages in your heart are stable or whether there's the possibility of heart damage with exercise that's too strenuous. The main thing is not to overexert yourself and get chest pain or shortness of breath.

- **High blood pressure.** Check with your doctor to make sure your blood pressure is sufficiently well controlled before you start exercising; you shouldn't begin an exercise program if you have uncontrolled high blood pressure. Blood pressure that's not quite perfect usually isn't an issue, and as you begin to exercise it will start to improve. If you're taking high blood pressure medication, there is the possibility that it will make your blood pressure go too low, especially if you've reduced your salt intake and lost weight since starting the Best Life program. This could cause dizziness or lightheadedness. Your doctor may need to reduce your medication in this case.

- **Retinal disease.** Sudden or severe increases in blood pressure inside the eye can cause vessels to rupture, worsening retinopathy. If you have significant retinopathy, do not lift heavy weights because this will cause the pressure in those vessels to increase. You should also avoid contact sports because of the risk of retinal detachment. Aerobic physical activities are usually fine, but your doctor may recommend brisk walking rather than running or jogging because of the jarring that can occur, possibly causing the delicate retinal blood vessels to leak blood or fluid.

- **Peripheral neuropathy.** If you have loss of sensation in your feet, you can injure your feet and not be aware of it. Be certain that you are wearing the proper kind of shoes for the exercise you're doing and that the shoes fit well. If the shoes are new, break them in gradually. Keep your toenails properly trimmed. Examine your feet after you exercise to make sure there are no areas of redness, swelling, or ulceration. If there are, stop exercising until you can discuss with your doctor or podiatrist what the cause may be and how to correct it. Again, brisk walking may be safer than running or jogging. Swimming or water aerobics may be good choices for someone who has severe peripheral neuropathy.

- **Kidney disease.** There aren't as many specific concerns about exercise and kidney disease. Certain kinds of intense exercise will increase creatinine production by the muscles and cause some albumin protein to appear in the urine. In both cases, these effects will make your kidney function appear worse than it is. Avoid having blood or urine tests for kidney function done within a couple of days of very intense exercise for this reason.

SEXUAL ISSUES

On the surface it seems as though people are more comfortable talking about sex than they used to be. Sometimes you get the feeling that every other ad on television is for a medication for erectile dysfunction, and the term "ED" is now part of our popular culture. But it's still not always an easy subject, and many times when people talk about sexual problems, they joke or skirt the real issues. We may think that doctors are immune to embarrassment regarding discussions about sex, but studies have shown that physicians ask their patients about sexual problems much less often than they should. You need to take the initiative here: talk to your doctor about any issues that you're having. The doctor should listen to your concerns and address them with the same seriousness as he or she would your diabetes or any other issue. Don't be reluctant to discuss sexual concerns because of your age. Though sexual performance isn't as vigorous as we age, it's perfectly normal for sexual desire and activity to continue as we get older. If your doctor doesn't seem sensitive to this, that's a big red flag: you may have to think about using somebody else as your caregiver.

Erectile dysfunction in men is the most common sexual problem in diabetes, and diabetes is high on the list of causes of ED. A generation ago, it was commonly thought that in most cases ED was caused by psychological problems, such as life stresses, anxiety, or depression. These things *are* sometimes to blame, but we now recognize that ED is usually a vascular disease; in other words, poor blood flow to the erectile tissues of the penis is the most common reason men have difficulty achieving or maintaining erections. Because insulin resistance and obesity cause diabetes, high blood pressure, and lipid abnormalities, all of which cause arterial blockage, it's no surprise that men with diabetes have such a high risk of ED. In fact, ED may be an early sign of widespread vascular disease. Many studies have shown a link between ED and heart disease, and it's not always in older men. For example, a study done by the Mayo Clinic that was reported in 2009 found that men between the ages of 40 and 49 with ED were twice as likely to have heart disease as those with no erectile problems.

Medications commonly contribute to ED. By far the most common are various blood pressure medications, including clonidine (brand name Catapres) and the many beta-blocker drugs, among others. Diuretics, which are often used in the treatment of hypertension, may also worsen ED. You might be reading this and saying, "Great! High blood pressure causes ED and the medicines used to treat high blood pressure cause ED. What am I supposed to do?" You can't let high blood pressure go untreated, because it will worsen your vascular disease overall, and increase your risk of heart attack and stroke. The goal is to find the medicines that are the least likely to worsen ED. Fortunately, ACEs and ARBs have a fairly low risk of causing ED.

If you watch TV, you know that there are now a variety of treatments for ED. The most widely used, of course, are drugs such as Viagra (sildenafil), Levitra (vardenafil), and Cialis (tadalafil). These drugs improve blood flow to the penis. If the drugs don't seem to work immediately, it may be worth continuing to use them because responsiveness improves somewhat with continued use. No one of these medications is superior to the others, but many people report that one or another works better for them. These drugs are very expensive; if you don't need the maximum strength, you can often save money by buying the highest dose and cutting the tablets. The drugs tend to lower blood pressure, and there can be a dangerous fall in blood pressure if they are used in combination with nitroglycerine, used to treat coronary heart disease, or longer-acting medicines in the same family. If your doctor has given you a prescription for nitroglycerine tablets to have "just in case," he may be reluctant to also give you a prescription for an ED medicine. Speak to your doctor if you don't use the nitroglycerine; he might decide you no longer really need the prescription. If you do take the ED medicine, avoid sexual activity that's too strenuous; this could cause chest pain or even a heart attack. Remember that the physical exertion of sex is like any other exercise: you need to build up your activity gradually. Talk to your doctor about using other drugs that lower blood pressure, including the alpha-blockers (Hytrin [terazosin], Cardura [doxazosin], Flomax [tamsulosin], and Uroxatral [alfuzosin]) that are used to treat prostate enlargement, in combination with Viagra, Levitra, or Cialis, as they can also cause dangerously low blood pressure.

There are other treatment options for ED. Alprostadil is a medication that improves blood flow to the penis and improves erections. It can be given either by injection (Caverject and other brands) at the base of the penis or by putting an alprostadil gel (brand name MUSE) directly into the urethra, using a thin tube and a little lubricant so it slides in easily. The medicine is absorbed from the lining of the urethra into the surrounding tissues. The shot is less appealing to most people, of course, but more effective. Vacuum devices can also be used to treat ED. A gentle vacuum pulls blood into the penis, and then a rubber band–type device placed at the base of the penis prevents the blood from flowing out. If other options are not successful, a penile implant can be placed surgically. And we shouldn't forget that intercourse with an erect penis isn't the only form of sexual intimacy. Some couples dealing with erectile dysfunction find that they can have a rich sex life even without full erections. A sex therapist or counselor can often be of help here.

Another major issue for men with diabetes may be lack of sexual desire. Obviously, there are a lot of things that interfere with sexual desire, including the stresses of dealing with a medical problem, but sometimes a lack of desire results from a low testosterone level. Testosterone is the main male sex hormone. A large percentage of men—as many as 25 percent in some studies—have testosterone levels that fall below the normal range, but a low blood level doesn't always mean that there is a problem. Many men have what appear to be low blood levels, but biologically the amount of testosterone in their systems is perfectly adequate. It's important to look not only at blood tests but also at whether the man has symptoms of low testosterone, such as a diminished sex drive, reduced muscle mass and stamina, depression, or irritability. Only about half of men with low testosterone levels report any symptoms, and the symptoms are not specific enough to be sure that the low testosterone causes the problem. Unless the blood level is very low, diagnosing a testosterone problem requires a careful evaluation by the doctor to exclude other causes of the man's symptoms. As you recall, type 1 diabetes can be associated with other autoimmune problems, including damage to the testes by the immune system resulting in a reduced testosterone level. Recent evidence suggests that men with type 2 diabetes may also be at higher risk of low testosterone levels.

If a careful evaluation by your doctor suggests that low testosterone is a problem, it can be treated by giving testosterone either topically, in the form of a gel that you rub into the skin or a patch, or by injection once weekly or once every couple of weeks. Men on testosterone treatment have to have regular follow-ups to make sure there are no problems with prostate enlargement or an increase in the red blood cell count.

Just as some medications reduce erectile function, others may actually diminish libido. Probably the most common are antidepressants in the selective serotonin reuptake inhibitor (SSRI) family: fluoxetine (Prozac), sertraline (Zoloft), escitalopram (Lexapro), and others. These drugs tend to lessen sex drive, and they can lead to difficulty with orgasms in both men and women. If the problem is significant, sometimes the addition of buproprion (Wellbutrin) will help, or a change in treatment may be necessary. Diabetic neuropathy, too, may diminish orgasms in either men or women if the neuropathy involves the genital area.

In addition to a lower libido in response to certain medicines, women have their own issues with sexual function and diabetes. Diabetes increases the likelihood of vaginal yeast infections, especially if the blood sugar levels are not well controlled. This can cause itching, burning, and pain. Although we don't think of "erectile dysfunction" as a female issue, poor blood flow to the clitoris and the vagina can contribute to lessened sexual responsiveness. Women with diabetes are at increased risk of urinary tract infections, both because high blood sugar levels predispose them to infection and because neuropathy may cause problems with urine incontinence and bladder emptying. A woman may be hesitant about engaging in sexual activity because of this risk.

Testosterone controls libido in women just as it does in men, and sometimes women have a low testosterone level as well. In women, testosterone is made both in the ovaries and in the adrenal glands. Women with type 1 diabetes are at increased risk of autoimmune problems involving either of these organs, sometimes leading to a fall in testosterone with an accompanying reduced sex drive. Treating a low testosterone level in women is a bit of a specialized problem, so if you're a woman who thinks her sex drive or sexual responsiveness is diminished, you should talk to your gynecologist or see an endocrinologist to discuss evaluation and treatment.

ISLANDS OF THE FUTURE

From the moment insulin became available, diabetes became a treatable disease, but our real goal is to prevent diabetes from ever developing or to restore the body's ability to make insulin in those who already have it. Type 1 diabetes is one of many autoimmune diseases awaiting more effective treatment to stop the body from attacking its own tissues. Our understanding of type 1 diabetes increases all the time, but the immune system is extraordinarily complex, and our tools for modifying it remain crude. Most drugs used to treat autoimmune disorders are highly toxic and suppress the immune system so broadly that the person becomes susceptible to serious infections. Prevention of type 1 diabetes will require the ability to identify those in the very early stages of the disease and treat them with highly targeted immune therapy that won't suppress the entire immune system.

Pancreas transplantation is sometimes used to restore insulin production in type 1 diabetes. This is a major surgical procedure with a high risk of complications, so it is done only in those people whose blood sugar levels absolutely can't be controlled by other means. The availability of organs is quite limited because they cannot be donated by a living person. We have only one pancreas and removing it causes serious problems. Even when a pancreas does become available from a deceased donor, there is a risk of rejection, as with all organ transplantation, so long-term success isn't guaranteed. In addition, the same autoimmune process that destroyed the insulin-producing beta cells in the person's own pancreas is likely to attack the cells in the transplanted pancreas. The majority of people who undergo pancreas transplantation also have kidney failure and need a kidney transplant. The kidney transplant has a higher likelihood of success, and the same drugs are used to prevent rejection of both the transplanted kidney and pancreas. Therefore, if a person needs a kidney transplant and there is a suitable pancreas available, it's much easier to justify the pancreas transplant than for someone who needs only the pancreas.

A less invasive way to restore insulin production in type 1 diabetes is with islet cell transplantation. The insulin-producing beta cells in the pancreas are scattered in little clusters called islets, or islands, and these cells can be extracted and purified from the pancreas of a deceased organ donor. Often two or three donor pancreases are required to yield sufficient numbers of cells for one transplantation, so the availability of donor pancreas tissue is an even more serious problem than with pancreas transplantation. The advantage of islet cell transplantation is that the insulin-producing cells are given to someone intravenously, via a vein to the liver, without the need for major surgery. The liver is more accessible than the pancreas, and the transplanted insulin-producing cells function perfectly well in the liver. Anti-rejection drugs are needed after islet cell transplantation because the body will try to reject the new cells even though they're not transplanted as a whole organ. Here, too, the autoimmune process that led to diabetes in the first place may attack the transplanted cells. In a study published in 2005, only about 10 percent of those who had received islet cell transplantation were off of insulin completely after five years, but many of those who still took insulin needed less and had much less volatility in their blood sugar levels. In some ways, they became a bit more like people with type 2 diabetes: they had some insulin in their bodies, just not enough to meet their needs completely.

In the minds of doctors, stem cell research holds the best promise for curing type 1 diabetes. Stem cells have the capability to become cells of different types given the proper environment and the correct chemical signals, and researchers have made excellent progress in turning stem cells into insulin-producing cells. The advantage of stem cells is that, at least in theory, they can be grown in large numbers in the laboratory for use in patients, rather than having to depend on cells from organ donors. Some people have objected to stem cell research, of course, because most early stem cells were obtained from human embryos. However, stem cells can also be obtained from other sources, including from adult tissues and maybe even from the individual seeking treatment. The hope for stem cell research is that cells can be obtained in a way that wouldn't pose any moral or ethical dilemma and grown in large quantities, coaxed into producing insulin like normal pancreatic beta cells, and then transplanted back into the person with diabetes. If the stem cells could be obtained from the individual with diabetes, there might not be a need to take anti-rejection drugs, though the problem of autoimmunity that caused the diabetes to begin with would remain. Some form of immunosuppressive treatment might overcome this, or the person might require periodic stem cell infusions. There is even evidence that stem cells reside in normal pancreas tissue, and there may be the possibility that these can be triggered to form new insulin-producing cells in those with either type 1 or type 2 diabetes. Like so much in medical research, the prospect seems close because we understand many of the fundamentals, but it is still far off because there are many daunting technical challenges. Still, stem cell research is just in its infancy, and we're optimistic that the ability to grow new cells and tissues will lead to treatments for diabetes that we can only dream of at present.

6

BEST LIFE DIABETES- FRIENDLY MEAL PLANS

WHEN YOU HAVE DIABETES, there are a lot of "don'ts" in your diet: don't eat too many carbs, don't eat too much saturated fat, don't consume too many calories. But this meal plan is full of "dos": do enjoy hearty meals, do have luxuriously rich-tasting food, and do have some chocolate and other treats. These are meals you'd be proud to share with guests, and many dishes will instantly become family favorites. In fact, we designed the meals with your family in mind; they're full of familiar dishes that will ensure that they can enjoy a way of eating that will prevent diabetes down the road. (Check out the "Family-Friendly Fare" box on page 251 for recipe ideas.)

The tastiness of the meals belies their carefully composed nutrition specs. For instance, the Summer Squash Whole Wheat Pasta Bake is the type of comfort food casserole that'll be a hit with the whole family. Pasta, especially whole grain pasta, is a low-glycemic-index food, and the addition of almonds and walnuts to this dish lowers the glycemic index even further. Meanwhile, each portion offers three vegetable servings, but as they're baked in with the pasta, even your picky eaters won't notice!

Nutritionally, the plan works out to about 38 to 42 percent of calories from carbohydrates, 21 to 26 percent from protein, and 36 to 42

FAMILY-FRIENDLY FARE

Looking to get your children to eat more nutritiously—whether it's because you'd like to help them lose weight, reduce their risk for pre-diabetes or diabetes, or simply eat healthier? Try these nutrient-packed recipes that are sure to please even the pickiest palates!

Vanilla Peanut Butter Smoothie (page 290)

White Bean Chili (page 298)

Hearty Beef Ragout over Barley (page 306) (If barley's too foreign for your child, try serving this over Barilla PLUS pasta, which does not taste like a high-fiber pasta)

Slow-Cooked Pork (page 308)

Ground Turkey Casserole (page 312)

BBQ Tofu (page 324)

Oat Cake (page 326)

Chocolate Mini-cakes (page 331)

Popcorn and Oat Cookies (page 332)

percent from fat, with a low 7 percent of calories from saturated fat. Our plan is high in fiber, averaging about 34 grams per day. We've found that this balance of carbohydrates, protein, and fat is easiest on your blood sugar—and your arteries. It's a little lower in carbohydrates than the 50-percent-carbohydrate-or-higher diets recommended by health authorities for the general population, but the general population doesn't have to worry about its blood sugar. It's a Mediterranean-style diet, rich in heart-healthy foods such as olive oil, nuts, vegetables, fish, and poultry. All the grains are whole grain or a mix of whole grain and fiber (such as Barilla PLUS pasta). We do include some red meat, sticking with the leanest cuts.

If you don't have much time to spend cooking, you'll be happy to know that the recipes have short ingredient lists, and most will have you in and out of the kitchen in 30 minutes—many take just 10 minutes to prepare. And if you do love to cook, you'll find many of these recipes a delicious departure from the same old dishes found in many health books. The meal plans use a mix of recipes, easily prepared food such as sandwiches, and some convenience foods, such as gardein frozen meals. Because you can exchange meals from different days, you can lean on the fastest meals when you're tight on time and prepare meals requiring more cooking when your schedule permits. Another bonus: most of these meals are very easy on the budget. For even more meal choices, go to www .thebestlife.com/diabetes.

Here's what you have to do to make this plan work for you:

- Pick a calorie level. Use the guidelines on pages 48 and 53 to help you find your level.

- Check the note under each meal to see if there are specific guidelines for your calorie level. If not, just eat the meal presented. The basic plan is 1,700 calories, so you won't see special notes for that calorie level.

- Add more calories if needed. If you need more calories because you're hungry much of the day due to a high exercise level (or because you simply have a great metabolism and can afford the extra calories), use the 2,250-calorie meal plan and tack on 100 calories each day until you hit a calorie level that keeps you satisfied, but doesn't pack on body fat. Gaining muscle is always okay—you'll know if you look more toned and lose inches! Start by simply eating a little more of the foods already on the 2,250-calorie plan. Just watch the carbs—the first 100 to 200 extra calories should be foods low in carbs, then you can add 50 to 100 calories of carbs, maxing out at about 200 carb calories; let your blood sugar be your guide. For instance, if you need to add 500 calories, up to 200 of them would come from high-carbohydrate foods and 300 from low-carbohydrate choices. (Some high-level exercisers need even more carbohydrates—see page 56 for details).

  Here are just a few ways to tack on 50 or 100 calories. For more ideas, turn to the charts listing servings from various food groups (see pages 59, 111, and 121):

Low-carb/no-carb foods

- 100 calories of nuts: 15 almonds, 17 peanuts, 7 walnut halves, 1 tablespoon plus 2 teaspoons of pine nuts, or 14 whole cashews (2 tablespoons cashew pieces)

- 50 calories of oil: 1 teaspoon olive oil, canola oil, or other oil

- 50 calories of healthy spread, such as 2 teaspoons Bestlife Buttery Spread

- 50 calories of fish, skinless poultry, or lean meat (about 1 ounce)

High-carb foods

- 50 calories of fat-free milk or soy milk with about 6 g carbohydrates (about ½ cup)

- 50 calories of bread with about 7 g carbohydrates (½ slice; check labels, as bread varies widely per slice in terms of calories and carbohydrates)

- 75 calories of cooked pasta with 14 g carbohydrates (⅓ cup)

- 50 calories of beans (such as black beans, white beans, garbanzo) with 9 g carbohydrates (¼ cup)

- 50 calories of hummus with 5 g carbohydrates: 2½ tablespoons

- 60 calories of fruit with 15 g carbohydrates (1 small apple, ⅔ cup blueberries, ½ cup grapes, or 1¼ cup strawberries)

- 25 calories of vegetables with 5 g carbohydrates (8 medium spears asparagus, 1 cup cauliflower, or ¾ cup chopped tomatoes)

- Swap meals if you'd like. Because all breakfasts have the same number of calories and carbohydrates, you can substitute any breakfast for any other. That also goes for lunches, dinners, and snacks. But you can't swap a breakfast for a lunch because the breakfasts don't have the same number of calories and carbs as the lunches or the dinners. As for the snacks, you can substitute any Snack 1 for another Snack 1, but you can't swap a Snack 1 for a Snack 2 or Snack 3. So, for instance, you could have a Day 1 breakfast with a Day 5 lunch, Day 10 dinner and Day 12 Snack 1, and Day 11 Snack 2.

■ Pick the right dessert for your calorie level. If you're on 1,700 calories per day, you're allowed a 100-calorie, 10-grams-carbohydrate treat. On 2,000 or 2,250 calories, you're allowed a 150-calorie, 15-gram-carbohydrate treat. There is no treat on 1,500 calories because there are no calories to spare!

■ Eat dessert at the end of the meal. It's best to eat your sweet at the end of your meal instead of by itself to take advantage of the blood-sugar-lowering effects of eating carbohydrates within a meal.

■ Don't worry about calculating carbs; we've done it for you. Below are the carbohydrate grams and calories per meal. Unless there's a special note on the meal, no matter what meal you choose, the carbs will be within 1 gram above or below what's written on the chart.

CALORIES/DAY	BREAKFAST	LUNCH	DINNER	SNACK 1	SNACK 2	SNACK 3	DESSERT
	Carbs/Cal	Carbs/Cal	Carbs/Cal	Carbs/Cal	Carbs/Cal	Carbs/Cal	Carbs/Cal
1,500	34/325	48/425	45/500	12/175	5/75	—	—
1,700	34/325	48/425	45/500	12/175	5/175	—	10/100
2,000	40/400	48/500	52/550	18/200	18/200	—	15/150
2,250	40/400	48/550	52/550	18/200	18/200	21/200	15/150

■ Start any day you'd like. Generally, there's more cooking involved on the weekends because you're likely to have more time to spend in the kitchen.

■ Make substitutions if you like. For instance, instead of 3 ounces of chicken, eat 3 ounces of fish. You can have ½ cup of raspberries instead of ½ cup strawberries. When substituting cereals, energy bars, and tortillas, make sure you pick products with the same amount of fiber, carbohydrates, sodium, and calories. You can exchange fat-free milk for soy, but be aware that fat-free milk has 12 grams of carbohydrates per cup and Silk, the soy milk recommended on this plan, has 11 grams per cup for regular and 8 grams for unsweetened. Some of the meals offer the option of milk or soy milk.

■ Add fiber if you'd like. This plan is designed to provide at least 25 grams of fiber, and many meal combinations will offer more. If you'd like more fiber, take a supplement; Benefiber carries the Best Life Seal of Approval, and we've used it in some of the meals to bolster fiber levels.

■ Look for low-sodium meals. Because diabetes puts you at higher risk for heart disease and high blood pressure is a risk factor for heart disease, we're helping you lower your blood pressure by keeping sodium levels low. The LS next to a meal means it's low sodium; no matter which LS meals you choose, you won't exceed the recommended 2,300 milligrams of sodium per day on the 1,500-, 1,700-, and 2,000-calorie-per-day plans. For the 2,250-calorie plan, the sodium content maxes out at 2,400; we went a little higher because it's difficult to keep sodium content lower when you're eating more calories, but it's still recommended by the U.S. Department of Agriculture. Here is how sodium is distributed in the meals marked LS:

Breakfast: No more than 450 mg

Lunch: No more than 600 mg

Dinner: No more than 750 mg

Snack 1: No more than 200 mg

Snack 2: No more than 200 mg

Snack 3 (for 2,250 calorie plan only): No more than 100 mg

Dessert: No more than 100 mg

■ Look for the V if you want a vegetarian meal. These meals contain no fish, red meat, or poultry. They may include dairy and eggs.

■ Stay hydrated. Water isn't mentioned on the meal plan because it would have to be mentioned at every meal! In order to get the six 8-ounce servings of water recommended on this program, you should drink water with every meal and in between. If you're on the go, a bottle of water is especially convenient. Look for the Best Life seal on Nestlé Pure Life Purified Water, a nationally available brand that is committed to using less plastic, which means it's kinder to the planet. If you want to add flavor, squirt a little lemon or lime juice into plain water.

A NOTE ON COMMON INGREDIENTS IN THE MEAL PLANS

"Healthy spread" means a spread that contains no partially hydrogenated oil and is about 60 to 80 calories per tablespoon, such as Bestlife Buttery Spread. Soy milk on this plan should contain no more than 110 calories and have at least 30 percent of the daily value for calcium per cup, like many of the Silk soy milks. A slice of whole wheat bread should be about 80 calories. Nuts that are incorporated into many of the meals should be unsalted. Use raw or dry-roasted nuts whenever possible. You can also toast your own nuts in the oven or toaster oven to make them more crunchy and flavorful. This can be done in a 350-degree oven, be aware that they burn quickly, so keep a close eye on them. The reduced-fat cheese used in the meal plans should have about 60 calories, 200 milligrams of sodium, and 1.5 grams of saturated fat per ounce, such as Cabot 75% Reduced Fat Cheddar. Low-sodium, low-fat cheese should have 5 to 35 milligrams of sodium and about 50 calories per ounce.

A NOTE ON BRAND NAMES

In many of the following recipes and meals, you'll notice brand-name suggestions for a variety of ingredients, including soy milk, whole grain crackers, and healthy spreads. Some of these recommended brands carry the Best Life Seal of Approval, meaning they're rich in good-for-you elements, such as whole grains, healthy fats, fiber, vitamins, calcium and other minerals, and phytonutrients. And you'll also see the Best Life's own Bestlife brand foods, which were introduced in 2010. As of the press time of this book, the two products available are Bestlife Buttery Spread and Bestlife Buttery Spray. Keep your eye out for more to come. In addition to the commonly used ingredients below, the following products are Best Life approved: Benefiber; gardein vegetarian entrées and meals; Hershey's cocoa and Extra Dark chocolate; and Nestlé Pure Life Purified Water. The California Table Grape Commission and Florida Grapefruit are also food partners. Bestlife foods and products carrying the Best Life seal or Best Life Treat seal are available in most supermarkets nationwide.

A NOTE ON SODIUM

In order to keep sodium in a healthy range, the recipes call for moderate amounts of salt; the meal plans don't call for any salt. Herbs and other flavorful ingredients are incorporated into recipes to provide great taste without using an excess of sodium. If you'd like a little more salt, add a few crystals to the food on your plate instead of adding it during preparation or cooking. The crystals hitting your tongue will give you a stronger salt sensation than if you'd used a lot more salt in cooking.

COMMONLY USED INGREDIENTS

Some healthful ingredients pop up frequently in recipes and meal plans. So as not to repeat the descriptions over and over, here's a one-stop explanation.

Beans: All of these recipes work with both boiled-from-scratch and canned beans. No particular brand was used consistently; we like the low-sodium Goya beans and the no-salt-added Eden Organic beans. If you have the choice, opt for either of these brands or any other no-salt-added or low-sodium (no more than 130 milligrams per ½ cup) variety. Otherwise, you can use regular canned beans, but drain them and rinse them well in a colander before adding to a recipe to rid them of excess sodium. Note that cooking times for recipes that contain beans assume that you're using canned beans; you'll have to factor in more time if you soak and boil them.

Crispbread: Recipes, meals, and snacks using this ingredient were developed with Wasa Multi-Grain, Light Rye, or other whole grain Wasa crispbreads carrying the Best Life seal.

Healthy spread: This refers to margarines or spreads made with no partially hydrogenated oil, such as Bestlife Buttery Spread.

Liquid eggs: The recipes were developed using AllWhites, which are 100% liquid egg whites, and Better'n Eggs, which are a fat-free, cholesterol-free replacement for whole eggs (98% liquid egg whites with vitamins added).

Mayonnaise: These recipes use mayonnaise that has no more than 50 calories per tablespoon. We relied on two Hellmann's varieties: Canola Cholesterol Free and Light, but other good choices are Kraft Light or Spectrum Light Canola Oil Mayonnaise.

Peanut butter: Smart Balance Omega Peanut Butter with omega-3 fats was used in recipes, meals, and snacks calling for peanut butter.

Soy milk: If a recipe calls for soy milk, it's the plain variety; otherwise, you'll notice that we've specified the flavor, such as unsweetened, vanilla, or chocolate. We used Silk Soymilk, which carries the Best Life seal.

Whole wheat or fiber-enriched pasta: Not everyone likes the grittiness of 100% whole wheat pasta, so we developed these recipes using two highly nutritious, fiber-rich Barilla pastas: Barilla Whole Grain, which is 51% whole grain, and Barilla PLUS (also protein-enriched).

Whole wheat wraps or flatbread: We used Flatout Healthy Grain Multi-Grain Flatbread throughout.

TWO WEEKS OF MEAL PLANS

DAY 1

BREAKFAST LS, V

- Steel-Cut Oats with Walnuts and Orange Zest (page 294)

- 1⅛ cups (1 cup plus 2 tablespoons) Silk Light Vanilla Soymilk

OPTION: Use 1 cup of nonfat milk instead of the soy milk.

(2,000 AND 2,250 CAL/DAY: Add 2 teaspoons of chopped unsalted walnuts to the oatmeal. Serve with 1⅔ cups Silk Light Vanilla Soymilk.)

OPTION: Use 1½ cups nonfat milk instead of the soy milk.

LUNCH LS

- Spinach salad: 3¼ cups fresh spinach, ½ cup cooked skinless chicken pieces (use leftover chicken or a rotisserie chicken), tossed with 5 sprays Wish-Bone Balsamic Salad Spritzer or Safeway Eating Right Balsamic Vinaigrette Spray

- Barley Salad with Parsley and Lemon (page 325)

- 1½ cups apple slices; ¾ large whole apple

(2,000 CAL/DAY: For the spinach salad, reduce the spinach to 2½ cups and add ½ tablespoon unsalted pumpkin seeds.)

(2,250 CAL/DAY: Make the spinach salad with 3 cups spinach tossed with ½ teaspoon olive oil and 10 sprays of Wish-Bone Balsamic Salad Spritzer. Add 1½ tablespoons unsalted pumpkin seeds to the salad.)

DINNER LS

- Flank Steak with Tomato Relish (page 307)

- Salad: 3½ cups salad greens, ⅓ cup canned, rinsed and drained artichoke hearts with no added salt (30–35 calories and 55–60 milligrams of sodium per ⅓-cup serving), tossed with 1¼ teaspoons olive oil, 1 teaspoon sherry vinegar

- ½ cup cooked grits seasoned with a pinch of salt and 1 tablespoon fresh chopped chives

- 1 cup whole strawberries

(2,000 AND 2,250 CAL/DAY: Make the salad with 2½ cups salad greens and add a scant ¼ cup cooked no-salt-added garbanzo beans. Serve with ¾ cup whole strawberries.)

SNACK 1 LS, V

- Hot herbal spiced tea: Steep Lipton Herbal Ginger Twist or Twinings Revive Herbal tea bag in 1 cup plain soy milk, such as Silk, and season with a small pinch of cinnamon and clove.

- 1½ tablespoons unsalted cashews, about ⅓ ounce

(2,000 AND 2,250 CAL/DAY: Make herbal spiced tea with 1⅓ cups plain soy milk. Serve with 1 tablespoon unsalted cashews, about ¼ ounce. Add ⅓ cup blackberries.)

SNACK 2 LS, V

- Sweet pepper gratin: Place ¼ cup sliced sweet pepper on an ovenproof dish, top with ¾ ounce grated reduced-fat cheddar cheese, and broil until the cheese is melted.

- 17 unsalted almonds, about ¾ ounce

(1,500 CAL/DAY: Make gratin with ¾ cup sliced sweet pepper and 1 ounce grated reduced-fat cheddar cheese. Omit the almonds.)

(2,000 AND 2,250 CAL/DAY: Make the gratin with ⅔ cup sliced sweet pepper and ½ ounce grated reduced-fat cheddar cheese. Add 1 Wasa Multi-Grain Crispbread and serve with 15 unsalted almonds, about ⅔ ounce total.)

SNACK 3 LS, V

(2,250 CAL/DAY ONLY: 2 cups air-popped unsalted popcorn [30 calories, 6 grams of carbohydrate, and 0 gram of saturated fat] tossed with 2 teaspoons olive oil and served with ¾ cup nonfat milk.)

TREAT LS, V

- Small cookie or half a small biscotti (45 calories, 7 grams carbohydrate, 1 gram saturated fat) such as ½ Nonni's Originali Biscotti biscotto

- 7 unsalted almonds, about ⅓ ounce

(1,500 CAL/DAY: Omit the treat.)

(2,000 AND 2,250 CAL/DAY: Have a larger cookie or biscotto: 90 calories, 14 grams carbohydrate, 1.5 grams saturated fat)

DAY 2

BREAKFAST LS, V

- ½ whole grain English muffin with 120 calories and 23 grams of carbohydrate per 1 whole muffin, such as Thomas's Hearty Grains Multi-Grain English Muffin, with 2½ teaspoons healthy spread, ¾ cup fat-free ricotta cheese, such as Sargento, mixed with 1½ teaspoons Benefiber, 2 sliced small strawberries (1-inch diameter), and a sprinkle of cinnamon

- 16 unsalted almonds, about ¾ ounce

(2,000 AND 2,250 CAL/DAY: 1 whole grain English muffin with 3 teaspoons healthy spread, and ¼ cup fat-free ricotta cheese mixed with 1 teaspoon Benefiber. Serve with 15 unsalted almonds (about ⅔ ounce, and add ½ cup nonfat milk.)

LUNCH LS ONLY IF USING NO-SALT-ADDED TUNA

- Tuna melt: Top 2 Wasa Multi-Grain Crispbreads with 4 ounces drained chunk light tuna canned in water (for a low-sodium meal, use no-salt-added or low-sodium tuna, such as Bumble Bee Chunk White Albacore Very Low Sodium in Water), 1½ teaspoons mustard, such as Gulden's (or other mustard with about 10 calories and 50–55 milligrams of sodium per teaspoon), and ¾ ounce shredded reduced-fat cheddar cheese. Place under broiler until the cheese is melted on top.

- Salad: 3½ cups mixed greens, ½ medium tomato, chopped, ½ cup sliced red pepper tossed with ¾ teaspoon olive oil and lime juice to taste

- 1 fresh orange, peeled (about ⅓ pound)

(2,000 CAL/DAY: Make the tuna melt with 4½ ounces drained chunk light tuna canned in water. For the salad, use 3 cups mixed greens and ⅔ cup sliced pepper and toss with 1¾ teaspoons olive oil.)

(2,250 CAL/DAY: Make the tuna melt with 5 ounces drained chunk light tuna, canned in water [or low-sodium chunk light tuna in water, drained], ¾ teaspoon mustard, and 1½ ounces reduced-fat cheddar cheese. For the salad, use 3 cups mixed greens, ¾ cup sliced peppers, and 2 teaspoons olive oil.)

DINNER LS

- White Bean Chili (page 298)

- Roasted Asparagus (page 327) with 1¼ teaspoons healthy spread

- ½ cup sliced mango

(2,000 AND 2,250 CAL/DAY: Serve the asparagus with 1½ teaspoons healthy spread and have ¾ cup mango with 1 teaspoon chopped walnuts.)

SNACK 1 LS, V

- Peanut butter yogurt: Serve ½ cup plain nonfat yogurt with 1 tablespoon plus ¼ teaspoon Smart Balance Omega Peanut Butter mixed in.

(2,000 AND 2,250 CAL/DAY: Make the peanut butter yogurt with ¾ cup plain nonfat yogurt.)

SNACK 2 LS, V (LS for 1,500/1,700 cal/day snacks only)

- Cream cheese dip: Mix 1¼ ounces (about 2½ tablespoons) nonfat cream cheese with 2 tablespoons fresh chives or ½ teaspoon dried oregano and a pinch of salt-free garlic seasoning, such as Mrs. Dash salt-free garlic and herb seasoning, 1 tablespoon nonfat plain yogurt, and 1 tablespoon olive oil. Serve the dip with ¾ cup sliced cucumbers.

(1,500 CAL/DAY: Make the dip with ¾ teaspoon olive oil and serve with
½ cup sliced cucumbers.)

(2,000 AND 2,250 CAL/DAY: Make the dip with 1¼ ounces
[2½ tablespoons] nonfat cream cheese, 1½ teaspoons olive oil, and
1½ tablespoons nonfat plain yogurt, and add 2 teaspoons sesame seeds.
Serve with 1 cup sliced cucumbers and 1 Wasa Multi-Grain Crispbread.)

SNACK 3 LS, V

(2,250 CAL/DAY ONLY: 1 low-sodium brown rice cake, such as Lundberg,
spread with 1 tablespoon fat-free sour cream, such as Breakstone's, and
topped with ¼ cup sliced avocado and 1 medium slice of tomato; drizzle
with 1¼ teaspoons olive oil.)

TREAT LS, V

- 2 Hershey's Extra Dark Pure Dark Chocolate tasting squares: Any
  flavor except Pomegranate, due to its higher carbohydrate content

(1,500 CAL/DAY: Omit the treat.)

(2,000 AND 2,250 CAL/DAY: 3 Hershey's Extra Dark Pure Dark Chocolate
tasting squares: Any flavor except Pomegranate, due to its higher
carbohydrate content.)

DAY 3

BREAKFAST V

- Tofu Spinach Scramble (page 291)

- 1½ cups plain soy milk, such as Silk

OPTION: Use 1¼ cups nonfat milk instead of soy milk. Use 1 teaspoon
canola oil to coat the pan for the Tofu Spinach Scramble instead of
vegetable oil cooking spray.

(2,000 AND 2,250 CAL/DAY: Add ⅔ cup sliced red pepper and
3 tablespoons shredded low-sodium, low-fat cheddar cheese to the Tofu
Spinach Scramble. Serve with 1¾ cups plain soy milk, such as Silk.)

OPTION: Include 1½ cups total nonfat milk instead of soy milk and use
1¼ teaspoons canola oil to coat the pan for the Tofu Spinach Scramble
instead of vegetable oil cooking spray.

LUNCH LS

- gardein Santa Fe Good Stuff, 1 breast
- Creamy Celery Salad (page 330)
- 1½ cups pear slices

(2,000 CAL/DAY: Melt ½ ounce reduced-fat cheese over gardein Santa Fe Good Stuff. Add ½ tablespoon sesame oil to each serving of Creamy Celery Salad.)

(2,250 CAL/DAY: Add 1 tablespoon sesame seeds and 2 teaspoons sesame oil to each serving of Creamy Celery Salad. Serve with 2 cups apple slices.)

DINNER LS

- Trout with Roasted Vegetables (page 314)
- 3 tablespoons dry whole wheat couscous (½ cup cooked), cooked according to package directions, with 2¼ teaspoons olive oil and 1 tablespoon chopped fresh parsley mixed in
- ½ cup fresh raspberries

(2,000 AND 2,250 CAL/DAY: Mix 2¾ teaspoons olive oil into the cooked couscous and serve with 1 cup raspberries.)

SNACK 1 LS, V

- Warm ¾ cup lowfat 1% milk and serve with a large pinch of ground cinnamon.
- 11 unsalted almonds, about ½ ounce

(2,000 AND 2,250 CAL/DAY: Use 1⅛ cups nonfat milk and serve with 14 unsalted almonds, about ⅔ ounce.)

SNACK 2 LS, V

- 1½ cups shredded romaine tossed with ½ teaspoon olive oil and 1 teaspoon red wine vinegar
- 11 unsalted walnut halves, about ¾ ounce

(1,500 CAL/DAY: Substitute the 1,700 cal/day snack with 3 medium celery stalks spread with 1½ teaspoons Smart Balance Omega Peanut Butter.)

(2,000 AND 2,250 CAL/DAY: Substitute the 1,700 cal/day snack with 6 small celery stalks and 1½ unsalted brown rice cakes (35 calories and 7 grams of carbohydrate per rice cake), spread with 1 tablespoon plus 1 teaspoon Smart Balance Omega Peanut Butter.)

SNACK 3 LS, V

(2,250 CAL/DAY ONLY: ½ cup nonfat plain yogurt with ½ cup strawberry halves and 2 tablespoons unsalted cashews, about ½ ounce, mixed in.)

TREAT LS, V

- 1 tablespoon of dark chocolate–covered raisins, such as Raisinets, mixed with 7 unsalted almonds, about ⅓ ounce

(1,500 CAL/DAY: Omit the treat.)

(2,000 AND 2,250 CAL/DAY: 1 tablespoon plus 1 teaspoon dark chocolate–covered raisins, such as Raisinets, mixed with 11 unsalted almonds, about ½ ounce.)

DAY 4

BREAKFAST LS, V

- Vanilla Peanut Butter Smoothie (page 290)

- 1 Wasa Multi-Grain Crispbread spread with 1¼ teaspoon healthy spread

(2,000 AND 2,250 CAL/DAY: Add ¼ cup nonfat milk (1¾ cups total) and 1¾ teaspoons Smart Balance Chunky Peanut Butter (1 tablespoon plus 1¾ teaspoons total) to the smoothie recipe.)

LUNCH V

- Veggie burger: Choose a burger with 130 calories, no more than 10 grams of carbohydrate, and no trans fats, such as Amy's California Veggie Burger, and top with ½ sliced medium tomato, ½ tablespoon

Hellmann's Canola Cholesterol Free Mayonnaise or Kraft Light Mayonnaise, and 1 ounce low-fat, low-sodium cheddar cheese.

- 1 small whole wheat pita bread (4-inch diameter, 75 calories, 15 grams carbohydrate per 1 pita)

- Salad: 2 cups fresh spinach with sections from one small orange tossed with 10 sprays Wish-Bone Red Wine Salad Spritzer or Newman's Own Tuscan Italian Natural Salad Mist and 1¼ teaspoons olive oil

- ½ cup halved strawberries

(2,000 CAL/DAY: Top the burger with 2½ ounces low-fat, low-sodium cheddar cheese. Make the salad with 3¼ cups total fresh spinach and toss with 10 sprays of Wish-Bone dressing and 1½ teaspoons olive oil. Serve ⅓ cup halved strawberries.)

(2,250 CAL/DAY: Top the burger with 1 tablespoon Hellmann's Canola Cholesterol Free Mayonnaise and 3 ounces low-fat, low-sodium cheddar cheese.)

DINNER LS

- Ground Turkey Casserole (page 312)

- 1 whole grain dinner roll (about 1 ounce), served with 1 teaspoon olive oil

- ¾ cup fresh pineapple chunks or frozen, unsweetened pineapple chunks, thawed or canned in juice sprinkled with 1½ teaspoons Benefiber

(2,000 AND 2,250 CAL/DAY: Serve 1¼ whole grain dinner rolls [about 1½ ounces] and 1 cup pineapple chunks sprinkled with 1½ teaspoons Benefiber.)

SNACK 1 LS, V

- Hot chocolate: 1 cup plain soy milk, such as Silk, heated with 2 teaspoons Hershey's Cocoa and 1 packet of Splenda (or add to taste)

- ⅓ ounce unsalted peanuts

(**2,000 AND 2,250 CAL/DAY:** For the hot chocolate, use 1¼ cups Silk Vanilla Soymilk and 1 tablespoon Hershey's cocoa.)

SNACK 2 LS, V

- ¼ cup sliced avocado mashed with 1½ teaspoons olive oil and served with 2½ small (5-inch-long) celery stalks for dipping

- 4 unsalted walnut halves

(**1,500 CAL/DAY:** Mix avocado with ⅛ teaspoon olive oil and serve with 4 small [5-inch-long] celery stalks for dipping. [Omit the walnuts.])

(**2,000 AND 2,250 CAL/DAY:** Use ⅓ cup avocado and mash with ¾ teaspoon olive oil. For dipping, use 5 small [5-inch-long] celery stalks and add 1 Wasa Multi-Grain Crispbread. Serve with 3 unsalted walnut halves, about ¼ ounce.)

SNACK 3 LS, V

(**2,250 CAL/DAY ONLY:** 6 baked tortilla chips [½ ounce, any brand, with about 110 calories and 20 grams of carbohydrates per 1 ounce], with 3½ tablespoons fat-free sour cream, such as Breakstone's, seasoned with chili powder for dipping.)

TREAT LS, V *(LS for 1,700-cal treat only)*

- 1 Chocolate Mini-cake (page 331)

(**1,500 CAL/DAY:** Omit the treat.)

(**2,000 AND 2,250 CAL/DAY:** Add ⅓ cup nonfat milk.)

DAY 5

BREAKFAST LS, V

- Cocoa Granola (page 293)

- 4 ounces nonfat plain yogurt with 1 teaspoon Benefiber mixed in

(**2,000 AND 2,250 CAL/DAY:** Serve the granola with 6 ounces nonfat plain yogurt with 1½ teaspoons Benefiber mixed in, and add 1½ teaspoons unsalted pumpkin seeds.)

LUNCH V

- Mustardy Sardine Salad (page 304)

- ⅓ cup cooked brown rice (quick-cooking is fine if you're short on time, or use leftover rice)

- 1 small pear, about 5.2 ounces

(**2,000 CAL/DAY**: Use ½ cup cooked brown rice and add 2 tablespoons plus 1 teaspoon unsalted slivered almonds to the rice. Serve with ½ small pear, 2.6 ounces.)

(**2,250 CAL/DAY**: Add 1 tablespoon plus 1 teaspoon Hellman's Canola Cholesterol Free Mayonnaise to each serving of Mustardy Sardine Salad.)

DINNER LS, V

- BBQ Tofu (page 324)

- Garlicky Broccoli and Eggplant (page 328)

- ⅓ cup cooked grits (1¼ tablespoons dry grits, cooked according to the package directions) topped with 1¾ teaspoons healthy spread

- ½ cup blackberries

(**2,000 AND 2,250 CAL/DAY**: Use ½ cup grits total [2 tablespoons dry grits, cooked according to package directions] topped with 2½ teaspoons healthy spread. Serve ⅔ cup blackberries.)

SNACK 1 LS, V

- Hot chocolate: ¾ cup plain soy milk, such as Silk, heated with 2 teaspoons Hershey's Cocoa and 1 packet of Splenda (or add to taste)

- 2 tablespoons unsalted sunflower seed kernels, about ½ ounce

(**2,000 AND 2,250 CAL/DAY**: For the hot chocolate, use 1½ cups soy milk and 1 tablespoon plus 1 teaspoon Hershey's Cocoa. Serve with 2 teaspoons unsalted sunflower seed kernels, about ⅛ ounce.)

SNACK 2 LS, V

- ⅓ cup cherry tomatoes

- 12 unsalted walnut halves, about ¾ ounce

(1,500 CAL/DAY: Serve ½ cup cherry tomatoes with 5 unsalted walnut halves.)

(2,000 AND 2,250 CAL/DAY: Serve 1⅛ cups cherry tomatoes and 8 unsalted walnut halves, about ½ ounce, and add low-fat soy crisps with about 70 calories and 9 grams of carbohydrate per one 18-gram serving, such as Glenny's Low-Fat Lightly Salted Soy Crisps.)

SNACK 3 LS, V

(2,250 CAL/DAY ONLY: ¾ roasted medium sweet potato, about 3.2 ounces, topped with 2 teaspoons healthy spread and 1 tablespoon plus 1 teaspoon unsalted chopped pecans.)

TREAT LS, V

- 2 Hershey's Extra Dark Tasting Squares: Any flavor except Pomegranate, due to its higher carbohydrate content

(1,500 CAL/DAY: Omit the treat.)

(2,000 AND 2,250 CAL/DAY: 3 Hershey's Extra Dark Tasting Squares: Any flavor except Pomegranate, due to its higher carbohydrate content.)

DAY 6

BREAKFAST LS, V *(LS for 1,500/1,700 cal/day only)*

- Scrambled egg whites with toast: Coat a frying pan with 1¾ teaspoons olive oil and scramble 2 egg whites or ¼ cup AllWhites with ⅛ cup shredded low-fat, low-sodium cheddar cheese and ⅓ cup chopped tomato. Serve the egg white mixture on 1 slice of toasted whole grain bread that has about 70 calories and 13 grams of carbohydrates per slice.

- 1⅓ cup Silk Vanilla Soymilk with 2 teaspoons Benefiber mixed in.

(2,000 AND 2,250 CAL/DAY: Coat a frying pan with ½ tablespoon olive oil and scramble 3 egg whites or ½ cup AllWhites with ¼ cup shredded low-fat, low-sodium cheddar cheese and ⅓ cup chopped tomato. Serve with 1⅔ cups Silk Vanilla Soymilk with 2 teaspoons Benefiber mixed in.)

LUNCH LS

- Lentil Turkey Soup (page 299)

- 2 Wasa Multi-Grain Crispbreads with 1½ teaspoons healthy spread

- 1 cup blackberries

(**2,000 CAL/DAY**: Add ¼ cup shredded low-fat, low-sodium cheese to the soup and spread the crispbreads with 2½ teaspoons healthy spread.)

(**2,250 CAL/DAY**: Add ½ cup shredded low-sodium, low-fat cheese to the soup.)

DINNER LS

- Spinach-Stuffed Chicken (page 309)

- Wild rice salad: ½ cup cooked wild rice tossed with 2 teaspoons olive oil, 1 cup sliced tomatoes, 2 teaspoons balsamic vinegar, and 2 tablespoons finely chopped basil

- ¾ cup fresh blueberries

(**2,000 AND 2,250 CAL/DAY**: For the wild rice salad, use ¾ cup wild rice tossed with 2¾ teaspoons olive oil with 2 teaspoons Benefiber mixed in, ¼ cup sliced tomatoes, 2½ teaspoons balsamic vinegar, and 2 tablespoons finely chopped basil.)

SNACK 1 LS, V

- 1 cup plain soy milk, such as Silk, with 1½ tablespoons unsalted cashews, about ⅓ ounce

(**2,000 AND 2,250 CAL/DAY**: Add ½ small orange, peeled, about 5 whole oranges per 1 pound.)

SNACK 2 LS, V

- 1½ cups fresh spinach and 2 tablespoons unsalted pine nuts tossed with 1 teaspoon olive oil and 1 teaspoon balsamic vinegar

(**1,500 CAL/DAY**: Use 3 cups fresh spinach, 2 teaspoons unsalted pine nuts, and ¼ teaspoon olive oil.)

(**2,000 AND 2,250 CAL/DAY:** Use 3 cups fresh spinach, 1 tablespoon unsalted pine nuts, ¾ teaspoon olive oil, and 2 teaspoons balsamic vinegar. Serve with 1 cup nonfat milk.)

SNACK 3 LS, V

(**2,250 CAL/DAY ONLY:** 2 cups air-popped unsalted popcorn [30 calories, 6 grams of carbohydrate, and 0 gram of saturated fat] tossed with 2 teaspoons olive oil. Serve with ¾ cup nonfat milk.)

TREAT LS, V

- 2 graham crackers with 20 calories, 4 grams of carbohydrate, and 0 gram of saturated fat per cracker, such as Health Valley Original Oat Bran Graham Crackers, with 2 teaspoons Smart Balance Creamy Peanut Butter

(**1,500 CAL/DAY:** Omit the treat.)

(**2,000 AND 2,250 CAL/DAY:** Use 3½ graham crackers with 2½ teaspoons Smart Balance Creamy Peanut Butter.)

DAY 7

BREAKFAST V

- Quinoa Pancake (page 297) topped with 1 tablespoon plus 1 teaspoon healthy spread and 2 teaspoons maple-flavored syrup that contains about 100 calories and 25 grams of carbohydrate per ¼ cup, such as Mrs. Butterworth's Lite or Hungry Jack Lite

- ⅔ cup Silk Vanilla Soymilk with 1 teaspoon Benefiber and ½ teaspoon cinnamon mixed in

(**2,000 AND 2,250 CAL/DAY:** Top pancake with just 1 tablespoon healthy spread and add ⅔ cup 1% low-fat cottage cheese with no sodium added [any brand with about 80 calories, 3 grams of carbohydrate, and 0.7 gram or less of saturated fat per ½-cup serving]).

LUNCH LS

- Chicken and pasta salad: 3 ounces cooked skinless chicken pieces (use leftover chicken or pull from a rotisserie chicken), tossed with 1¼ ounces (½ cup plus ⅛ cup cooked) Barilla PLUS Penne cooked according to box directions, ½ cup grated carrots, 3 cups shredded romaine lettuce, 1½ teaspoons olive oil, 1 tablespoon red wine vinegar, ⅛ teaspoon salt, and black pepper to taste

- ½ medium banana or 1 whole small banana

(**2,000 CAL/DAY**: Make the salad with only ¼ cup grated carrots, use 2½ teaspoons olive oil total, and add 1½ tablespoons low-sodium Parmesan cheese [20–25 calories and 5–25 milligrams of sodium per tablespoon]).

(**2,250 CAL/DAY**: Make the salad with 1 tablespoon plus ½ teaspoon olive oil and 2 tablespoons Parmesan cheese.)

DINNER LS

- Roasted Cod Cooked with Spring Onions and Topped with Avocado and Celery Compote (page 318)

- 1 cup mashed roasted butternut squash with 2½ teaspoons healthy spread and ¼ teaspoon finely chopped fresh rosemary mixed in. (To cook squash, cut in half lengthwise, remove seeds, and coat with vegetable oil spray. Place on a sheet tray, cut-side down, in a 375-degree oven until soft, about 20 minutes.)

- 1½ cups sliced peeled cucumber tossed with ¾ teaspoon olive oil and the juice of ½ fresh lemon

- 1 small plum, about 7 plums per pound

(**2,000 AND 2,250 CAL/DAY**: Use 1¼ cups cooked mashed butternut squash and serve 2 cups cucumber slices tossed with 1¼ teaspoons olive oil.)

SNACK 1 LS, V

- ½ cup nonfat yogurt with 2 tablespoons unsalted chopped pecans, about ½ ounce, mixed in

(**2,000 AND 2,250 CAL/DAY:** Have 1 cup nonfat plain yogurt with 1½ tablespoons unsalted chopped pecans, about ⅓ ounce, mixed in.)

SNACK 2 LS, V

■ Sweet pepper gratin: ¼ cup sliced sweet red pepper topped with ¾ ounce reduced-fat cheddar cheese; melt the cheese under the broiler

■ 17 unsalted almonds, about ¾ ounce

(**1,500 CAL/DAY:** For the gratin, use ¾ cup sliced sweet red pepper and 1 ounce grated reduced-fat cheddar cheese melted under the broiler. Omit the almonds.)

(**2,000 AND 2,250 CAL/DAY:** For the gratin, use ⅓ cup sliced sweet pepper and 1 ounce low-fat, low-sodium cheese drizzled with ¾ teaspoon olive oil melted under the broiler. Serve with 1½ cups Silk Light Vanilla Soymilk. Omit the almonds.)

SNACK 3 LS, V

(**2,250 CAL/DAY ONLY:** Apple with cottage cheese: 1 small apple, cored [about ¼ pound] stuffed with ¾ cup low-fat, low-sodium cottage cheese [80 calories, 3 grams of carbohydrate, less than 0.7 gram of saturated fat, and 15–20 milligrams of sodium per ½-cup serving; measure out ¾ cup] sprinkled with 1 teaspoon chopped walnuts and a pinch of cinnamon)

TREAT V

■ 1 cup air-popped, no-salt, no-butter-added popcorn drizzled with 1½ teaspoons melted healthy spread and served with ½ cup plain soy milk, such as Silk

(**1,500 CAL/DAY:** Omit the treat.)

(**2,000 AND 2,250 CAL/DAY:** 1¼ cup air-popped popcorn drizzled with 2½ teaspoons melted healthy spread and served with ¾ cup Silk Light Vanilla Soymilk.)

DAY 8

BREAKFAST LS, V

- 1½ whole grain frozen waffles with 190 calories per 2 waffles and 30 grams of carbohydrate, such as Van's All Natural Multigrain Waffles, topped with ½ cup low-fat, plain yogurt, 2 tablespoons raspberries, and 2 tablespoons chopped pecans.

(**2,000 AND 2,250 CAL/DAY:** Have ⅔ cup yogurt, 3 tablespoons raspberries, and 3 tablespoons chopped pecans.)

LUNCH

- gardein Beefless Tips, 1 serving, 3½ ounces
- Spinach salad: 3¼ cups fresh spinach with ½ cup sliced tomatoes, ⅓ cup corn (from frozen or canned, no salt added) tossed with 1 tablespoon walnut oil or another heart-healthy oil, such as canola, olive oil, peanut, sunflower, or flaxseed oil, and 2 teaspoons red wine vinegar
- 1½ cups fresh cantaloupe, cubed

(**2,000 CAL/DAY:** Add 2 tablespoons walnuts to the salad.)

(**2,250 CAL/DAY:** Add 3 tablespoons walnuts to the salad and have a total of 1¼ cups cantaloupe.)

DINNER LS, V

- Broiled Wild Salmon with Fennel and Red Onion (page 319)
- Oat Cake (page 326)
- 1 cup fresh cauliflower, roasted, topped with 1¼ teaspoons healthy spread (To roast cauliflower, preheat oven to 375 degrees, place the cauliflower on a sheet tray and lightly spray with vegetable oil spray. Roast until tender, about 10 minutes.)
- ¾ cup blueberries

(2,000 AND 2,250 CAL/DAY: Use 1¼ cups cauliflower, 2½ teaspoons healthy spread. Serve 1 cup blueberries.)

SNACK 1 LS, V

- 1 cup soy milk, such as Silk Vanilla Soymilk

- 1½ tablespoons unsalted cashews, about ⅓ ounce

(2,000 AND 2,250 CAL/DAY: Have 1⅓ cups Silk Vanilla Soymilk.)

SNACK 2 LS, V *(LS for 1,500/1,700 cal/day only)*

- Cream Cheese Dip: 1¼ ounces nonfat cream cheese mixed with 2 tablespoons fresh chives or ½ teaspoon dried oregano and a pinch of salt-free garlic seasoning, such as Mrs. Dash salt-free garlic and herb seasoning, 1 tablespoon nonfat plain yogurt, and 1 tablespoon olive oil, served with ¾ cup sliced cucumbers

(1,500 CAL/DAY: Make the dip with ¾ teaspoon olive oil and serve with ½ cup sliced cucumbers.)

(2,000 AND 2,250 CAL/DAY: Make the dip with 1½ tablespoons nonfat plain yogurt, and 1½ teaspoons olive oil, add 2 teaspoons sesame seeds, and serve with 1 cup sliced cucumbers and 1 Wasa Multi-Grain Crispbread.)

SNACK 3 V

(2,250 CAL/DAY ONLY: 3 tablespoons hummus mixed with ½ teaspoon olive oil and spread on 1 Wasa Light Rye Crispbread. Serve with ⅔ cup plain soy milk, such as Silk.)

TREAT LS, V

- 1 Skinny Cow Mini Fudge Pop with 3 unsalted walnuts halves, about ¼ ounce

(1,500 CAL/DAY: Omit the treat.)

(2,000 AND 2,250 CAL/DAY: 1 Skinny Cow Mini Fudge Pop with 5 walnut halves, about ⅓ ounce.)

DAY 9

BREAKFAST LS, V

- ¾ cup Special K Protein Plus cereal combined with ¼ cup Fiber One cereal

- ⅔ cup nonfat milk

- 10 unsalted walnut halves, about ¾ ounce

OPTION: Use 1 cup plain soy milk, such as Silk, and 7 unsalted walnut halves, about ½ ounce.

(2,000 AND 2,250 CAL/DAY: With the cereal use 1 cup nonfat milk and 14 unsalted walnut halves, about 1 ounce.)

OPTION: Use 1¼ cups plain soy milk, such as Silk, and 10 unsalted walnut halves, about ¾ ounce.

LUNCH LS

- Black-eyed Pea Salad with Turkey Bacon (page 301)

- 2 kiwifruits

(2,000 CAL/DAY: For the salad, use 1½ tablespoons unsalted pine nuts and serve with 1¾ kiwifruits.)

(2,250 CAL/DAY: For the salad, use 2 tablespoons plus 1 teaspoon unsalted pine nuts and serve with 1¾ kiwifruits.)

DINNER LS

- Hearty Beef Ragout over Barley (page 306) with ½ ounce (2 tablespoons) shredded reduced-fat cheddar cheese melted on top

- 1 small tangerine, about 2¼ inches in diameter

(2,000 AND 2,250 CAL/DAY: Use ¼ ounce [1 tablespoon] reduced-fat cheddar cheese and add 1 Wasa Light Rye Crispbread spread with 2 teaspoons healthy spread.)

SNACK 1 LS, V

- Hot chocolate: 1 cup plain soy milk, such as Silk, heated with ½ tablespoon Hershey's Cocoa and 1 packet of Splenda (or add to taste)

- 1 tablespoon plus 1 teaspoon unsalted peanuts

(2,000 AND 2,250 CAL/DAY: For hot chocolate, use 1¼ cup total Silk Vanilla Soymilk and 1 tablespoon Hershey's Cocoa. Serve with 1 tablespoon plus ½ teaspoon unsalted peanuts.)

SNACK 2 LS, V

- ¼ cup sliced avocado, mashed, with 1½ teaspoons olive oil and a pinch of salt and served with 2½ small stalks of celery for dipping and 4 unsalted walnut halves, about ¼ ounce.

(1,500 CAL/DAY: Mix the avocado with ⅛ teaspoon olive oil and serve with 4 small stalks of celery for dipping. Omit the walnuts.)

(2,000 AND 2,250 CAL/DAY: Use ⅓ cup sliced avocado, mashed, with ¾ teaspoon olive oil and a pinch of salt. Omit the celery and include 12 baked, unsalted tortilla chips with 118–120 calories and 23 grams of carbohydrate per ounce, such as Tostitos Baked Scoops or Guiltless Gourmet Unsalted Yellow Corn Tortilla Chips. Serve with 2 unsalted walnut halves, about ⅛ ounce.)

SNACK 3 V

(2,250 CAL/DAY ONLY: ½ whole grain English muffin that contains 120 calories and 23 grams of carbohydrate per 1 whole muffin, such as Thomas's Hearty Grains Multi-Grain English Muffin, spread with 1 tablespoon Smart Balance Omega Peanut Butter. Serve with ½ cup nonfat milk.)

TREAT LS, V

- Popcorn and Oat Cookie (page 332)

(1,500 CAL/DAY: Omit the treat.)

(2,000 AND 2,250 CAL/DAY: Add ½ tablespoon unsalted cashews [about ⅛ ounce] and ⅓ cup nonfat milk.)

DAY 10

BREAKFAST LS, V

- ½ toasted whole grain English muffin with 120 calories and 23 grams of carbohydrate per 1 whole muffin, such as Thomas's Hearty Grains Multi-Grain English Muffin, topped with 1¼ teaspoons healthy spread and ⅔ cup low-fat, no-sodium-added cottage cheese (any brand with 80 calories, 3 grams of carbohydrate, and about 15 milligrams of sodium per ½-cup serving) sprinkled with 1 tablespoon chopped scallions

- 1⅓ cups Silk Vanilla Soymilk with 2 teaspoons Benefiber mixed in

(**2,000 AND 2,250 CAL/DAY:** 1 whole grain English muffin topped with 2 teaspoons healthy spread and ¾ cup low-fat, no-sodium-added cottage cheese sprinkled with 1½ tablespoons chopped scallions. Serve with 1 cup Silk Vanilla Soymilk with 1 teaspoon Benefiber mixed in.)

LUNCH LS, V

- Salmon Salad with Creamy Hummus Dressing (page 305)

- ½ Flatout Healthy Grain Multi-Grain Flatbread (save the other half for Day 11's lunch)

- 1 cup grapes

(**2,000 CAL/DAY:** Use 1 tablespoon olive oil in the Salmon Salad with Creamy Hummus Dressing.)

(**2,250 CAL/DAY:** Use 1 tablespoon plus 1¼ teaspoons olive oil in the Salmon Salad with Creamy Hummus Dressing.)

DINNER LS

- Slow-Cooked Pork (page 308)

- Cabbage slaw: 1 cup fresh shredded cabbage and ½ cup chopped apple dressed with 1½ tablespoons Hellmann's Canola Cholesterol Free Mayonnaise or Spectrum Light Canola Oil Mayonnaise and 1½ teaspoons cider vinegar

- One medium whole wheat roll (2½ inches in diameter with about 95–100 calories and 18 grams of carbohydrate)

- ½ cup fresh raspberries

(**2,000 AND 2,250 CAL/DAY**: Make the cabbage slaw with 1¾ cups shredded cabbage, ¾ cup chopped apples, and 2 tablespoons mayonnaise.)

SNACK 1 LS, V

- Hot chocolate: 1 cup plain soy milk, such as Silk, heated with 2 teaspoons Hershey's Cocoa Powder and 1 packet of Splenda (or add to taste)

- 1 tablespoon plus 1 teaspoon, about ⅓ ounce, unsalted peanuts

(**2,000 AND 2,250 CAL/DAY**: For the hot chocolate, use 1½ cups Silk Vanilla Soymilk and 2 teaspoons unsalted peanuts, about ⅔ ounce.)

SNACK 2 LS, V *(LS for 1,500 cal/day only)*

- Spicy cream cheese dip: 3 tablespoons, about 1½ ounces, nonfat cream cheese with 1 tablespoon olive oil, ½ teaspoon paprika, and cayenne to taste and 2 romaine outer lettuce leaves for dipping

(**1,500 CAL/DAY**: 2 tablespoons, about 1 ounce, nonfat cream cheese with ¾ teaspoon olive oil, ¼ teaspoon paprika, and cayenne to taste and 3 romaine outer lettuce leaves for dipping.)

(**2,000 AND 2,250 CAL/DAY**: 4 tablespoons, about 2 ounces, nonfat cream cheese with 2 teaspoons olive oil, ½ teaspoon paprika, and cayenne to taste plus 4 romaine lettuce leaves and 1 Wasa Multi-Grain Crispbread for dipping.)

SNACK 3 V

(**2,250 CAL/DAY ONLY**: ½ toasted whole grain English muffin with 120 calories and 23 grams of carbohydrate per 1 whole muffin, such as Thomas's Hearty Grains Multi-Grain English Muffin with 1 tablespoon plus ½ teaspoon Smart Balance Peanut Butter and 4 medium (7½–8-inch-long) celery stalks.)

TREAT LS, V

- Small cookie or half a small biscotti (45 calories, 7 grams carbohydrate, 1 gram saturated fat)

- 7 unsalted almonds, about ⅓ ounce

(1,500 CAL/DAY: Omit the treat.)

(2,000 AND 2,250 CAL/DAY: Have a larger cookie or biscotti: 90 calories, 14 grams carbohydrate, 1.5 grams saturated fat)

DAY 11

BREAKFAST V

- Almond Butter Spice Smoothie (see page 290)

- 1 slice toasted whole grain bread (about 65–70 calories per slice, 13 grams of carbohydrate, and 1–2 grams of fiber per slice)

- 1½ teaspoons healthy spread

(2,000 AND 2,250 CAL/DAY: Use 1¾ cups total Silk Vanilla Soymilk and 1 tablespoon plus 1½ teaspoons total Smart Balance Chunky Peanut Butter in the smoothie. Use 1 teaspoon healthy spread on the bread.)

LUNCH LS

- Chicken salad: 3¼ cups thinly sliced fresh cabbage (preshredded packaged is fine), 4 ounces cooked skinless chicken pieces (use leftover chicken or pull from a rotisserie chicken), 1 teaspoon olive oil, 2½ teaspoons balsamic vinegar, a dash of salt, and pepper to taste

- 1 cup grapes

- ½ Flatout Healthy Grain Multi-Grain Flatbread (or any 100-calorie whole grain wrap or tortilla with at least 5 grams of fiber and no more than 17 grams of carbohydrate and 280 milligrams or less of sodium)

(2,000 CAL/DAY: For the chicken salad, use 2¾ teaspoons olive oil.)

(**2,250 CAL/DAY**: For the chicken salad, use 5 ounces chicken and 1 tablespoon olive oil.)

DINNER LS

- Poached Scallops with Leeks and Turkey Bacon (page 316) over ½ cup Barilla Whole Grain Thin Spaghetti (or any brand of pasta with about 200 calories, 6 grams of fiber, and 41 grams of carbohydrate per 2-ounce serving)

- ¾ cup fresh string beans roasted with 2¼ teaspoons olive oil

- ⅔ cup raspberries

(**2,000 AND 2,250 CAL/DAY**: 1 cup fresh string beans and add 2 teaspoons grated Parmesan cheese (any brand with about 15 calories and 55 milligrams of sodium per tablespoon) to the string beans. 1 cup of raspberries.)

SNACK 1 LS, V

- 1 cup plain soy milk, such as Silk, with 1½ tablespoons unsalted cashews, about ⅓ ounce

(**2,000 AND 2,250 CAL/DAY**: Add ½ small orange, peeled [about 5 whole oranges per pound].)

SNACK 2 LS, V

- Tomato gratin: ¼ cup sliced tomato topped with ¾ ounce grated reduced-fat cheddar cheese melted under the broiler

- 17 unsalted almonds, about ¾ ounce

(**1,500 CAL/DAY**: For the gratin, use ⅔ cup sliced tomato and 1 ounce grated reduced-fat cheddar cheese. Omit the almonds.)

(**2,000 AND 2,250 CAL/DAY**: For the gratin, use ⅔ cup sliced tomato and ½ ounce grated reduced-fat cheddar cheese. Serve with 15 unsalted almonds, about ⅔ ounce, and add 1 Wasa Multi-Grain Crispbread.)

SNACK 3

- Tuna on crackers: 3 ounces water-packed chunk light tuna, drained (for a lower-sodium option, try canned chunk light tuna with no salt added, such as Bumble Bee Chunk White Albacore Very Low Sodium in Water, mixed with 1 teaspoon Hellmann's Canola Cholesterol Free Mayonnaise and ⅛ cup chopped celery. Spread the tuna mixture on 3 Wasa Light Rye Crispbreads.

TREAT LS, V

- 2 Hershey's Extra Dark Tasting Squares: Any flavor with the exception of Pomegranate, due to its higher carbohydrate content

(1,500 CAL/DAY: Omit the treat.)

(2,000 AND 2,250 CAL/DAY: 3 Hershey's Extra Dark Tasting Squares: Any flavor with the exception of Pomegranate, due to its higher carbohydrate content.)

DAY 12

BREAKFAST LS, V

- Pumpkin Steel-Cut Oats (page 295)
- 1¼ cups plain soy milk, such as Silk

(2,000 AND 2,250 CAL/DAY: Add an additional ⅛ cup canned pumpkin and 2 teaspoons chopped unsalted pecans to the oatmeal; serve with 1⅔ cups plain soy milk.)

OPTION: 1,500 and 1,700 cal/day: Serve with ¾ cup nonfat milk and add an additional 1 tablespoon plus 1 teaspoon unsalted pecans to the oatmeal.

(2,000 AND 2,250 CAL/DAY: Use 1 cup total nonfat milk and add an additional 2 tablespoons plus ½ teaspoon unsalted pecans to the oatmeal [no additional pumpkin].)

LUNCH LS, V

- 1 cup canned lentil or other bean-based soup with about 180 calories, 25 grams of carbohydrate, and 300 milligrams of sodium or less per 1-cup serving, such as Amy's Kitchen Light in Sodium Organic Lentil Soup

- 1 small whole wheat dinner roll (2 inches × 2 inches), sliced in half, toasted, and dipped in 1 tablespoon plus ½ teaspoon olive oil

- ½ small grapefruit, approximately 3½ inches in diameter

(2,000 CAL/DAY: Add ⅛ cup shredded low-fat, low-sodium cheese to the soup and serve the roll with 4¾ teaspoons olive oil for dipping.)

(2,250 CAL/DAY: Add ¼ cup shredded low-fat, low-sodium cheese to the soup and serve the roll with 1¾ tablespoons olive oil for dipping.)

DINNER LS, V

- Summer Squash Whole Wheat Pasta Bake (page 323)

- ⅔ cup fresh strawberry halves

(2,000 AND 2,250 CAL/DAY: Add ½ small [4-inch] whole wheat pita spread with ¾ teaspoon healthy spread.)

SNACK 1 LS, V

- Hot chocolate: ¾ cup plain soy milk, such as Silk, with 2 teaspoons Hershey's Cocoa and 1 packet of Splenda (or add to taste)

- 2 tablespoons unsalted sunflower seed kernels (without the shell), about ½ ounce

(2,000 AND 2,250 CAL/DAY: With the hot chocolate have 1 tablespoon plus 2 teaspoons unsalted, dry-roasted sunflower seed kernels, about ⅓ ounce, and add 1 cup air-popped, unsalted popcorn [about 30 calories, 6 grams of carbohydrate, 0 gram saturated fat per 1 cup popcorn].)

SNACK 2 LS, V

- Cheesy Spinach: 3 cups fresh spinach tossed with 1 ounce shredded low-fat, low-sodium cheddar cheese, drizzled with 2 teaspoons olive oil and 2 teaspoons balsamic vinegar and sprinkled with 1 teaspoon sesame seeds, then placed under the broiler for 2 minutes

(1,500 CAL/DAY: For the Cheesy Spinach, use 3½ cups fresh spinach drizzled with 1 teaspoon balsamic vinegar. Omit the olive oil and sesame seeds.)

(2,000 AND 2,250 CAL/DAY: For the Cheesy Spinach use 2¼ cups fresh spinach tossed with ¼ cup finely chopped red pepper, 1½ teaspoons olive oil, and 2 teaspoons balsamic vinegar. Omit the sesame seeds. Add 3 small low-fat graham crackers with 20 calories, 4 grams of carbohydrate, and 0 gram of saturated fat per cracker, such as Health Valley Oat Bran Graham Crackers.)

SNACK 3 V

(2,250 CAL/DAY ONLY: 1 Slim-Fast High Protein Peanut Granola Meal Bar)

TREAT LS, V

- 1 Skinny Cow Mini Fudge Pop and 1 tablespoon, about 3, unsalted walnut halves

(1,500 CAL/DAY: Omit the treat.)

(2,000 AND 2,250 CAL/DAY: Skinny Cow French Vanilla Truffle Bar and 3 unsalted walnut halves served with 4 small whole strawberries [1 inch in diameter each].)

DAY 13

BREAKFAST LS, V

- ¾ cup Special K Protein Plus cereal combined with ¼ cup Fiber One cereal

- ⅔ cup nonfat milk

- 10 unsalted walnut halves, about ¾ ounce

OPTION: Use 1 cup plain soy milk, such as Silk, and 7 unsalted walnut halves, about ½ ounce.

(2,000 AND 2,250 CAL/DAY: Use 1 cup total nonfat milk and 1 ounce unsalted walnut halves [about 14 walnut halves].)

OPTION: Use 1¼ cups plain soy milk, such as Silk, and 10 unsalted walnut halves, about ¾ ounce.

LUNCH LS

- Open-face turkey bacon, lettuce, and tomato sandwich: Assemble sandwich on 2 slices of toasted whole wheat bread (about 70 calories and 12 grams of carbohydrate per slice). Spray a frying pan with vegetable oil cooking spray and fry 2 medium slices reduced-sodium turkey bacon (about 25 calories, 0.5 gram of saturated fat, and 135 milligrams of sodium per slice). Top the toasted bread with cooked turkey bacon, 1 outer romaine lettuce leaf sliced in half, 2 medium slices of tomato (¼-inch thick each), and 1 teaspoon Hellmann's Canola Cholesterol Free Mayonnaise.

- Carrot and raisin sauté: In a frying pan, sauté ⅓ cup fresh carrot strips or slices and 1 tablespoon plus 1 teaspoon raisins with 1 tablespoon olive oil. Sauté for 2 minutes or until the carrots are soft and cooked through.

- 1 medium peach, about ¼ pound

(2,000 CAL/DAY: For the carrot and raisin sauté, use 1 tablespoon plus 2 teaspoons olive oil.)

(2,250 CAL/DAY: For the carrot and raisin saute, use 1½ tablespoons olive oil. Fry the turkey bacon in ½ tablespoon olive oil instead of cooking spray.)

DINNER LS

- Shrimp and Quinoa Jambalaya (page 321)

- 3½ cups fresh arugula tossed with 2 teaspoons fresh lemon juice and 2½ teaspoons olive oil

- ¾ cup blackberries

(2,000 AND 2,250 CAL/DAY: Add 1 tablespoon unsalted sunflower seed kernels, about ¼ ounce, to the arugula and toss with 2¼ teaspoons olive oil. Serve with 1⅛ cups blackberries.)

SNACK 1 LS, V

- Peanut butter milk shake: In a blender, combine ¾ cup Silk Light Vanilla Soymilk, 1 tablespoon plus ½ teaspoon Smart Balance Peanut Butter, and 2 ice cubes. Blend until smooth.

(2,000 AND 2,250 CAL/DAY: For the shake, use 1½ cups Silk Light Vanilla Soymilk. Omit the peanut butter. Add 1 tablespoon plus 2 teaspoons unsalted peanuts, about ½ ounce.)

SNACK 2 LS, V

- 1 small (2⅖ inches in diameter) tomato, sliced and dressed with 1 teaspoon olive oil and ¼ cup low-sodium Parmesan cheese (about 115 calories and 15 milligrams of sodium per ¼ cup)

(1,500 CAL/DAY: Use 1 medium [2⅗ inches in diameter] tomato and 2½ tablespoons low-sodium Parmesan cheese. Omit the olive oil.)

(2,000 AND 2,250 CAL/DAY: Use 3½ tablespoons low-sodium Parmesan cheese and add 2 Wasa Light Rye Crispbreads.)

SNACK 3 V

- ½ small baked potato (about 3 whole potatoes per pound) with 2 tablespoons fat-free sour cream, such as Breakstone's, mixed with 1½ tablespoons plain nonfat yogurt and 1 ounce shredded reduced-fat cheese, drizzled with ¾ teaspoon olive oil

TREAT LS, V

- Popcorn and Oat Cookie (page 332)

(1,500 CAL/DAY: Omit the treat.)

(2,000 AND 2,250 CAL/DAY: Add ½ tablespoon unsalted cashews, about ⅛ ounce, and ⅓ cup nonfat milk.)

DAY 14

BREAKFAST V

- Cheesy Corn Bread (page 296)

- 1 link vegetarian breakfast sausage such as Morningstar Farms Veggie Sausage Links

- ¾ cup Silk Plus Fiber Vanilla Soymilk

(**2,000 AND 2,250 CAL/DAY**: Use 2 sausage links and 1⅓ cups Silk Plus Fiber Soymilk.)

LUNCH LS

- Fish Wrap (page 317)

- ½ medium tomato (2⅗ inches in diameter), chopped and tossed with 1 teaspoon lime juice and ¾ teaspoon olive oil

- ½ cup peeled fresh mango slices

(**2,000 CAL/DAY**: Add ½ teaspoon mayonnaise to the Fish Wrap and use 2½ teaspoons olive oil in the tomato dressing.)

(**2,250 CAL/DAY**: Use 4 teaspoons olive oil in the tomato dressing.)

DINNER LS

- Chicken Curry (page 310)

- ⅓ cup cooked brown rice with ¾ tablespoon olive oil, 1 tablespoon fresh chopped mint, and 1 tablespoon fresh chopped parsley

- ¾ cup grapes

(**2,000 AND 2,250 CAL/DAY**: Use ½ cup total brown rice with 2¾ teaspoons olive oil. Serve with ⅔ cup grapes.)

SNACK 1 LS, V

- Creamy Vanilla Orange Tea: 1 bag Lipton Herbal Orange or Tetley Orange Peach Herbal Tea steeped in ¾ cup Silk Light Vanilla Soymilk. Serve with 15 unsalted almonds, about ⅔ ounce

(**2,000 AND 2,250 CAL/DAY**: Use 1½ cups Silk Light Vanilla Soymilk and 8 unsalted almonds, about ⅓ ounce.)

SNACK 2 LS, V

- ⅓ cup artichoke hearts packed in oil, drained and tossed with ⅓ cup shredded romaine lettuce, 1½ teaspoons unsalted pine nuts, and 2¼ teaspoons olive oil

(1,500 CAL/DAY: Use ⅓ cup artichoke hearts packed in oil, drained, and serve with 1½ teaspoons unsalted pine nuts. Omit the romaine lettuce and olive oil.)

(2,000 AND 2,250 CAL/DAY: Use ⅓ cup artichoke hearts packed in oil, drained, and serve with 1½ teaspoons unsalted pine nuts and 1 teaspoon olive oil. Add 8 baked potato chips with about 150 calories and 23 grams of carbohydrate per one 32-gram serving, such as Baked Lay's.)

SNACK 3 LS, V

(2,250 CAL/DAY ONLY: Chopped salad: Combine 3 cups of shredded romaine with 2 tablespoons garbanzo beans, 3 tablespoons fresh (or canned and drained, no-salt-added) corn, ¼ cup fresh chopped tomato, and ¼ cup fresh cucumber slices. Toss with 2¼ teaspoons olive oil and 2 teaspoons red wine vinegar.)

TREAT LS, V

- Melt one Hershey's Extra Dark Pure Dark Chocolate tasting square (any flavor with the exception of Pomegranate, due to its higher carbohydrate content) over a double boiler or in a microwave-safe bowl in the microwave for 10 seconds or until melted and dip 1 slice (1 linear inch) of peeled fresh banana (16 grams) into the melted chocolate. Roll in 2½ teaspoons of chopped walnuts.

(1,500 CAL/DAY: Omit the treat.)

(2,000 AND 2,250 CAL/DAY: Use ¼ cup sliced banana dipped into 1 melted Hershey's Extra Dark Pure Dark tasting square rolled in 1½ tablespoons chopped walnuts.)

7

BEST LIFE
RECIPES

THE FOOD EXCHANGES POSTED for each recipe (such as "grain/starchy vegetables" or "fat") will help you fit our recipes into your daily calorie plan outlined on page 54. In some cases, our exchanges differ a little from the typical ones. For instance, under the traditional system, peanut butter is classified as a high-fat meat serving. We classify each tablespoon of peanut butter as a "high-protein" serving and a "fat" serving. With our protein servings, calories are as important as grams of protein. That's why you get 1½ ounces of a low-calorie food—such as skinless chicken—but just one ounce of a higher calorie protein-rich food, such as red meat or salmon. The exact portions constituting servings of high-carbohydrate foods are listed in tables starting on page 59 and in the Carb Counts appendix (page 343). Servings of protein-rich foods start on page 112; fat servings are listed on pages 121 to 122.

BREAKFAST

Vanilla Peanut Butter Smoothie

SERVES 1

THIS BREAKFAST CAN BE made quickly, tastes deliciously decadent, and keeps you going all morning.

1½ cups fat-free milk

2 teaspoons Benefiber

½ teaspoon vanilla extract

1 tablespoon chunky peanut butter, such as Smart Balance Chunky Peanut Butter

Combine all the ingredients in a blender and blend until smooth, about 2 minutes.

PREP TIME: 5 minutes   TOTAL TIME: 5 minutes

PER SERVING, ABOUT: Calories: 250 Protein: 16 g Carbohydrate: 25 g Dietary Fiber: 4 g Sugars: 20 g Total Fat: 9 g Saturated Fat: 1.7 g Cholesterol: 7 mg Calcium: 452 mg Sodium: 246 mg

EXCHANGES: ¼ grain/starchy vegetable serving; 1½ milk/yogurt servings; 1 protein-rich serving; 1 fat serving

Almond Butter Spice Smoothie

SERVES 1

ADJUST THE SPICES IN this smoothie recipe to fit your taste or experiment with a favorite spice or spice combination of your own.

1¼ cups Silk Vanilla Soymilk

⅛ teaspoon ground cinnamon

Pinch of ground nutmeg

Pinch of ground clove

1 tablespoon almond butter (with preferably no more than 75 milligrams of sodium per tablespoon)

2 teaspoons Benefiber

Combine all the ingredients in a blender and blend until smooth, about 2 minutes.

PREP TIME: 5 minutes   **TOTAL TIME:** 5 minutes

PER SERVING, ABOUT: Calories: 244 Protein: 10 g Carbohydrate: 20 g Dietary Fiber: 5 g Sugars: 10 g Total Fat: 14 g Saturated Fat: 1.6 g Cholesterol: 0 mg Calcium: 424 mg Sodium: 192 mg

EXCHANGES: ¼ grain/starchy vegetable serving; 1¼ milk/yogurt servings; 2 fat servings

Tofu Spinach Scramble

SERVES 1

EVEN IF YOU'RE NOT usually a fan of tofu, this wrap is easy to love. The tofu takes on the flavors of the onions and spinach and adds a pleasant texture to this portable breakfast.

Vegetable oil cooking spray

1 tablespoon finely chopped onion

3 ounces soft tofu, crumbled

1 cup roughly chopped fresh spinach

1 whole wheat 100-calorie wrap, tortilla, or flatbread with at least 5 grams of fiber and no more than 17 grams of carbs, such as Flatout Multi-Grain Flatbread

Black pepper to taste

1 Heat a medium skillet over medium heat and coat with the cooking spray. Add the onion and cook until translucent, about 3 minutes.

2 Place the tofu in a small bowl and lightly coat with the cooking spray. Place the tofu in the skillet with the onions and cook until lightly browned, stirring frequently, about 5 minutes. Add the spinach, stir, and remove the skillet from the heat.

3   Roll up the tofu-onion mixture in a room-temperature or warmed
    flatbread and serve immediately.

    PREP TIME: 5 minutes   **TOTAL TIME:** 15 minutes

    PER SERVING, ABOUT: Calories: 176 Protein: 18 g Carbohydrate: 21 g Dietary Fiber:
    8 g Sugars: 1 g Total Fat: 6 g Saturated Fat: 0 g Cholesterol: 0 mg Calcium: 162 mg
    Sodium: 353 mg

    EXCHANGES: 1 grain/starchy vegetable serving; ½ nonstarchy vegetable serving;
    1 protein-rich serving

Sweet Potato Frittata

SERVES 1

THIS TASTY SCRAMBLE IS elegant enough for a weekend breakfast with
guests and simple enough for an any-day breakfast. The sweet potatoes add
a delicious, unexpected flavor to your morning meal.

1 tablespoon finely chopped
onion

½ medium sweet potato,
thinly sliced into rounds

Vegetable oil cooking spray

1 tablespoon finely chopped
fresh basil or parsley

½ cup liquid eggs, such as
Better'n Eggs

1   Heat the oven to broiling temperature.

2   Lightly coat the onion and sweet potato with the cooking spray and
    cook on a sheet tray in the oven until tender, about 5 minutes.
    Meanwhile, heat a 9-inch heavy-bottomed ovenproof skillet over
    medium heat.

3   Coat the skillet with the cooking spray and immediately spread the
    sweet potato and onion evenly over the bottom of the skillet. Sprinkle
    the chopped herbs on top and pour the liquid eggs over the herbs.

Cook until the edges start to look firm, about 2 minutes. Place the skillet under the broiler until the top is golden brown, about 2 minutes.

PREP TIME: 5 minutes   **TOTAL TIME:** 15 minutes

PER SERVING, ABOUT: Calories: 121 Protein: 13 g Carbohydrate: 16 g Dietary Fiber: 2 g Sugars: 5 g Total Fat: 0 g Saturated Fat: 0 g Cholesterol: 0 mg Calcium: 226 mg Sodium: 276 mg

EXCHANGES: 1 grain/starchy vegetable serving; trace of nonstarchy vegetable serving; 1 protein-rich serving

Cocoa Granola

SERVES 4

MAKE A BATCH OR double batch of this granola to have on hand for a busy morning. It's delicious with yogurt, milk, or soy milk.

¼ cup liquid egg whites, such as AllWhites or 1 egg white

2 tablespoons olive oil

¼ teaspoon vanilla extract

1½ cups old-fashioned rolled oats

3 tablespoons unsalted pumpkin seeds

3 tablespoons unsalted sunflower seeds

1 tablespoon ground cinnamon

1 teaspoon unsweetened cocoa powder, such as Hershey's Natural Cocoa

¼ teaspoon baking powder

1   Preheat the oven to 350 degrees.

2   Whisk together the egg whites, oil, and vanilla in a large mixing bowl. Add the remaining ingredients and combine thoroughly.

3   Place the mixture on a baking sheet and bake for 30 minutes.

4   Serve immediately or store in an airtight container for up to 1 week.

PREP TIME: 5 minutes   **TOTAL TIME:** 35 minutes

PER SERVING, ABOUT: Calories: 269 Protein: 10 g Carbohydrate: 24 g Dietary Fiber: 4 g Sugars: 1 g Total Fat: 16 g Saturated Fat: 2.4 g Cholesterol: 0 mg Calcium: 48 mg

EXCHANGES: 1½ grain/starchy vegetable servings; trace of protein-rich serving; 3 fat servings

Steel-Cut Oats with Walnuts and Orange Zest

SERVES 4

STEEL-CUT OATS HAVE a low glycemic index; a bowl will keep you satisfied until lunchtime.

3 cups water

⅛ teaspoon salt

¾ cup raw steel-cut oats
  (regular or quick-cooking)

½ teaspoon vanilla extract

1 tablespoon orange zest

½ cup plus 4 teaspoons
  chopped walnuts

1   Bring the water to a boil in a medium pot. Add the salt and stir in the oats and vanilla.

2   Cook the oatmeal according to the package directions.

3   Divide into serving bowls and top with orange zest and walnuts.

PREP TIME: 5 minutes   TOTAL TIME: 7 to 30 minutes, depending on whether you use quick-cooking or regular oats

PER SERVING, ABOUT: Calories: 237 Protein: 7 g Carbohydrate: 23 g Dietary Fiber: 7 g Sugars: 0 g Total Fat: 14 g Saturated Fat: 1 g Cholesterol: 0 mg Calcium: 32 mg Sodium: 73 mg

EXCHANGES: 1½ grain/starchy vegetable servings; 2⅓ fat servings

Pumpkin Steel-Cut Oats

SERVES 4

IF YOU EAT PUMPKIN only during the fall, it's time to break this veggie out of the seasonal rut. Pumpkin adds a unique, rich flavor to oatmeal's nutty taste. Not to mention that it's loaded with the antioxidant beta-carotene, which helps protect your eyes. Use plain canned pumpkin here, *not* pumpkin pie filling.

3 cups water	Pinch of ground clove
⅛ teaspoon salt	Pinch of ground ginger
¾ cup raw steel-cut oats (regular or quick-cooking)	Pinch of ground nutmeg
½ cup canned pumpkin	⅛ teaspoon ground cinnamon
	⅓ cup chopped pecans

1   Bring the water to a boil in a medium pot. Add the salt and stir in the oats.

2   Cook the oatmeal according to the package directions. Once the oatmeal is done, stir in the pumpkin and spices and continue cooking until the mixture is hot throughout, about 2 minutes.

3   Divide into serving bowls and top with pecans.

PREP TIME: 5 minutes   TOTAL TIME: 7 to 30 minutes, depending on whether you use quick-cooking or regular oats

PER SERVING, ABOUT: Calories: 199 Protein: 6 g Carbohydrate: 24 g Dietary Fiber: 8 g Sugars: 1 g Total Fat: 9 g Saturated Fat: 0.6 g Cholesterol: 0 mg Calcium: 73 mg Sodium: 74 mg

EXCHANGES: 1⅔ grain/starchy vegetable servings; 1⅓ fat servings

Cheesy Corn Bread

SERVES 4

ON PAGE 286 OF the meal plan, this comforting corn bread is paired with vegetarian sausage links and fat-free milk for a healthy makeover of a classic diner breakfast.

⅓ cup cornmeal, preferably whole grain

3 tablespoons whole wheat flour

2 teaspoons healthy spread, such as Bestlife Buttery Spread, melted

½ tablespoon baking powder

¼ teaspoon baking soda

⅓ cup nonfat buttermilk

¼ cup liquid eggs, such as Better'n Eggs

3 tablespoons fat-free milk

3¼ ounces low-sodium, low-fat cheese (with about 50 calories and no more than 35 milligrams of sodium per 1 ounce)

Vegetable oil cooking spray

1 Preheat the oven to 375 degrees.

2 Combine all the ingredients except for the cooking spray in a large mixing bowl and mix well.

3 Spray a 9-inch heavy-bottomed skillet with the cooking spray. Pour the mix into the skillet and bake until springy to the touch, about 15 minutes. This tastes best served right out of the oven.

PREP TIME: 5 minutes   TOTAL TIME: 20 minutes

PER SERVING, ABOUT: Calories: 170 Protein: 11 g Carbohydrate: 22 g Dietary Fiber: 3 g Sugars: 2 g Total Fat: 4 g Saturated Fat: 1.7 g Cholesterol: 6 mg Calcium: 327 mg Sodium: 340 mg

EXCHANGES: 1 grain/starchy vegetable serving; trace of milk/yogurt serving; 1 protein-rich serving; ¼ fat serving

Quinoa Pancake

SERVES 4

THE QUINOA IN THIS pancake provides a nutty flavor, and the whole grains offer a number of nutritional benefits. The batter can be stored in the refrigerator for up to two days.

⅓ cup plus 1 tablespoon uncooked quinoa, rinsed

1¼ cups liquid eggs, such as Better'n Eggs

½ cup nonfat buttermilk

¼ teaspoon baking powder

⅛ teaspoon baking soda

⅓ cup plus 1½ tablespoons whole wheat flour

Vegetable oil cooking spray

1 Place the quinoa in a pot and cover with water. Bring to a boil, then reduce heat to a simmer. Cook, stirring regularly, for 10 minutes.

2 Combine the liquid eggs, buttermilk, baking powder, and baking soda in a large mixing bowl. Mix until combined.

3 Drain the quinoa.

4 Add the flour to the liquid egg mixture and mix until just incorporated. Add the quinoa and mix until just incorporated.

5 Heat a large heavy-bottomed skillet over medium heat. Coat the skillet with the cooking spray. Pour ¼ of the batter into the skillet to form a pancake; repeat three more times. Cook until golden brown, about 2 minutes, and then flip the pancakes. Cook until golden brown, about 2 more minutes. Serve immediately.

PREP TIME: 5 minutes   TOTAL TIME: 25 minutes

PER SERVING, ABOUT: Calories: 155 Protein: 12 g Carbohydrate: 23 g Dietary Fiber: 3 g Sugars: 3 g Total Fat: 2 g Saturated Fat: 0 g Cholesterol: 1 mg Calcium: 192 mg Sodium: 256 mg

EXCHANGES: 1¼ grain/starchy vegetable servings; trace of milk/yogurt serving; ⅔ protein-rich serving

SOUPS/CHILI

White Bean Chili

SERVES 4

THIS WARM DISH WILL be a hit with diners of all ages. You can enjoy it right after it's prepared or after it's been stored in the refrigerator for up to five days, or it can also be frozen.

1 tablespoon olive oil

½ large onion, chopped

3 cloves garlic, minced

4 cups water

2 cups fresh or canned no-salt-added tomatoes

⅛ teaspoon ground cayenne or more to taste

½ teaspoon ground cumin

1 bay leaf

2 tablespoons chili powder

1 tablespoon cocoa powder

½ teaspoon salt

1½ pounds skinless, boneless chicken breast

¾ cup canned no-salt-added white beans, drained and rinsed

4 cups chard

4 tablespoons nonfat sour cream

1   Heat a large heavy-bottomed stockpot over medium heat and coat with the oil. Add the onion and garlic and cook until golden brown, stirring regularly, about 8 minutes.

2   Add the remaining ingredients except the sour cream. Stir and bring to a boil.

3   Reduce the heat and simmer for 30 minutes. Remove the bay leaf and garnish with the sour cream before serving.

PREP TIME: 15 minutes   TOTAL TIME: 1 hour

PER SERVING, ABOUT: Calories: 323 Protein: 46 g Carbohydrate: 20 g Dietary Fiber: 6 g Sugars: 4 g Total Fat: 7 g Saturated Fat: 1.5 g Cholesterol: 100 mg Calcium: 119 mg Sodium: 534 mg

EXCHANGES: ²⁄₃ grain/starchy vegetable serving; 1³⁄₄ nonstarchy vegetable servings; 4 protein-rich servings; ³⁄₄ fat serving

Lentil Turkey Soup

SERVES 4

LENTILS ARE NUTRITIONAL SUPERSTARS: they're virtually fat-free, high in fiber, and packed with minerals and protein. In addition, they are the quickest-cooking members of the legume family; red lentils are even quicker than other varieties. (See the vegan option at the end of the recipe.)

Vegetable oil cooking spray

½ onion, sliced

1 pound 95% lean ground turkey

5 cups water

⅓ cup red lentils (if you use another type of lentil, cooking time will increase by 10 to 30 minutes)

½ cup chopped fresh herbs, such as basil, rosemary, sage, and thyme

1 cup peeled and chopped carrot

⅛ teaspoon salt

1 Heat a heavy-bottomed stockpot over medium heat and coat with the cooking spray. Add the onion and cook until translucent, about 5 minutes.

2 Add the turkey and cook, stirring frequently, until browned, about 5 minutes.

3 Add the water, lentils, and herbs. Bring the soup to a boil and reduce the heat to a simmer. Cook for 5 minutes.

4 Add the carrot and cook for an additional 5 minutes.

5 Add the salt just before serving.

PREP TIME: 15 minutes   TOTAL TIME: 35 minutes

PER SERVING, ABOUT: Calories: 241 Protein: 24 g Carbohydrate: 13 g Dietary
Fiber: 3 g Sugars: 2 g Total Fat: 10 g Saturated Fat: 2.6 g Cholesterol: 90 mg
Calcium: 38 mg Sodium: 203 mg

EXCHANGES: ²/₃ grain/starchy vegetable serving; ²/₃ nonstarchy vegetable serving;
2²/₃ protein-rich servings

> Make it vegan by replacing the turkey with 1 pound firm tofu, drained
> and crushed with the back of a fork, and using ¼ cup chopped carrot
> and ¼ small onion. Instead of cooking spray, coat pan with
> 2 tablespoons canola oil.

NUTRITION ANALYSIS FOR THE VEGAN VERSION: Calories: 224 Protein: 14 g
Carbohydrate: 14 g Dietary Fiber: 2 g Sugars: 1 g Total Fat: 12 g Saturated Fat: 0.5 g
Cholesterol: 0 mg Calcium: 162 mg Sodium: 80 mg

EXCHANGES: ²/₃ grain/starchy vegetable serving; ¼ nonstarchy vegetable serving;
1³/₄ protein-rich servings; 1½ fat servings

Tofu Minestrone

SERVES 4

MINESTRONE LITERALLY MEANS "big soup," and this vegetarian version
is sure to satisfy.

1 cup whole grain penne, such as
Barilla Whole Grain Penne

Vegetable oil cooking spray

1 onion, finely chopped

1 cup peeled and chopped
carrot

4 cloves garlic, peeled and
chopped

1 tablespoon finely chopped
fresh rosemary or thyme

24 ounces firm tofu, drained and
crumbled

1 cup chopped fresh or canned
no-salt-added tomatoes

½ cup canned no-salt-added
cannellini beans, or another
variety of white bean, drained
and rinsed

2 stalks celery, chopped

½ cup zucchini, chopped

6 cups water

³/₄ teaspoon salt

Freshly ground black pepper to
taste

1   Cook the pasta according to the package directions; set
    aside.

2   Spray a large heavy-bottomed stockpot with cooking spray. Add
    the onion, carrot, and garlic and cook, stirring frequently, for 5
    minutes.

3   Add the herbs, tofu, tomato, beans, celery, zucchini, and water. Bring to
    a boil. Reduce heat and simmer for 15 minutes.

4   Right before serving, add the pasta, salt, and pepper.

    PREP TIME: 10 minutes   **TOTAL TIME:** 35 minutes

PER SERVING, ABOUT: Calories: 271 Protein: 20 g Carbohydrate: 29 g Dietary
Fiber: 5 g Sugars: 5 g Total Fat: 7 g Saturated Fat: 0 g Cholesterol: 0 mg Calcium:
273 mg Sodium: 480 mg

EXCHANGES: 1½ grain/starchy vegetable servings; 2 nonstarchy vegetable servings;
2 protein-rich servings

SALADS

Black-eyed Pea Salad with Turkey Bacon

SERVES 4

THE TURKEY BACON, black-eyed peas, and pecans all play their part in
making this a memorable, rich, and satisfying salad.

2 cups canned no-salt-added
  black-eyed peas, drained and
  rinsed

1½ cups chopped fresh
  tomatoes

2½ tablespoons olive oil

¼ cup cider vinegar

¼ teaspoon salt

8 medium slices turkey bacon

12 cups shredded romaine
  lettuce

⅓ cup chopped pecans

1   Heat a large heavy-bottomed skillet over medium heat.

2   Combine the black-eyed peas, tomatoes, oil, vinegar, and salt in a large mixing bowl. Set aside.

3   Cook the bacon in the skillet until crispy, about 3 minutes on each side. Remove the bacon from the skillet and let it cool. Once the bacon is cool, slice it into ¼-inch pieces and mix it into the black-eyed pea mixture.

4   Gently toss the lettuce and pecans with the black-eyed pea mixture and serve immediately.

PREP TIME: 5 minutes   **TOTAL TIME:** 10 minutes

PER SERVING, ABOUT: Calories: 332 Protein: 10 g Carbohydrate: 26 g Dietary Fiber: 9 g Sugars: 7 g Total Fat: 22 g Saturated Fat: 3.4 g Cholesterol: 25 mg Calcium: 178 mg Sodium: 504 mg

EXCHANGES: 1 grain/starchy vegetable serving; 1½ nonstarchy vegetable servings; 1⅓ protein-rich servings; 3 fat servings

Spicy Chicken Noodle Salad

SERVES 4

FEEL FREE TO ADJUST the heat in this very quick, family-friendly recipe depending on your personal taste. And try the vegan option outlined at the bottom of this recipe.

3 ounces (about 1 1/2 cups cooked) angel hair or thin spaghetti, such as Barilla PLUS Thin Spaghetti

2 tablespoons sesame tahini

1 tablespoon seasoned rice wine vinegar with no more than 240 milligrams of sodium per 1 tablespoon

2 tablespoons water

1/4 teaspoon honey

1/8 teaspoon salt

Ground cayenne to taste

3/4 pound rotisserie chicken, skin removed, meat removed from the bone and roughly chopped (this is the approximate yield of a 3 1/4-pound chicken)

1 cup frozen shelled edamame, thawed

1 cup shredded carrots

1 cup sliced cucumber

1/2 cup sliced button mushrooms

2 tablespoons finely chopped spring onions

1   Cook the pasta according to the package directions. Set aside.

2   Combine the tahini, vinegar, water, honey, salt, and cayenne in a medium-sized bowl to make the dressing. Set aside.

3   Combine the chicken, edamame, pasta, carrots, cucumber, mushrooms, and spring onions in a large bowl.

4   Gently toss the dressing with the salad ingredients and serve immediately.

PREP TIME: 5 minutes   TOTAL TIME: 15 minutes

PER SERVING, ABOUT: Calories: 333 Protein: 36 g Carbohydrate: 25 g Dietary Fiber: 5 g Sugars: 5 g Total Fat: 9 g Saturated Fat: 1.7 g Cholesterol: 72 mg Calcium: 100 mg Sodium: 238 mg

EXCHANGES: 1½ grain/starchy vegetable servings; ¾ nonstarchy vegetable serving; 2¾ protein-rich servings; ¾ fat serving

Turn this into a vegan recipe by replacing the chicken with 1 pound tofu, drained and cut in ½-inch cubes. Skip the carrots, and decrease the pasta to 2 ounces (about 1 cup cooked). Also, add 1 tablespoon plus 1 teaspoon sesame oil to dressing mixture.

NUTRITION ANALYSIS FOR THE VEGAN VERSION: Calories: 294 Protein: 18 g Carbohydrate: 21 g Dietary Fiber: 3 g Sugars: 3 g Total Fat: 15 g Saturated Fat: 1.5 g Cholesterol: 0 mg Calcium: 220 mg Sodium: 150 mg

EXCHANGES FOR THE VEGAN VERSION: 1 grain/starchy vegetable serving; ¼ nonstarchy vegetable serving; 2 protein-rich servings; 1¾ fat servings

Mustardy Sardine Salad

SERVES 1

SARDINES HAVE SO MUCH going for them—they're rich in omega-3 fatty acids, environmentally sustainable, very low in mercury, and reasonably priced. The mustard in this fuss-free recipe is a complement to the richly flavored fish.

1 teaspoon stone-ground mustard

¼ teaspoon red wine vinegar

1 can (3.75 ounces) sardines packed in olive oil, drained

¾ cup sliced celery

1 tablespoon finely chopped red onion

3 cups mixed greens

1   Whisk together the mustard and red wine vinegar in a medium-sized bowl.

2   Gently mix in the sardines, celery, and onion.

3   Serve over the mixed greens.

PREP TIME: 5 minutes   **TOTAL TIME:** 5 minutes

PER SERVING, ABOUT: Calories: 246 Protein: 26 g Carbohydrate: 9 g Dietary Fiber: 4 g Sugars: 2 g Total Fat: 11 g Saturated Fat: 1.5 g Cholesterol: 131 mg Calcium: 474 mg Sodium: 623 mg

EXCHANGES: 1½ nonstarchy vegetable servings; 3¾ protein-rich servings

Salmon Salad with Creamy Hummus Dressing

SERVES 1

CANNED SALMON IS A nutritious, affordable alternative to fresh. The hummus in the dressing creates a creamy, richly flavored salad.

3 tablespoons hummus	3 cups mixed greens
1 teaspoon olive oil	1 cup sliced cucumber
1 teaspoon fresh lemon juice	½ cup grated carrot
2 tablespoons finely chopped spring onion	3 ounces canned wild pink salmon, drained and broken into chunks
1 tablespoon water	

1   Combine the hummus, oil, lemon juice, onion, and water in a food processor and whip until smooth, about 1 minute.

2   Place the greens, cucumber, carrot, and salmon in a large mixing bowl. Dress with the hummus mixture and toss gently. Serve immediately.

PREP TIME: 5 minutes   **TOTAL TIME:** 5 minutes

PER SERVING, ABOUT: Calories: 310 Protein: 23 g Carbohydrate: 24 g Dietary Fiber: 8 g Sugars: 6 g Total Fat: 15 g Saturated Fat: 2 g Cholesterol: 47 mg Calcium: 155 mg Sodium: 237 mg

EXCHANGES: ½ grain/starchy vegetable serving; 3 nonstarchy vegetable servings; 3 protein-rich servings; 1¾ fat serving

MAIN COURSES
Red Meat

Hearty Beef Ragout over Barley

SERVES 4

THIS RAGOUT, ANOTHER NAME for a well-seasoned meat sauce, is family friendly. If you have picky eaters, you can serve their portion over whole grain pasta instead of barley.

¾ cup barley

1 tablespoon olive oil

¾ teaspoon salt

Black pepper to taste

1 small yellow onion, chopped

1 cup sliced eggplant

1 red pepper, cored, seeded, and sliced

3 medium tomatoes, each cut into 4 pieces

1 tablespoon finely chopped fresh oregano

6 large cloves garlic, peeled and halved

1 cup water

1½ pounds 95% lean ground beef

1   Place the barley in a medium pot and cover with water. Bring to a boil and reduce the heat to a simmer. Cook until the barley is tender, about 30 minutes. Drain thoroughly, place in a medium bowl, and season with the oil, salt, and pepper.

2   Place the vegetables, oregano, garlic, and water in a large pot. Bring to a boil, then reduce to a simmer. Cook until the vegetables are cooked through, about 30 minutes.

3   Heat a heavy-bottomed skillet and cook the beef, stirring constantly, for about 5 minutes. Add the beef to the vegetable mixture.

4   Serve the barley covered with the vegetable ragout.

PREP TIME: 15 minutes   TOTAL TIME: 50 minutes

PER SERVING, ABOUT: Calories: 431 Protein: 43 g Carbohydrate: 36 g Dietary Fiber: 9 g Sugars: 6 g Total Fat: 13 g Saturated Fat: 4.5 g Cholesterol: 106 mg Calcium: 54 mg Sodium: 560 mg

EXCHANGES: 2 grain/starchy vegetable servings; 2 nonstarchy vegetable servings; 4 protein-rich servings; ³/₄ fat serving

Flank Steak with Tomato Relish

SERVES 4

THIS DISH WILL TASTE the best in the summer, when tomatoes are in season. Experiment with different types and varieties of tomatoes, as any ripe, delicious tomato will work perfectly in this recipe.

2 cups diced fresh tomatoes

1 tablespoon finely chopped red onion

1 tablespoon cider vinegar

1 tablespoon olive oil

1 cup finely chopped fresh herbs, such as basil, parsley, or Italian parsley

¹/₂ teaspoon salt (for the tomatoes) plus ¹/₈ teaspoon (for the steak)

Black pepper to taste

Vegetable oil cooking spray

1¹/₄ pounds flank steak, pierced repeatedly with a fork

1 Heat a large skillet over medium heat.

2 Combine the tomatoes, onion, vinegar, oil, herbs, ½ teaspoon salt, and pepper in a medium bowl. Set aside.

3 Coat the skillet with cooking spray. Cook the flank steak until browned on one side, about 3 minutes. Flip and cook until browned on the other side, about 3 more minutes.

4 Remove the steak from the pan and let rest for 5 minutes. Season with the remaining ⅛ teaspoon salt and pepper. Slice thinly against the grain.

5 Serve the sliced flank steak with the tomato relish.

PREP TIME: 10 minutes   TOTAL TIME: 25 minutes

PER SERVING, ABOUT: Calories: 264 Protein: 32 g Carbohydrate: 5 g Dietary Fiber: 2 g Sugars: 3 g Total Fat: 13 g Saturated Fat: 4.2 g Cholesterol: 60 mg Calcium: 71 mg Sodium: 457 mg

EXCHANGES: 1 nonstarchy vegetable serving; 5 protein-rich servings; ³/₄ fat serving

Slow-Cooked Pork

SERVES 4

COOKING IN A SLOW cooker is a bit like doing magic: you place raw ingredients in the pot and leave it alone without as much as a peek. After eight hours, you open the lid to uncover a fully cooked, tender, flavorful pork.

1½ pounds pork tenderloin

1 onion, chopped

4 tablespoons tomato paste

¼ cup cider vinegar

¼ cup water

1 teaspoon sugar

1 teaspoon freshly ground black pepper

¼ teaspoon salt

¼ teaspoon ground cinnamon

⅛ teaspoon ground clove

1   Place all the ingredients in a slow cooker. Cover and cook on low for 7 to 9 hours, until tender.

2   Remove the pork and shred with a fork. Serve with the sauce from the pot.

PREP TIME: 10 minutes   TOTAL TIME: 7 hours, 10 minutes

PER SERVING, ABOUT: Calories: 261 Protein: 36 g Carbohydrate: 6 g Dietary Fiber: 1 g Sugars: 4 g Total Fat: 9 g Saturated Fat: 3.2 g Cholesterol: 112 mg Calcium: 24 mg Sodium: 247 mg

EXCHANGES: 1 nonstarchy vegetable serving; 6 protein-rich servings

Poultry

Spinach-Stuffed Chicken

SERVES 4

THIS DISH TAKES A little bit longer to prepare than most in this book, but the majority of the time is unsupervised cooking time. And besides, it's worth the wait—this chicken is incredibly tender and full of flavor.

1 large onion, minced

3 cups chopped fresh spinach

2 cloves garlic, minced

1 tablespoon extra-virgin olive oil

1 1/2 teaspoons finely chopped fresh sage or 3/4 teaspoon dried

1 teaspoon ground cinnamon

1/4 teaspoon plus 1/8 teaspoon salt

Black pepper to taste

1 whole chicken (about 28 ounces)

1   Heat the oven to 375 degrees. Heat a large heavy-bottomed skillet over medium heat.

2   Mix together the onion, spinach, garlic, oil, sage, cinnamon, salt, and pepper in a medium bowl. Set aside.

3   To remove the skin from the chicken, place the chicken with the back facing up and cut through the skin the length of the chicken's back. Using a paper towel to help you grip, peel the skin off the chicken. Wash the chicken in cold water and pat dry.

4   Stuff the chicken with the spinach mixture.

5   Place the chicken in a medium-sized roasting pan. Cover the chicken with foil and bake until the meat separates easily from the bone, about 1 hour, 15 minutes.

6   Remove the foil and cook for an additional 10 minutes. Serve.

PREP TIME: 20 minutes   TOTAL TIME: 1 hour, 50 minutes

PER SERVING, ABOUT: Calories: 236 Protein: 36 g Carbohydrate: 4 g Dietary Fiber: 1 g Sugars: 1 g Total Fat: 8 g Saturated Fat: 1.6 g Cholesterol: 111 mg Calcium: 58 mg Sodium: 364 mg

EXCHANGES: 1 nonstarchy vegetable serving; 1²/₃ protein-rich servings; ³/₄ fat serving

Chicken Curry

SERVES 4

READY TO SPICE THINGS UP? Give this recipe a try. You can play with the amounts of spices and cayenne pepper to customize it to your taste. Or, make it vegan as we describe at the end of the recipe.

Vegetable oil cooking spray

1 small onion, sliced

2 cloves garlic, minced

1 tablespoon minced fresh
   ginger

1 teaspoon ground cumin

¼ teaspoon ground cayenne
   (optional)

1 medium tomato, sliced, or
   1 cup canned no-salt-added
   tomatoes

4½ cups water

¼ cup red lentils

1 teaspoon ground turmeric

¼ teaspoon salt

Black pepper to taste

1½ pounds boneless, skinless
   chicken breast cut into
   ¼-inch strips

¾ cup chopped fresh
   cauliflower

⅓ cup fresh peas (or frozen,
   if fresh are not available)

4 cups fresh spinach

⅓ cup plain nonfat yogurt

1   Heat a heavy-bottomed stockpot over medium heat and coat with the vegetable oil spray. Add the onion and cook until translucent, about 5 minutes.

2   Add the garlic, ginger, cumin, and cayenne, if desired. Cook for 2 more minutes, stirring constantly.

3 Add the tomato, water, lentils, turmeric, salt, and pepper. Cook until the lentils are tender, about 20 minutes.

4 Add the chicken and cauliflower and cook for an additional 10 minutes. Add the peas and spinach and cook until the soup returns to a low boil. Simmer for about 2 minutes. Garnish with the yogurt and serve.

PREP TIME: 15 minutes **TOTAL TIME:** 55 minutes

PER SERVING, ABOUT: Calories: 282 Protein: 46 g Carbohydrate: 17 g Dietary Fiber: 6 g Sugars: 3 g Total Fat: 3 g Saturated Fat: 0.7 g Cholesterol: 99 mg Calcium: 112 mg Sodium: 300 mg

EXCHANGES: ²/₃ grain/starchy vegetable serving; 1¼ nonstarchy vegetable servings; trace of milk/yogurt serving; 4 protein-rich servings

Curry lends itself well to tofu, so instead of the chicken, use 1 pound firm tofu, drained and cut into ¼-inch strips. Also use a total of 3 tablespoons red lentils instead of ¼ cup, and ½ medium tomato instead of a whole one. Coat the stockpot with 2 tablespoons canola oil instead of the vegetable oil spray.

NUTRITION ANALYSIS FOR THE VEGAN VERSION: Calories: 243 Protein: 16 g Carbohydrate: 17 g Dietary Fiber: 5 g Sugars: 3 g Total Fat: 12 g Saturated Fat: 0.6 g Cholesterol: 0 mg Calcium: 233 mg Sodium: 188 mg

EXCHANGES FOR THE VEGAN VERSION: ½ grain/starchy vegetable serving; 1 nonstarchy vegetable serving; trace of milk/yogurt serving; 1⅓ protein-rich servings

Ground Turkey Casserole

SERVES 4

CASSEROLES ARE CLASSIC COMFORT dishes. Using ground turkey gives this one high-quality, low-fat protein, and the spices lend unique flavors. Use another healthy protein—tofu—in the vegan version at the end of the recipe.

1 onion, thinly sliced

Vegetable oil cooking spray

1½ pounds 93% lean ground turkey

4 cloves garlic, minced

1 tablespoon fresh oregano

½ teaspoon ground cinnamon

½ teaspoon ground cumin

⅛ teaspoon salt

Black pepper to taste

3½ cups chard, well washed and chopped, or other leafy greens, such as kale, collards, or turnip

1 cup prepared tomato sauce with no more than 500 milligrams of sodium per ½ cup, such as Barilla Marinara Sauce

¼ cup water

1 small tomato, sliced

1   Preheat the oven to 375 degrees. Heat a large heavy-bottomed skillet over medium heat.

2   Coat the onion with the cooking spray and cook in the skillet for 5 minutes, stirring often.

3   Add the turkey and garlic. Cook until browned, stirring often, about 5 minutes. Stir in the oregano, cinnamon, cumin, salt, and pepper. Mix in the chard.

4   Coat a 9-inch-square pan with the cooking spray. Pour in ½ cup tomato sauce and top with half of the turkey mixture. Pour in the remaining ½ cup tomato sauce and top with the remaining half of the turkey mixture. Pour the water around the edges.

5   Spray the tomato slices with the cooking spray. Top the casserole with tomatoes.

6   Bake in the oven for 40 minutes. Serve immediately.

PREP TIME: 10 minutes   **TOTAL TIME:** 1 hour

PER SERVING, ABOUT: Calories: 320 Protein: 32 g Carbohydrate: 13 g Dietary Fiber: 3 g Sugars: 5 g Total Fat: 15 g Saturated Fat: 3.9 g Cholesterol: 134 mg Calcium: 89 mg Sodium: 533 mg

EXCHANGES: 2¼ nonstarchy vegetable servings; 4 protein-rich servings

Make this a vegan casserole by replacing the turkey with 1½ pounds tofu, drained and crushed with the back of a fork. Also, instead of the cooking spray, coat the frying pan with 2 tablespoons canola oil. Skip the onion and reduce tomato sauce to ¾ cup.

NUTRITION ANALYSIS FOR THE VEGAN VERSION: Calories: 259 Protein: 17 g Carbohydrate: 13 g Dietary Fiber: 2 g Sugars: 3 g Total Fat: 14 g Saturated Fat: 0.6 g Cholesterol: 0 mg Calcium: 274 mg Sodium: 315 mg

EXCHANGES FOR THE VEGAN VERSION: 1⅓ nonstarchy vegetable servings; 2 protein-rich servings; 1½ fat servings

Fish and Seafood

Trout with Roasted Vegetables

SERVES 4

TROUT IS AN EXCELLENT fish choice because it's environmentally sustainable, is a good source of omega-3 fatty acids, contains very low levels of contaminants, and is reasonably priced. This dish will taste best during the warm months, when the eggplant, pepper, and summer squash are in season.

1 onion, sliced

2 cups sliced eggplant

4 cloves garlic, peeled and cut into 4 pieces

2 cups sliced summer squash

1 sweet red pepper, sliced, cored, and seeds removed

1 tablespoon and 1 teaspoon healthy spread, such as Bestlife Buttery Spread, melted

1/4 teaspoon salt (1/8 teaspoon for the vegetables, 1/8 teaspoon for the trout)

Black pepper to taste

Vegetable oil cooking spray

1 cup nonfat yogurt

1 cup roughly chopped fresh basil

1 1/2 pounds trout, cut into 4 pieces (about 6 ounces each)

1   Preheat the oven to 375 degrees.

2   Combine the onion, eggplant, garlic, squash, and red pepper in a large bowl. Toss the vegetables with the healthy spread, 1/8 teaspoon salt, and black pepper.

3   Place the vegetables on 2 sheet trays coated with the cooking spray and bake in the oven for 30 minutes, stirring every 10 minutes.

4   Combine the yogurt and basil in a small bowl. Set aside.

5   Heat a heavy-bottomed skillet over medium heat. Once the skillet is hot, coat with the cooking spray. Place the trout in the skillet and cook until browned, about 3 minutes. Flip and cook until the other side is browned, about 2 minutes.

6 Remove the trout from the skillet, season with ⅛ teaspoon salt and black pepper to taste and serve with the vegetables. Top with yogurt.

PREP TIME: 15 minutes **TOTAL TIME:** 45 minutes

PER SERVING, ABOUT: Calories: 273 Protein: 34 g Carbohydrate: 14 g Dietary Fiber: 3 g Sugars: 4 g Total Fat: 9 g Saturated Fat: 2.5 g Cholesterol: 142 mg Calcium: 191 mg Sodium: 329 mg

EXCHANGES: 2½ nonstarchy vegetable servings; ⅓ milk/yogurt serving; 6 protein-rich servings

Shrimp with Lime and Avocado

SERVES 4

THE RICHNESS OF THE avocado and the tartness of lime work in concert to highlight the slightly sweet flavor of the shrimp. If you are a fan of spicy foods, use a little extra cayenne pepper.

1½ pounds shrimp, cooked and shelled

4 cups chopped romaine lettuce

1 avocado, skin and pit removed, flesh sliced

1 tablespoon olive oil

1 tablespoon freshly squeezed lime juice

Pinch of cayenne pepper (or more to taste)

1 tablespoon finely chopped red onion

¼ teaspoon salt

Black pepper to taste

Combine all the ingredients in a large bowl. Let sit for 5 minutes at room temperature, or up to 1 hour refrigerated, before serving.

PREP TIME: 10 minutes **TOTAL TIME:** 10 minutes

PER SERVING, ABOUT: Calories: 277 Protein: 36 g Carbohydrate: 7 g Dietary Fiber: 3 g Sugars: 1 g Total Fat: 12 g Saturated Fat: 1.8 g Cholesterol: 259 mg Calcium: 110 mg Sodium: 404 mg

EXCHANGES: ¼ nonstarchy vegetable serving; 4 protein-rich servings; 2¼ fat servings

Poached Scallops with Leeks and Turkey Bacon

SERVES 4

THE TURKEY BACON ADDS a rich flavor to this nutritious seafood dish.

Vegetable oil cooking spray	1/2 cup white wine
1 cup thinly sliced leeks	1 cup water
4 slices turkey bacon, chopped	1 3/4 pounds bay scallops

1   Heat a heavy-bottomed skillet over medium heat and coat with the cooking spray. Add the leeks and cook until translucent, about 5 minutes.

2   Add the turkey bacon and cook, stirring constantly, for 5 minutes. Add the wine and water and bring to a boil.

3   Turn the heat down to a low simmer and cook for 5 minutes. Add the scallops, cover, and cook for an additional 2 minutes.

4   Portion the scallops and broth into individual bowls and serve.

PREP TIME: 10 minutes   **TOTAL TIME:** 35 minutes

PER SERVING, ABOUT: Calories: 248 Protein: 36 g Carbohydrate: 9 g Dietary Fiber: 0 g Sugars: 1 g Total Fat: 4 g Saturated Fat: 0.9 g Cholesterol: 78 mg Calcium: 69 mg Sodium: 495 mg

EXCHANGES: 1/2 nonstarchy vegetable serving; trace of alcohol; 5 protein-rich servings

Fish Wrap

SERVES 1

LOOKING FOR MORE WAYS to fit fish into your diet? Try this quick, delicious wrap.

Vegetable oil cooking spray

¾ cup shredded cabbage

1 tablespoon mayonnaise with no more than 50 calories per tablespoon, such as Hellmann's Canola Cholesterol Free Mayonnaise or Spectrum Light Canola Oil Mayonnaise or Kraft Light

1 teaspoon fresh lemon juice

5 ounces Pacific cod

1 tablespoon cornmeal

1 whole wheat 100-calorie wrap, tortilla, or flatbread with at least 5 grams of fiber and no more than 17 grams of carbohydrate and 280 milligrams of sodium, such as Flatout Healthy Grains Multi-Grain Flatbread

1   Heat a heavy-bottomed skillet over medium heat and coat with the cooking spray.

2   Combine the cabbage, mayonnaise, and lemon juice in a large bowl. Set aside.

3   Sprinkle the cod with cornmeal. Place the fish in the skillet and cook until browned, about 3 minutes. Flip the fish and cook until the other side is browned, about 2 minutes.

4   Roll the fish and cabbage in the wrap and serve.

PREP TIME: 5 minutes   **TOTAL TIME:** 10 minutes

PER SERVING, ABOUT: Calories: 328 Protein: 37 g Carbohydrate: 32 g Dietary Fiber: 11 g Sugars: 3 g Total Fat: 9 g Saturated Fat: 0.2 g Cholesterol: 52 mg Calcium: 55 mg Sodium: 485 mg

EXCHANGES: 1½ grain/starchy vegetable servings; ⅔ nonstarchy vegetable serving; 2½ protein-rich servings; 1 fat serving

Roasted Cod Cooked with Spring Onions and Topped with Avocado and Celery Compote

SERVES 4

THE CREAMINESS OF THE avocado compote pairs nicely with the moist flakiness of the fish. Use Pacific cod if possible—it's free of contaminants and more sustainable than Atlantic cod.

1½ ripe avocados, cut into ½-inch cubes

2 cups sliced celery

2 tablespoons fresh lime juice

½ cup fresh cilantro leaves

1 tablespoon olive oil

¾ teaspoon salt (¼ teaspoon for the compote, ½ teaspoon for the fish)

Black pepper to taste

Vegetable oil cooking spray

1 cup chopped spring onions

1½ pounds Pacific cod, cut into 4 pieces (about 6 ounces each)

1   Heat a large heavy-bottomed skillet over medium heat.

2   Gently toss the avocados, celery, lime juice, cilantro, oil, ¼ teaspoon salt, and pepper in a large bowl.

3   Coat the skillet with cooking spray. Add the onions and cook for 3 minutes, stirring often. Add the fish and cook until browned, about 3 minutes. Flip the fish and cook for about 2 more minutes, until the fish just begins to flake but the center is still translucent. The fish will continue to cook when it is removed from the pan.

4   Season the fish with the remaining ½ teaspoon salt. Serve topped with the avocado compote.

PREP TIME: 5 minutes   TOTAL TIME: 15 minutes

PER SERVING, ABOUT: Calories: 281 Protein: 32 g Carbohydrate: 10 g Dietary Fiber: 5 g Sugars: 3 g Total Fat: 12 g Saturated Fat: 1.7 g Cholesterol: 63 mg Calcium: 51 mg Sodium: 604 mg

EXCHANGES: 1 nonstarchy vegetable serving; 3 protein-rich servings; 4 fat servings

Broiled Wild Salmon with Fennel and Red Onion

SERVES 4

WILD SALMON, WHICH IS available fresh from the spring through September, is loaded with heart-healthy omega-3 fatty acids and essential vitamins and minerals. In this dish, the distinctive flavor of fennel complements the flavorful salmon.

1 red onion, sliced

3 cups sliced fennel

Vegetable oil cooking spray

1/4 teaspoon salt (1/8 teaspoon for the vegetables, 1/8 teaspoon for the fish)

Freshly ground black pepper to taste

3/4 cup roughly chopped fresh basil

Juice from 1 lemon

1 1/2 pounds Pacific wild salmon (or farm-raised salmon, if wild salmon is not available), cut into 4 pieces (about 6 ounces each)

1 Heat the oven to broiling temperature.

2 Place the onion and fennel in a large bowl and coat with the cooking spray. Toss with 1/8 teaspoon salt and pepper.

3 Place the fennel mixture on a sheet pan and broil until browned, stirring every 3 minutes, for about 6 minutes total. Remove the fennel from the oven, add basil and lemon juice, and set aside.

4 Place the salmon on a sheet tray and coat with the cooking spray. Broil until the top is lightly browned and the fish is cooked halfway through, about 3 minutes. Flip the fish and cook for slightly less time than the first side, about 2 minutes.

5 Season the fish with the remaining 1/8 teaspoon salt. Spoon the fennel mixture onto individual plates and place the salmon on top.

PREP TIME: 5 minutes   TOTAL TIME: 20 minutes

PER SERVING, ABOUT: Calories: 278 Protein: 35 g Carbohydrate: 9 g Dietary Fiber: 3 g Sugars: 1 g Total Fat: 11 g Saturated Fat: 1.7 g Cholesterol: 94 mg Calcium: 72 mg Sodium: 255 mg

EXCHANGES: 2 nonstarchy vegetable servings; 6 protein-rich servings

Baked Arctic Char with Tomatoes and Black Olives

SERVES 4

WRAPPING THIS OMEGA-3-RICH FISH in foil infuses it with the flavors of the ingredients it's cooked with, resulting in a unique and delicious meal. You can use salmon or cod, if Arctic char is not available.

¼ cup pitted black olives

2 cloves garlic, crushed

Pinch of red pepper flakes (optional)

¼ cup roughly chopped fresh basil

1 tablespoon olive oil

4 cups cherry tomatoes

Juice from ½ lemon

⅛ teaspoon salt

Freshly ground black pepper to taste

1 pound Arctic char

1   Put the olives, garlic, red pepper flakes, basil, and oil in a large bowl. Cut the cherry tomatoes in half and add to the bowl. Add the lemon juice, salt, and pepper. Set aside.

2   Preheat the oven to 425 degrees.

3   Cut a long piece of aluminum foil and place ½ of the tomatoes and marinade in the center of the foil. Place the fish on top of the tomatoes and season with pepper. Tightly wrap the fish with the foil, sealing in the liquid.

4   Bake for about 20 minutes. Remove the fish from the oven and let it sit for about 5 minutes before opening.

5   Divide the fish into 4 portions and serve with the remaining uncooked tomatoes and marinade.

PREP TIME: 5 minutes   TOTAL TIME: 30 minutes

PER SERVING, ABOUT: Calories: 305 Protein: 24 g Carbohydrate: 9 g Dietary Fiber: 2 g Sugars: 4 g Total Fat: 15 g Saturated Fat: 2.2 g Cholesterol: 27 mg Calcium: 35 mg Sodium: 242 mg

Shrimp and Quinoa Jambalaya

SERVES 4

ENJOY THIS HEALTHY TWIST on a classic Cajun dish. If you prefer, you can make your own spice mixture by blending garlic, cayenne, paprika, chili powder, dried mustard, and ground clove. As an alternative, try the vegan rendition at the end of the recipe.

1½ pounds raw shrimp, peeled and deveined

½ teaspoon salt

Black pepper to taste

½ teaspoon no-salt-added Cajun or Creole spice (or more to taste)

¾ cup quinoa

Vegetable oil cooking spray

1 onion, chopped

1 sweet red pepper, stem and seeds removed, chopped

1 cup chopped celery

2 cloves garlic, minced

1 cup fresh chopped tomato or 2 cups canned no-salt-added tomatoes

1 tablespoon fresh thyme leaves

3 tablespoons finely chopped fresh Italian parsley

3 tablespoons finely chopped green onion

1   Place the shrimp in a large bowl. Add the salt, pepper, and Cajun spice and toss to coat. Set aside.

2   Place the quinoa in a pot and cover with water. Bring to a boil and then reduce heat to a simmer. Cook until the quinoa just pops open, about 10 minutes. Drain and set aside.

3   Heat a heavy-bottomed skillet over medium-high heat. Coat the skillet with the cooking spray and add the onion, sweet red pepper, and celery. Cook until tender, about 5 minutes. Turn the heat down to medium and add the garlic. Cook for 1 to 2 minutes, stirring to keep the garlic

from browning. Add the shrimp and cook until the shrimp just begins to turn pink, about 5 minutes.

4 Add the tomato, thyme, and 1 tablespoon each of the parsley and green onion to the skillet. Cook on medium-high heat until the sauce is hot. Add the quinoa.

5 To serve, sprinkle the remaining 2 tablespoons each of parsley and green onion over the jambalaya.

PREP TIME: 10 minutes **TOTAL TIME:** 35 minutes

PER SERVING, ABOUT: Calories: 332 Protein: 40 g Carbohydrate: 31 g Dietary Fiber: 4 g Sugars: 4 g Total Fat: 5 g Saturated Fat: 0.8 g Cholesterol: 259 mg Calcium: 141 mg Sodium: 576 mg

EXCHANGES: 1⅓ grain/starchy vegetable servings; 1¾ nonstarchy vegetable servings; 4 protein-rich servings

Turn it into a vegan dish by replacing the shrimp with 1½ pounds tofu, drained and cut into ½-inch cubes. Instead of the cooking spray, coat pan with 1 tablespoon plus 1 teaspoon canola oil. Also, use ½ small onion, ½ medium sweet red pepper, and ½ cup chopped celery.

NUTRITION ANALYSIS FOR THE VEGAN VERSION: Calories: 334 Protein: 20 g Carbohydrate: 31 g Dietary Fiber: 3 g Sugars: 2 g Total Fat: 13 g Saturated Fat: 0.6 g Cholesterol: 0 mg Calcium: 260 mg Sodium: 313 mg

EXCHANGES FOR THE VEGAN VERSION: 1⅓ grain/starchy vegetable servings; 1 nonstarchy vegetable serving; 2 protein-rich servings; 1 fat serving

Vegetarian

Summary Squash Whole Wheat Pasta Bake

SERVES 4

LOTS OF FRESH VEGETABLES, two kinds of nuts, and whole grain pasta add up to comfort food that is truly healthy.

Vegetable oil cooking spray

¾ cup raw unsalted almonds

¾ cup raw unsalted walnuts

1 onion, thinly sliced

2 cloves garlic, minced

1 cup fresh basil leaves

⅛ teaspoon ground nutmeg

1 teaspoon salt

Black pepper to taste

½ cup water

½ cup whole grain rotini, such as Barilla Whole Grain Rotini, cooked according to the package directions

3 cups thinly sliced summer squash

3 fresh tomatoes, chopped

1½ tablespoons olive oil

1 Heat the oven to 375 degrees. Coat a 9-inch-square (or a 10-inch × 8-inch) pan with the cooking spray.

2 Combine the nuts, onion, garlic, basil, nutmeg, salt, pepper, and water in a food processor and pulse until smooth, about 1 minute.

3 Combine the nut mixture, pasta, squash, tomatoes, and oil in a large bowl. Place the mixture in the pan.

4 Bake for 40 minutes. Turn the oven to broil and broil until top is browned, about 2 minutes. Serve.

PREP TIME: 15 minutes   **TOTAL TIME:** 1 hour 5 minutes

PER SERVING, ABOUT: Calories: 465 Protein: 14 g Carbohydrate: 37 g Dietary Fiber: 10 g Sugars: 8 g Total Fat: 32 g Saturated Fat: 3 g Cholesterol: 0 mg Calcium: 133 mg Sodium: 444 mg

EXCHANGES: ¾ grain/starchy vegetable serving; 2⅔ nonstarchy vegetable servings; 7 fat servings

BBQ Tofu

SERVES 4

IN THIS DISH YOU get classic barbecue flavor without the fat, cholesterol, or sodium.

Vegetable oil cooking spray

1 onion, finely chopped

1 large sweet pepper, stem and seeds removed, finely chopped

24 ounces firm tofu, drained

1¼ cups chopped fresh or canned no-salt-added tomatoes

⅓ cup canned no-salt-added kidney beans, drained and rinsed, mashed with the back of a fork

4 tablespoons tomato paste

4 tablespoons cider vinegar

⅛ teaspoon ground clove

¼ teaspoon ground cinnamon

½ teaspoon brown sugar

¾ teaspoon salt

Black pepper to taste

1   Heat a large skillet over medium heat. Spray with the cooking spray and add the onion and sweet pepper. Cook for 3 minutes, stirring.

2   Crumble in the tofu and cook until browned. Keep breaking it apart with a spoon for about 4 minutes.

3   Stir in the tomatoes, beans, tomato paste, vinegar, clove, cinnamon, brown sugar, salt, and pepper. Cook for an additional 4 minutes. Serve.

PREP TIME: 8 minutes   TOTAL TIME: 20 minutes

PER SERVING, ABOUT: Calories: 220 Protein: 18 g Carbohydrate: 19 g Dietary Fiber: 4 g Sugars: 7 g Total Fat: 7 g Saturated Fat: 0 g Cholesterol: 0 mg Calcium: 244 mg Sodium: 459 mg

EXCHANGES: ¼ grain/starchy vegetable serving; 2 nonstarchy vegetable servings; 2 protein-rich servings

SIDE DISHES

Barley Salad with Parsley and Lemon

SERVES 4

BARLEY HAS A VERY low glycemic index. You can serve this versatile side dish in place of rice with virtually any entrée, from Slow-Cooked Pork (page 308) to BBQ Tofu (page 324).

½ cup barley

¾ cup shredded carrots

1 cup finely chopped fresh parsley

1 tablespoon olive oil

2 tablespoons fresh lemon juice

¼ plus ⅛ teaspoon salt

Black pepper to taste

1 Place the barley in a medium saucepan and cover with water. Bring to a boil and reduce to a simmer. Cook until the barley is soft, about 15 minutes. Drain the barley and place in a medium bowl.

2 Toss the barley with the carrots, parsley, oil, lemon juice, salt, and pepper. Serve.

PREP TIME: 5 minutes   TOTAL TIME: 20 minutes

PER SERVING, ABOUT: Calories: 128 Protein: 4 g Carbohydrate: 21 g Dietary Fiber: 5 g Sugars: 2 g Total Fat: 4 g Saturated Fat: 0.6 g Cholesterol: 0 mg Calcium: 37 mg Sodium: 246 mg

EXCHANGES: 1⅓ grain/starchy vegetable servings; ¾ nonstarchy vegetable serving; ¾ fat serving

Oat Cake

SERVES 4

THIS IS AN UNEXPECTED use of oatmeal that is surprisingly delicious. Although this side can be served with a large variety of main dishes, it's a memorable match with roasted poultry.

1 cup uncooked thick-cut oatmeal	1 tablespoon finely chopped fresh rosemary
1 tablespoon olive oil	Black pepper to taste
¼ plus ⅛ teaspoon salt	Vegetable oil cooking spray

1 Cook the oatmeal according to the package directions. Immediately stir in the oil, salt, rosemary, and pepper.

2 Coat a 9-inch-square baking dish with the cooking spray. Pour the oats into the prepared dish.

3 Let the oats cool. Slice into 4 wedges.

4 Heat a heavy-bottomed skillet over medium heat and coat with the cooking spray. Cook the oat cakes until browned, about 3 minutes per side. Serve.

PREP TIME: 5 minutes   **TOTAL TIME:** 20 to 30 minutes depending on whether you use traditional or quick-cooking oats

PER SERVING, ABOUT: Calories: 105 Protein: 3 g Carbohydrate: 14 g Dietary Fiber: 2 g Sugars: 0 g Total Fat: 5 g Saturated Fat: 0.7 g Cholesterol: 0 mg Calcium: 11 mg Sodium: 219 mg

EXCHANGES: 1 grain/starchy vegetable serving; ¾ fat serving

Roasted Asparagus

SERVES 4

THESE DAYS, IT'S POSSIBLE to buy fresh asparagus year-round, but for a real treat, prepare this recipe in the spring, when asparagus is in season. If possible, buy it from a good farmers' market to ensure it was just picked. For the best flavor and texture, take care not to overcook the asparagus, especially if it's superfresh.

1¾ pounds asparagus	⅛ teaspoon salt
Vegetable oil cooking spray	2 teaspoons fresh lemon juice
2 cloves garlic, minced	⅓ cup shelled pistachios, chopped
Black pepper to taste	

1　Preheat the oven to 400 degrees. Break the ends off the asparagus at the point where they break easily and naturally. Lay the asparagus on a sheet tray and lightly coat with the cooking spray. Season with the garlic and pepper.

2　Place the asparagus in the oven and cook for 2 to 6 minutes, depending on the thickness of the stalks. Asparagus is best if it's still crunchy and barely cooked.

3　Remove the asparagus and season with the salt. Drizzle with the lemon juice, top with pistachios, and serve.

PREP TIME: 5 minutes　**TOTAL TIME:** 10 minutes

PER SERVING, ABOUT: Calories: 101 Protein: 7 g Carbohydrate: 11 g Dietary Fiber: 5 g Sugars: 5 g Total Fat: 5 g Saturated Fat: 0.7 g Cholesterol: 0 mg Calcium: 62 mg Sodium: 78 mg

EXCHANGES: 1½ nonstarchy vegetable servings; 1⅓ fat servings

Garlicky Broccoli and Eggplant

SERVES 4

ROASTING IS AN IDEAL preparation for a wide variety of vegetables; in fact, you can use almost any other vegetable in place of the broccoli and eggplant.

3 cups thinly sliced eggplant

¼ cup olive oil

2½ cups roughly chopped broccoli

4 cloves garlic, finely chopped

Vegetable oil cooking spray

1 tablespoon balsamic vinegar

⅛ teaspoon salt

Black pepper to taste

1   Preheat the oven to 375 degrees. Place the eggplant in a large bowl, pour in the oil, and toss to coat lightly. Place the eggplant on a baking sheet and bake for 5 minutes.

2   Place the broccoli and garlic in the same large bowl and coat lightly with the cooking spray. Add the broccoli and garlic to the baking sheet with the eggplant and cook for 5 minutes. (The eggplant will be in the oven for 10 minutes.)

3   Test the vegetables to see if they are firm but tender. Either leave in for an additional 2 to 5 minutes or remove. Place in the same large bowl, dress with balsamic vinegar, salt, and pepper, and serve.

PREP TIME: 5 minutes   **TOTAL TIME:** 20 minutes

PER SERVING, ABOUT: Calories: 161 Protein: 2 g Carbohydrate: 9 g Dietary Fiber: 4 g Sugars: 3 g Total Fat: 14 g Saturated Fat: 1.9 g Cholesterol: 0 mg Calcium: 38 mg Sodium: 94 mg

EXCHANGES: 1½ nonstarchy vegetable servings; 3 fat servings

Cucumber with Yogurt and Mint

SERVES 4

COOL CUCUMBERS AND CREAMY yogurt are perfect partners in this side dish. If you have space for a small garden, mint is one of the easiest edible plants to grow. Do so, and you'll be rewarded with a delicious, inexpensive herb that adds a fresh flavor to many foods.

1 cup nonfat yogurt

1 clove garlic, crushed

1 tablespoon olive oil

1/2 cup finely chopped fresh mint

1/4 teaspoon salt

Black pepper to taste

4 cups sliced cucumbers, peeled if not organic and seeds removed if they are large

1 Mix together the yogurt, garlic, olive oil, mint, salt, and pepper in a medium bowl until fully incorporated.

2 Add the cucumbers and combine. Serve immediately or refrigerate for up to 24 hours before serving.

PREP TIME: 10 minutes   TOTAL TIME: 10 minutes

PER SERVING, ABOUT: Calories: 84 Protein: 5 g Carbohydrate: 8 g Dietary Fiber: 2 g Sugars: 2 g Total Fat: 4 g Saturated Fat: 0.6 g Cholesterol: 1 mg Calcium: 163 mg Sodium: 198 mg

EXCHANGES: 1 nonstarchy vegetable serving; 1/3 milk/yogurt serving; 3/4 fat serving

Creamy Celery Salad

SERVES 4

TAHINI, OR SESAME PASTE, is available in most grocery stores as well as Middle Eastern specialty stores. It gives a boost of protein and a creamy texture to salad dressings and dips.

3 tablespoons sesame tahini

1 tablespoon cider vinegar

1 tablespoon water

2 tablespoons sesame oil

1 tablespoon fresh lemon juice

Ground cayenne to taste

12 stalks celery, cut into ¼-inch slices

1   Combine the tahini, vinegar, water, oil, lemon juice, and cayenne in a small bowl. Mix until smooth.

2   Place the celery in a large bowl and dress with the tahini mixture. Serve immediately or store in the refrigerator for up to 24 hours.

PREP TIME: 10 minutes   TOTAL TIME: 10 minutes

PER SERVING, ABOUT: Calories: 143 Protein: 3 g Carbohydrate: 7 g Dietary Fiber: 3 g Sugars: 2 g Total Fat: 12 g Saturated Fat: 1.8 g Cholesterol: 0 mg Calcium: 96 mg Sodium: 105 mg

EXCHANGES: ¾ nonstarchy vegetable serving; 2⅔ fat servings

TREATS/DESSERTS

Chocolate Mini-cakes

MAKES 4 MINI-CAKES

SURPRISED TO FIND CAKE in a diet book? This healthful version replaces butter with heart-healthy oil, a measured amount of sugar, and just a little whole wheat flour so it's very tender and moist, almost like a flourless chocolate cake.

Vegetable oil cooking spray

3 tablespoons soy milk, such as Silk

¼ teaspoon apple cider vinegar

2 tablespoons sugar

2 tablespoons olive or canola oil

½ teaspoon vanilla extract

¼ cup whole wheat flour

1½ tablespoons cocoa powder, such as Hershey's Natural Cocoa

Scant ¼ teaspoon baking soda

⅛ teaspoon baking powder

1   Preheat the oven to 350 degrees. Line four cupcake cups with paper liners or spray with cooking spray. Put two tablespoons of water in the remaining cups so the tin won't burn. Whisk together the soy milk and vinegar in a large bowl and set aside for a few minutes.

2   Add the sugar, oil, and vanilla to the milk mixture and mix until incorporated.

3   Add the dry ingredients and mix until just combined.

4   Divide into 4 cupcake cups and bake for 20 minutes. Serve.

PREP TIME: 5 minutes   TOTAL TIME: 25 minutes

PER SERVING, ABOUT: Calories: 108 Protein: 1 g Carbohydrate: 11 g Dietary Fiber: 1 g Sugars: 7 g Total Fat: 7 g Saturated Fat: 1.1 g Cholesterol: 0 mg Calcium: 26 mg Sodium: 100 mg

EXCHANGES: ¾ grain/starchy vegetable serving; trace of milk/yogurt serving; 1½ fat servings

Popcorn and Oat Cookies

MAKES 4 COOKIES

THIS IS NOT A traditional use of popcorn, but after you taste this cookie, it may become your favorite way to enjoy it.

1 cup air-popped popcorn

¼ cup uncooked old-fashioned
   rolled oats

1½ tablespoons sugar

½ teaspoon baking powder

2 tablespoons olive oil

½ tablespoon soy milk

Pinch of salt

Vegetable oil cooking spray

1   Preheat the oven to 350 degrees.

2   Combine all the ingredients except the cooking spray in a mixer or food processor and mix until the popcorn and oats break up, about 2 to 3 minutes.

3   Coat a cookie sheet with the cooking spray. Divide the dough evenly to make 4 individual cookies and place on the sheet tray. Wet your palm with a little water and flatten the cookies with your palm.

4   Bake until golden brown, about 8 minutes. Serve.

PREP TIME: 10 minutes   TOTAL TIME: 20 minutes

PER SERVING, ABOUT: Calories: 105 Protein: 1 g Carbohydrate: 10 g Dietary Fiber: 1 g Sugars: 5 g Total Fat: 7 g Saturated Fat: 1 g Cholesterol: 0 mg Calcium: 39 mg Sodium: 62 mg

EXCHANGES: ⅔ grain/starchy vegetable serving; trace of milk/yogurt serving; 1½ fat servings

Baked Cinnamon Apple

SERVES 1

IN MANY PARTS OF the country and during much of the year, apples are the only available local fruit. Fortunately, they are healthy, delicious, and versatile. You can enjoy them raw as a snack or try this warm end-of-a-meal treat.

2 tablespoons ground walnuts	Large pinch of ground cinnamon
¼ teaspoon honey	½ small apple, cored
Tiny squirt of fresh lemon juice	

1 Preheat the oven to 350 degrees.

2 Combine the walnuts, honey, lemon juice, and cinnamon in a small bowl.

3 Fill in the spot where the core was with the walnut mixture.

4 Place the apple on a baking dish and bake for 20 minutes. Serve warm or at room temperature.

PREP TIME: 5 minutes TOTAL TIME: 25 minutes

PER SERVING, ABOUT: Calories: 102 Protein: 2 g Carbohydrate: 11 g Dietary Fiber: 3 g Sugars: 7 g Total Fat: 7 g Saturated Fat: 0.6 g Cholesterol: 0 mg Calcium: 27 mg Sodium: 1 mg

EXCHANGES: ½ fruit serving; 2 fat servings

APPENDIX 1:
THE BEST LIFE
DIABETES
MANAGEMENT LOG

To develop the best diet, exercise, and medication regimens, you have to track how the three factors affect your blood sugar. Keep a log, and you'll start to see the connections: "When I eat fruit for breakfast, my blood sugar level is a little high" or "If I stay under 40 grams of carbohydrate for lunch, my blood sugar level is fine" or "If I lower my insulin dose by 3 units before getting on the treadmill, my blood sugar level won't drop too low." That's what the Best Life Diabetes Management Log is for—it's a place to track your food intake, exercise, medication dose, and blood sugar level, and figure out those all-important patterns.

Don't panic when you see all those columns! As we explained in Phase One (page 35), most people don't have to track their blood sugar level all day long. If you have type 1 diabetes or are taking several daily shots of insulin, you will need to check your blood sugar level much more frequently—perhaps at every meal and before and after exercising. But for most of you, testing once or twice a day—such as before a meal and two hours after, or before exercise and thirty to sixty minutes afterward, will be enough. Vary the times you test so that you get a sense of how your blood sugar level varies not only by meal but by time of day. You'll need to check more often whenever you make changes to your lifestyle, such as increasing your exercise or medication. Your doctor might suggest a testing schedule, or you can use our model on page 44.

We've also included an abbreviated log called the Doctor's Log for you to fill out and take along on your next doctor's visit. This log basically contains a space to record your blood sugar levels and mealtimes; that's likely all your doctor will need to see. The full log may be helpful if you see a certified diabetes educator.

Here's how to use the log:

- Make photocopies of the log on pages 340–341, or go to www.thebestlife.com/diabetes to print out a copy. You can tailor the online log to your needs—for instance, you can start the day at a different time or give yourself more room to write in meals. Even better, join www.thebestlife.com to get access to a more interactive log. Plus, when you are a member, all your information will be stored online so you can access it whenever you need to.

- For the next week, fill out at least one "before and after" time period a day (for instance, your blood sugar levels before and two hours after a meal). Some days you might want to test two time periods. The most important time periods to check your blood sugar include:

  - Upon waking and two hours after breakfast

  - Before lunch, snacks, or dinner and two hours after any of these meals

  - Before exercise and thirty to sixty minutes afterward

  - Anytime you think you're having a low-blood-sugar reaction or you don't feel well

  - Before bedtime (record any snack you might have had two hours before bedtime) and three hours after going to sleep (you'll have to set an alarm).

- If you've taken medication during the time period tested—for instance, if you took short-acting insulin before a meal— record the exact dosage.

- There are two ways to record cardiovascular (aerobic) physical activity: either by minutes or, if you're wearing a pedometer, by steps. For instance, if you took a 25-minute power walk with your pedometer attached, you can record either the steps or the 25 minutes, but not both—that's double-dipping! As for weight-training sessions, write down the number of exercises you did along with the number of sets and reps. For instance, if you did 3 different types of arm exercises (arm curls, lateral pulls, and flies) and three 3 types of leg exercises (squats, lunges, and leg curls) and did 12 repetitions of each exercise 2 times, you'd record: "6 strength-training exercises, 2 sets each, 12 reps."

- For each time period tested, record any food you've eaten. Be specific; for instance, make sure to include precise amounts of food (¾ cup fat-free milk, 1 slice whole wheat toast spread with 2 teaspoons of peanut butter).

- Record carbohydrates for the entire meal using food labels and our tables starting on pages 59 and 343. (If you belong to www.thebestlife.com, you can look up the carbohydrate content of thousands of foods with the help of the handy and easy-to-use database.) For instance, if you had a salad made of 3 cups lettuce (5 grams of carbohydrate), ½ cup grapes (8 grams of carbohydrate), ⅔ cup chicken strips (0 gram of carbohydrate), and olive oil and lemon juice (0 gram of carbohydrate), along with two Wasa Sourdough Crispbreads (18 grams of carbohydrate), your carbohydrate tally would be 5 + 8 + 18, or 31 grams of carbohydrate for that meal.

- After recording for a week, decide which time periods are most important to test the next week, using the advice on pages 44 to 47 as a guide.

- Remember also to record your blood sugar levels in the Doctor's Log. Not only is this useful during your appointments, but seeing a week or more of numbers on one sheet will also help you discern patterns that you might not notice on the more complex log, such as "My blood sugar is always high when I wake up."

The Best Life Doctor's Log

DATE	BEFORE BREAKFAST	2 HOURS AFTER BREAKFAST	BEFORE LUNCH	2 HOURS AFTER LUNCH	BEFORE DINNER	2 HOURS AFTER DINNER	BEDTIME	OVERNIGHT (2 A.M. TO 3 A.M.)

The Best Life Diabetes Management Log

DATE: _____

TIME	BLOOD SUGAR	MEDICATION	CARBOHYDRATE GRAMS	
5–6 A.M.				
6–7 A.M.				
7–8 A.M.				
8–9 A.M.				
9–10 A.M.				
10–11 A.M.				
11 A.M.–12 P.M.				
12–1 P.M.				
1–2 P.M.				
2–3 P.M.				
3–4 P.M.				
4–5 P.M.				
5–6 P.M.				
6–7 P.M.				
7–8 P.M.				
8–9 P.M.				
9–10 P.M.				
10–11 P.M.				
11 P.M.–12 A.M.				
12–1 A.M.				
1–2 A.M.				
2–3 A.M.				
3–4 A.M.				
4–5 A.M.				

FOOD (time/amount)	Hunger Scale Before/After Eating	Physical Activity (time/min. OR steps)

APPENDIX 2:
CARBOHYDRATE
COUNTS

Turn to this list whenever you need to check the carbohydrate count of a food. We've also provided numbers for other important nutrients. You'll notice that some foods also have a glycemic index (GI) value. The GI hasn't been calculated for every food yet; in fact, most brand-name items don't have one. So just because you don't see a GI number next to a food, that does *not* mean that food is not healthful.

This list is by no means complete—it's just a sampling of some of the more common carbohydrate-containing foods. You can look up thousands of foods on our Web site—www.thebestlife.com—or on the U.S. Department of Agriculture's site, www.nal.usda.gov/fnic/foodcomp/search.

FOODS	WEIGHT (oz. unless noted)	PORTION SIZE (cups unless noted)	CARBOHYDRATES (g)	FIBER (g)	CALORIES	FAT (g)	SAT. FAT (g)	SODIUM (mg)	GI
Breakfast cereal			GRAINS (APPROX. 15 G CARBOHYDRATE SERVING)						
All-Bran	0.73	1/3	15	7	53	0	0	53	49
All-Bran Bran Buds	0.80	1/4	18	10	53	0	0	150	58
Multi-Bran Chex	0.50	1/4	13	2	53	1	0	103	58
Bran Flakes	0.75	1/2	14	3	72	0	0	66	74
Cheerios	0.75	3/4	15	2	75	2	0	142	74
Corn Flakes, dry	0.58	2/3	14	0	64	0	0	168	86
Cream of Wheat, dry	0.75	2 tablespoons	16	1	78	0	0	2	66
Cream of Wheat, instant, dry	0.81	2 tablespoons	17	1	84	0	0	3	74
Oat Bran	1	1/3	17	3	114	2	1	3	59
Oatmeal, instant (1/4 cup dry = 1/2 cup prepared with water)	0.66	1/4 cup dry	14	2	75	1	0	0	82
Oatmeal, made from steel-cut oats (1/8 cup dry = 3/4 cup prepared with water)	0.66	1/8 cup dry	14	2	75	1	0	0	52
Raisin Bran	0.65	1/3	14	3	58	0	0	113	61
Shredded Wheat, spoon size	0.56	1/3	15	6	53	0	0	0	83
Special K Protein Plus	1	3/4	14	5	100	3	0.5	110	
Bread									
Bagel, 100% whole wheat	1	1/4 a typical (4 oz.) bagel	16	3	73	0	0	152	72

Bread dinner roll, whole wheat	1	1 roll (2" × 2")	14	2	75	1	0	134	70
Pancakes	1.4	3 small (3" each)	15	1	88	2	0	197	66
Pita bread, 100% whole wheat	1	1 small (4" pita)	16	3	74	0	0	106	63
Pumpernickel bread	1	1	14	2	71	1	0.1	190	50
Raisin toast	1	1 slice	14	1	75	1	0.1	102	63
Rye bread	1	1 slice	14	2	73	1	0	187	76
Rye bread—reduced calorie	1	1 slice	12	3	58	1	0	115	68
Sourdough bread	1	1 slice	16	1	82	1	0.1	184	54
Thomas's English Muffins—Hearty Grains—Multi-Grain	1	½ muffin	12	2	60	0.5	0	110	
Tortilla, wheat	1	1 small tortilla	16	1	95	2	0	139	71
Waffles, Kashi GOLEAN—original	1.5	1 waffle	17	3	85	1.5	0	165	
Waffles, Van's Multi-Grain	1.3	1 waffle	15	3	95	3	0.2	153	
Whole grain bread	1	1 slice	13	1	65	1	0	160	71
Wonder White Low GI bread	1	1 slice	13	3	81	1	0	151	54
Cereal grains									
Barley, pearled, boiled	2	⅓	16	2	70	0	0	2	25
Bulgur, cooked	3.2	⅓	17	4	76	0	0	4	48
Couscous, cooked	1.8	⅓	12	1	58	0	0	3	65
Grits, corn, cooked	4.3	½	16	0	71	0	0	2	
Millet, boiled	2	⅓	14	1	68	1	0	0	71

FOODS	WEIGHT (oz. unless noted)	PORTION SIZE (cups unless noted)	CARBOHYDRATES (g)	FIBER (g)	CALORIES	FAT (g)	SAT. FAT (g)	SODIUM (mg)	GI
Cereal grains (cont.)									
Polenta, boiled	2.8	1/3	16	2	74	0	0	0	68
Quinoa, boiled	2	1/3	13	1	69	1	0	5	53
Rice and pasta									
Arborio risotto rice, white, boiled	1.64	1/4	18	0	80	0	0	0	69
Barilla PLUS Pasta	0.67 oz. dry	heaping 1/3 cup cooked	13	1	71	1	0	8	
Barilla Whole Grain Pasta	0.67 oz. dry	heaping 1/3 cup cooked	14	2	68	1	0	0	
Basmati rice, white, dry	0.7	1 3/4 tablespoons	15	0	66	0	0	0	58
Egg noodles	0.6 oz. dry	1/3 cup cooked	13	1	72	1	0	4	40
Soba noodles	0.6 oz. dry	1/3 cup cooked	14	0	63	0	0	149	59
Spaghetti, white durum wheat	0.6 oz. dry	1/3 cup cooked	14	0	69	0	0	1	58
Spaghetti, whole wheat	0.6 oz. dry	1/3 cup cooked	14	1	66	0	0	2	42
Udon noodles	0.6	1/3	12	1	63	1	0	220	
Uncle Ben's Converted white rice, boiled	2	1/3	15	1	71	0	0	191	50
Uncle Ben's Ready Rice, Original Long Grain (pouch)	1.9	1/3	14	0	63	0	0	192	48
Uncle Ben's Ready Rice, Whole Grain Brown (pouch)	2.4	1/3	16	1	77	1	0	211	48
Wild rice, boiled	1.9	1/3	12	1	53	1	0	2	57

STARCHY VEGETABLES (APPROX. 15 G CARBOHYDRATE SERVING)

Baked beans, canned	2.2	¼	13	3	60	0	0	210	49
Beets, canned	6	1 cup sliced	12	3	53	0	0	330	64
Black beans, boiled without salt	2	⅓	14	5	75	0	0	1	30
Black-eyed peas, boiled	1.9	½	17	4	80	0	0	188	42
Butter beans, boiled without fat or salt	2	⅓	13	4	70	0	0	1	36
Butter beans, canned	2.8	⅓	12	4	63	0	0	267	31
Butternut squash, boiled, mashed	5.5	⅔	14	4	59	1	0	288	51
Cannellini beans, small, dried, boiled	4	⅓	15	6	84	0	0	1	31
Chickpeas, canned in brine	2.7	⅓	18	3	94	1	0	237	40
Chickpeas, dried, boiled	1.9	⅓	16	4	97	1	0	4	28
Corn on the cob, boiled	2.5	1 small ear	14	2	63	1	0	11	48
Corn, whole kernel, canned, drained	2.8	½	15	1	66	1	0	265	48
Green plantain, peeled, boiled	1.5	¼ medium	14	1	55	1	0	2	39
Hummus*	3.1	6 tablespoons	13	5	149	9	1	341	
Kidney beans, red, canned	2.9	⅓	13	5	72	0	0	288	43
Kidney beans, red, dried, boiled without salt	2	⅓	13	4	74	0	0	1	28
Lentils, dried, boiled without salt	2.3	⅓	13	5	76	0	0	1	30
Lima beans, baby, frozen, reheated	2.4	⅓	13	4	71	0	0	20	32

*Counts as one grain/starchy vegetable serving and 1½ fat servings

FOODS	WEIGHT (oz. unless noted)	PORTION SIZE (cups unless noted)	CARBOHYDRATES (g)	FIBER (g)	CALORIES	FAT (g)	SAT. FAT (g)	SODIUM (mg)	GI
STARCHY VEGETABLES (APPROX. 15 G CARBOHYDRATE SERVING) *(CONT.)*									
Parsnips, pieces, boiled	2.75	½	13	3	55	0	0	188	52
Peas, green, frozen, boiled	2.8	½	11	4	62	0	0	58	48
Potato, baked, russet	2.4	½ small	15	2	67	0	0	10	75
Pumpkin, boiled, mashed	8.6	1	12	3	50	0	0	2	66
Sweet potato, baked, mashed	2.9	¼	15	2	62	0	0	22	46
Yam, peeled, boiled	2	½	19	3	79	0	0	5	54
FRUIT (APPROX. 15 G CARBOHYDRATE SERVING)									
Apple	4	1 small	15	3	55	0	0	1	38
Apricots, fresh	4	3 fruits	12	2	50	0	0	1	57
Apricots, halves, dried	0.7	⅛	12	2	50	0	0	1	30
Banana	2	½ medium	14	2	53	0	0	1	52
Blueberries	4.5	⅔	14	4	55	0	0	0	53
Cantaloupe	6	1 cup balls	14	2	60	0	0	28	65
Cherries, pitted, fresh	4	¾	14	2	58	0	0	3	63
Dates	0.5	2	13	1	47	0	0	0	45
Grapefruit	7	1 small	16	2	64	0	0	0	25
Grapes	3	1	16	1	58	0	0	1	53
Kiwifruit	4	1½ fruits	17	3	70	0	0	3	53
Mango	3	½ cup slices	14	1	55	0	0	2	51
Orange	4	1 medium	15	2	62	0	0	0	62

Papaya	5	1 small	15	3	60	0	0	5	59
Peach	5.5	1 large	15	2	61	0	0	0	42
Pear	3.6	½ large	16	3	61	0	0	1	38
Pineapple	4	¾ cup diced	15	2	56	0	0	1	59
Plums	4.6	2 fruits	15	2	61	0	0	0	39
Raisins	0.6	⅛ (2 tablespoons)	14	1	54	0	0	2	64
Raspberries	4	1	15	8	64	0	0	1	
Strawberries	6	1¼ cups whole	14	4	58	0	0	2	40
Watermelon	7	1¼ cups diced	14	1	57	0	0	2	76

NONSTARCHY VEGETABLES (APPROX. 5 G CARBOHYDRATE SERVING)

Artichoke hearts, whole, boiled and drained	1.5	¼ cup hearts	5	2	21	0	0	40	
Asparagus, raw	5	1	5	3	34	0	0	3	
Avocado	1.8	⅓ cup sliced	5	2	83	7	0.8	0	
Bean sprouts, raw	3	¾	5	1	47	0	0	2	
Bok choy, cooked	6	1	4	2	24	0	0	3	
Broccoli, flowerets, raw	2.5	1	5	2	24	0	0	23	
Brussels sprouts, raw	2	⅔	5	2	25	0	0	15	
Cabbage, green, raw	2.4	1 cup shredded	4	1	17	0	0	13	
Cauliflower, raw	3.5	1	5	3	25	0	0	30	

FOODS	WEIGHT (oz. unless noted)	PORTION SIZE (cups unless noted)	CARBOHYDRATES (g)	FIBER (g)	CALORIES	FAT (g)	SAT. FAT (g)	SODIUM (mg)	GI
NONSTARCHY VEGETABLES (APPROX. 5 G CARBOHYDRATE SERVING) (*CONT.*)									
Carrots, raw	1.5	1 medium, 1/3 cup chopped, 1/2 cup grated, or 1/2 cup chopped, cooked	4	1	17	0	0	30	35
Celery, raw	5.6	4 medium stalks	5	3	22	0	0	128	
Cucumber, raw	7	1 medium, peeled	4	1	24	0	0	4	
Eggplant, raw	3	1 cup cubes	5	3	20	0	0	2	
Fennel, raw	2	3/4	5	2	20	0	0	34	
Lettuce, iceberg	6	2 1/2 cups shredded	5	2	25	0	0	18	
Lettuce, romaine	5	3 cups shredded	5	3	24	0	0	11	
Mushrooms, raw, sliced	4.3	1 3/4	4	1	27	0	0	6	
Parsley, raw	2.1	1	4	2	22	0	0	34	
Peppers, green, sweet, raw	3	3/4 cup chopped, 1 1/4 cups sliced, 1 medium pepper	4	2	18	0	0	3	
Peppers, red, sweet, raw	2.6	1/2 cup chopped, 3/4 cup sliced, 1 small pepper	5	2	23	0	0	3	
Snow peas, raw	2	1 cup whole	5	2	27	0	0	3	
Spinach, raw	4	4	4	3	28	0	0	95	

Tomato paste	1.1	2 tablespoons	6	1	26	0	0	31–260 (depending on added salt)
Tomato puree, canned, no salt added	2	¼	6	1	24	0	0	18
Tomato, raw	4	1 medium	5	1	22	0	0	6
Tomatoes, cherry	5	1	6	2	27	0	0	7
Turnips, boiled and drained	6	1	5	3	28	0	0	4
Zucchini, raw	6	1 cup chopped, ½ large	5	2	26	0	0	16

DAIRY AND SOY PRODUCTS (APPROX. 12 G CARBOHYDRATE SERVING)

Skim milk	8	1	12	0	86	0	0	127
Whole milk	8	1	12	0	146	8	4.5	98
Yogurt, low-fat plain	6	1, 6 oz. container	12	0	108	3	1.7	119
Yogurt, nonfat plain	6	1, 6 oz. container	13	0	95	0	0	130

CONVENIENCE FOODS (APPROX. 15 G CARBOHYDRATE SERVING)

Crackers and snack foods

Baked potato chips, low-fat	0.6	10 chips	14	1	88	3	0.5	191
Baked tortilla chips, low-fat	0.6	8 chips	16	1	81	1	0	82
Glenny's Soy Crisps—lightly salted	0.9	10 crisps	14	2	105	2	0	225
Health Valley Original Oat Bran Graham Crackers	0.7	4 crackers	15	2	80	2	0	53
Lundberg brown rice cake, low-sodium	0.6	1 cake	15	1	70	0	0	55

FOODS	WEIGHT (oz. unless noted)	PORTION SIZE (cups unless noted)	CARBOHYDRATES (g)	FIBER (g)	CALORIES	FAT (g)	SAT. FAT (g)	SODIUM (mg)	GI
Crackers and snack foods (cont.)									
Popcorn, plain, air-popped	0.5	2	13	2	62	1	0	1	72
Potato chips	1	1 single-serve bag	14	1	153	11	3	147	51
Pretzels, fat-free	0.6	15 bite-size pretzels	14	1	68	0	0	244	83
Rice cakes, brown rice	0.6	2 rice cakes	15	1	70	1	0	59	82
Rice crackers	0.6	6 crackers	13	0	70	1	0	140	91
Rye crispbread	0.7	2 crispbreads	16	3	73	0	0	53	63
Stoned Wheat Thins crackers	0.7	5 crackers	13	1	95	4	1	159	67
Water crackers	0.7	5 crackers	14	1	85	2	0	149	63
Candy, cookies, muffins, and treats									
Angel food cake	0.8	1/2 of a 1/12 piece of a 10" diam. cake	15	0	64	0	0	127	67
Blueberry muffin (commercially made)	1	1/2 small	16	1	130	6	1.1	104	59
Bran muffin (commercially made)	1.2	1/2 large	14	2	87	3	1	120	60
Carrot cake, without icing	1.2	1/2 of a 1/10 piece of a 9" diam. cake	14	1	121	7	0.9	59	36
Chocolate brownies	0.9	11/2"	15	1	105	5	2	62	42
Chocolate chip cookies	0.8	11/2 cookies	13	1	103	5	1.6	73	43
Chocolate, dark	0.8	4 pieces	14	2	125	8	4.6	0	41

Chocolate, milk	1	3 pieces	15	0	131	8	4.6	15	41
Frozen yogurt	2	⅓	13	0	71	1	0.6	40	
Ice cream, low-fat	1.5	⅓	11	0	62	1	0.8	27	
Ice cream, regular	1.7	⅓	11	0	121	8	5	30	
Jelly beans	0.6	15 pieces	15	0	62	0	0	8	78
Licorice	0.5	10 bite-size pieces	13	0	53	0	0	7	78
Oatmeal cookies	0.8	3" diam.	16	1	113	5	1.2	79	54
Rice Krispies Treat	0.75	1½" square	17	0	90	3	1	105	63
Shortbread	0.75	3 small	14	0	105	5	1.2	96	64
Skittles	0.5	1 fun-size package	14	0	61	1	0	2	70
Sponge cake	0.8	1 individual dessert shell	15	0	70	1	0	60	46
Vanilla wafers	0.7	5 medium wafers	15	0	88	3	0.7	62	77

BEST LIFE APPROVED BRANDS CONTAINING CARBS (NOTE: CARBOHYDRATE GRAMS VARY)

Barilla PLUS Pasta (see page 346)	125 g							
Barilla Whole Grain Pasta (see page 346)	125 g							
Barilla Marinara Sauce	125 g	½	12	2	70	1.5	0	460
Barilla Tomato and Basil Sauce	125 g	½	12	2	60	1	0	460
Benefiber	3.5 g	2 teaspoons	4	3	15	0	0	0

FOODS	WEIGHT (oz. unless noted)	PORTION SIZE (cups unless noted)	CARBOHYDRATES (g)	FIBER (g)	CALORIES	FAT (g)	SAT. FAT (g)	SODIUM (mg)	GI
BEST LIFE APPROVED BRANDS CONTAINING CARBS (CONT.)									
Flatout Healthy Grain Multi-Grain Flatbread	53 g	1 wrap	17	8	100	2.5	0	280	
Silk Light Vanilla Soymilk	240 mL	1	10	1	80	2	0	95	
Silk Plain Soymilk	240 mL	1	8	1	100	4	0.5	120	
Silk Plus Fiber Vanilla Soymilk	240 mL	1	14	5	100	3.5	0.5	95	
Silk Unsweetened Soymilk	240 mL	1	4	1	80	4	0.5	85	
Silk Vanilla Soymilk	240 mL	1	10	1	100	3.5	0.5	95	
Wasa Crispbread—Fiber	10 g	1 slice	8	2	35	0.5	0	60	
Wasa Crispbread—Multi-Grain	14 g	1 slice	10	2	45	0	0	80	
Best Life Approved Brands—Treats									
Hershey's Extra Dark Pure Dark Chocolate squares	40 g	4 squares	21	4	180	14	9	0	
Hershey's Extra Dark Pure Dark Chocolate with cranberries, blueberries, and almonds	40 g	4 squares	21	4	190	14	9	0	

APPENDIX 3:
TWELVE-WEEK
FITNESS PLAN

You can use this gradual, manageable workout program whether you're a beginner or a regular exerciser. In most cases, you're adding just 5 more minutes of cardio, which includes walking, an aerobics class at the gym, or other aerobic activity, every 2 weeks. It's very important that you start at your *current* Activity Level (see page 83)—don't skip a level or you may overexert or injure yourself. For instance, if you've been sedentary, start Week 1 at Activity Level 1, not at Level 2 or 3. And get your doctor's okay before starting this or any other exercise program.

The program runs 12 weeks, but you can repeat it all year long, either staying at the level that you initially worked up to, or continuing to move up. For instance, if you're currently at Level 1 but eventually want to reach Level 3, then start Week 1 at Level 1. As you can see, you'll switch to Level 2 by the fifth week, finishing off the 12 weeks at Level 2. Ready for Level 3? Then go ahead and start the 12-week cycle at Level 3 this time. Need a few more weeks at Level 2? Start the cycle at Level 2 again.

If you start the program at Level 4, assume Week 5 is your starting point and go for the full 12 weeks. While we show you how to make the transition from Level 4 to 5, this program isn't for Level 5 exercisers. At Level 5, you're an athlete with a routine that is beyond the scope of this program.

At every level you should be maintaining a proper intensity (meaning you're breathing deeply, and although you're still able to talk, you would prefer not to; see page 93 for more on intensity levels). We don't require lots of cardio minutes because we assume you'll be making the most of those minutes with an intense workout. If medical problems prevent you from working out vigorously, ask your doctor if you can add more minutes, which will partly compensate for the lower intensity.

At Level 3, you'll add strength training; make sure to work all the major muscle groups, including chest, triceps, biceps, back, and legs. The "Basic Eight," described on pages 178 and 179, is a great example of a routine that gives you a complete body workout. Remember, choose a weight that's challenging enough so it's tough to complete the last few reps of the set, but not so heavy that you can't use proper form. And note that you'll need a different weight for different moves.

WEEK	CARDIO			STRENGTH TRAINING		
	BEGINNER	INTERMEDIATE	ADVANCED	BEGINNER	INTERMEDIATE	ADVANCED
1 to 2	Level 1	Level 2	Level 3	None	None	Level 3
	20 minutes (or as much as you can do), at least 3 days per week	40 minutes, 3 days per week	45 minutes, 5 days per week			6 to 8 strength-training moves; 1 to 2 sets of 8 to 10 repetitions, 2 days per week
3 to 4	Level 1	Level 2	Level 3	None	None	Level 3
	Add 5 more minutes of cardio to each workout for a total of 25 minutes, at least 3 days per week	Add 5 more minutes of cardio to each workout for a total of 45 minutes, 3 days per week	Add 5 more minutes of cardio to each workout for a total of 50 minutes, 5 days per week			Repeat routine from weeks 1 and 2

Congratulations, you are moving up to the next level! If moving up is too challenging, stay at your current level until you feel comfortable moving up. You'll know you're ready when your workout feels challenging but is no longer difficult.

WEEK	CARDIO			STRENGTH TRAINING		
	BEGINNER	INTERMEDIATE	ADVANCED	BEGINNER	INTERMEDIATE	ADVANCED
5 to 6	Level 2	Level 3	Level 4	None	Level 3	Level 4
	Add 5 more minutes of cardio to each workout for a total of 30 minutes, 3 days per week	Do only 30 minutes of cardio **BUT** add 2 days for a total of 5 days per week	Add 5 more minutes of cardio to each workout for a total of 55 minutes, 5 days per week		6 strength-training moves; 1 to 2 sets of 8 to 10 repetitions, 2 days per week	Add 2 more strength-training moves for a total of 8 to 10; 3 sets of 8 to 10 repetitions, 3 days per week
7 to 8	Level 2	Level 3	Level 4	None	Level 3	Level 4
	Add 5 more minutes of cardio to each workout for a total of 35 minutes, 3 days per week	Add 5 more minutes of cardio to each workout for a total of 35 minutes, 5 days per week	Add 5 more minutes of cardio to each workout for a total of 60 minutes, 5 days per week		Repeat the routine from weeks 5 and 6	Repeat the routine from weeks 5 and 6

WEEK	CARDIO			STRENGTH TRAINING		
	BEGINNER	INTERMEDIATE	ADVANCED	BEGINNER	INTERMEDIATE	ADVANCED
9 to 10	Level 2	Level 3	Level 4	None	Level 3	Level 4
	Add 5 more minutes of cardio to each workout for a total of 40 minutes, 3 days per week	Add 10 more minutes of cardio to each workout for a total of 45 minutes, 5 days per week	Add 5 more minutes of cardio to each workout for a total of 65 minutes, 5 days per week		6 to 8 strength-training moves; 3 sets of 8 to 10 repetitions, 2 days per week	8 to 10 strength-training moves; 3 sets of 8 to 10 repetitions, 3 days per week
11 to 12	Level 2	Level 3	Level 5	None	Level 3	Level 5
	Add 10 minutes of cardio to each workout for a total of 50 minutes, 3 days per week	Add 5 more minutes of cardio to each workout for a total of 50 minutes, 5 days per week	(This is to demonstrate what it's like to reach level 5. If you're not prepared for the greater exercise commitment, then stay at Level 4.) Add 10 more minutes of cardio to each workout for a total of 75 minutes, 5 days per week		6 to 8 strength-training moves; 3 sets of 8 to 10 repetitions, 3 days per week	(The same caveat about reaching level 5 as described in cardio applies here.) A minimum of 10 strength-training moves; 3 sets of 8 to 10 repetitions, at least 3 days per week

Congratulations! You can now move up to the next activity level or stay right where you are until you are more comfortable. Remember to keep challenging yourself, but don't move up before you are ready. This isn't a rush to the finish line—this is a lifelong commitment to yourself.

GENERAL INDEX

RECIPE INDEX

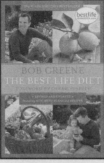
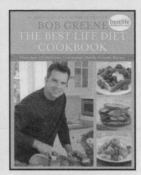
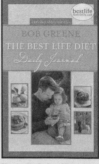
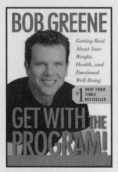
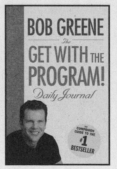
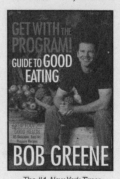
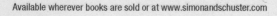